Releasing the Self
The Healing Legacy of Heinz Kohut

For Rosamond

Releasing the Self
The Healing Legacy
of Heinz Kohut

PHIL MOLLON PHD

Psychoanalyst (British Psychoanalytical Society),
Psychotherapist (Tavistock Society),
and Clinical Psychologist,
Lister Hospital, Stevenage

W
WHURR PUBLISHERS
LONDON AND PHILADELPHIA

© 2001 Whurr Publishers
First published 2001 by
Whurr Publishers Ltd
19b Compton Terrace, London N1 2UN, England and
325 Chestnut Street, Philadelphia PA 19106, USA

Reprinted 2003

British Library Cataloguing in Publication Data
A catalogue record for this book is available from the
British Library.

ISBN: 1 86156 229 2

Contents

Preface

> . . . the basis for my whole theoretical outlook . . . is characterised by
> the attempt to reconstruct inner experience . . . attempting to look at the
> psychological universe, as it were, via introspection and empathy and to bring
> order into the inner experience of man.
>
> (Kohut's Chicago lecture, 23 May 1975 – Kohut, 1996: 350)

The study of the mysterious unconscious mind has been a source of
endless fascination to me – ever since my first captivation by the writings
of Freud at the age of fourteen. Continually evolving, psychoanalysis is
profoundly absorbing, yet elusive and difficult, tantalizing and
frustrating. There is interest and value in all variants of psychoanalytic
theorizing, but all seem to carry a danger. This is that they will be
mistaken for the 'truth', the last word, the ultimate understanding. What
begins as a novel perspective, illuminating an area of mental life in a fresh
way, rapidly becomes a dogma – imprisoning rather than freeing the mind
of both patient and analyst. The radical and subversive insights of psychoanalysis give rise to the paradox of a psychoanalytic 'establishment'.

Many different psychoanalytic theories can provide plausible and
liberating formulations that facilitate the analytic process. Nevertheless,
'Ultimate Reality' (Bion, 1970) will always be greater than any particular
theory or interpretation, since it contains all possible points of view:

> However thorough an analysis is, the person undergoing it will be only partially
> revealed; at any point in the analysis the proportion of what is known to what is
> unknown is small. Therefore the dominant feature of a session is the unknown
> personality and not what the analysand or analyst thinks he knows. All psycho-
> analytic progress exposes a need for further investigation. There is a
> 'thing-in-itself', which can never be known.
>
> (Bion, 1970: 87)

Kohut appears to have been what Bion (1970) described as a 'creative mystic', who 'formally claims to conform to or even fulfil the conventions of the Establishment that governs his group' (1970: 74), before going on to develop new ideas which fundamentally challenge those conventions. His roots were in mainstream American psychoanalysis – and indeed his place at the centre of the establishment was indicated by his nickname as 'Mr Psychoanalysis' (Cocks, 1994). He himself remained committed to that Freudian tradition (Rubovits-Seitz, 1999), even whilst questioning some of its very foundations:

> . . . my own psychoanalytic knowledge and experience was obtained almost exclusively under the aegis of classical analysis and . . . an adequate appreci-ation of my work is impossible without a thorough knowledge of traditional theory and practice.
>
> (Kohut, 1984: 221)

What were these perspectives that Kohut bequeathed to the psychoana-lytic community? Essentially, he recognized the psychoeconomic dimension of mental life – the need to manage states of arousal, whether these are excessively high or low. He saw, for example, that an empathic-ally correct interpretation can be traumatic insofar as it is overstimulating in the fulfilment of a wish to be understood. In other instances he pointed out how states of understimulation and of enfeeblement or imminent fragmentation of the experience of self might lead to the compulsive engagement in certain kinds of sexual activity. Kohut grasped that a person's mental (and, to some extent, physical) state may depend on the empathic activity (or lack of it) of an other person's mind. In these ways, he anticipated by a number of years the current understanding of issues of attachment and affect regulation (Schore, 1994; Taylor, Bagby and Parker, 1997). Nevertheless, he was neither an 'object relations' nor an attachment theorist. He recognized that, at the level of *function*, minds are not separate, but his focus was consistently upon the *individual's* experience and mental activity as determined by the respon-siveness of the other.

In an earlier book – *The Fragile Self* (1993) – I attempted to place Kohut's work in the context of a spectrum of theories of narcissism. It was possible to see that Kohut had pointed to a whole range of disturbances in the experience of self that had not previously been coherently formu-lated; I listed these in a 'taxonomy' of seven categories. In working with a number of patients who had suffered severe interpersonal trauma and betrayal in childhood, I found that they tended to experience disturb-ances in all seven categories. Moreover, the repeatedly traumatized mind was often dissociated, such that its coherence and integrity could be profoundly compromised. These findings resulted in a further book: *Multiple Selves, Multiple Voices* (1996). The realization that repeated childhood trauma often seemed to be associated with pathology of autobiographical memory – discontinuities in the sense of self – led to *Remembering Trauma* (1998).

I have found that Kohut's work throws light into many dark areas of mental life, facilitating psychoanalytic engagement with patients who might otherwise appear too brittle or narcissistically vulnerable to tolerate the emotional stresses and injuries of psychoanalysis conducted not on a foundation of empathy for pathology of the self. However, it has seemed to me that Kohut's theories and insights have in many ways been eclipsed before they have been fully understood and integrated within psychoanalysis. This appears to have resulted from two post-Kohut trends: first, some of the writings *about* Kohut have simplified and distorted his ideas, denuding them of subtlety and wrenching them from their psychoanalytic roots and heritage; second, in the rush towards the field known as 'intersubjectivity' (in the USA) – a coalescence of thoughts and clinical perspectives partly, but not entirely, derived from self psychology – the original contribution of Kohut himself has in certain respects been lost. Therefore, my reason for writing the present book was to revisit in depth and detail Kohut's own accounts of his theory and clinical work and, in so doing, to interact with his ideas, linking them with other contemporary perspectives within psychoanalysis. I have done so not in order to present Kohut's theory as embodying a definitive truth, but, in a spirit of enquiry, to explore a valuable vantage point – to be considered alongside all the other potential vantage points that have been achieved in the past century, as well as those that emerge as psychoanalysis continues to evolve and blossom.

Psychoanalysis (in all its forms) is a special and precious thing:

> A friendly ear, an opportunity for ventilation and catharsis, helpful advice, simple or not so simple compassion – all of these can be obtained many places in the world outside an analyst's office. Nowhere else, however, can someone obtain a psychoanalysis.
>
> (Poland, 1996: 278)

A note on pronunciation

In Britain there is a curious tendency to pronounce Kohut's name incorrectly as 'Cahoot'. The correct pronunciation, as used by American colleagues, is simply Ko-(as in 'low')-hut.

A note on clinical material

Concern has increased in recent years regarding issues in relation to publication of clinical material (Gabbard, 2000; Michels, 2000; Scharff, 2000). At one time the usual practice was simply to disguise the description of the patient and assume that this comprised adequate safeguard of confidentiality. However, a new trend toward seeking explicit permission from patients is now emerging. Most of the clinical accounts presented in this book are Kohut's own, from his published work. Some are from other authors' published work. In the case of the discussions of 'Jo', 'Miss C', and 'Robert' in Chapter 8, the patients have been consulted and written permission has been obtained. Where very short illustrative vignettes are presented, these are generalized composites, inspired by a variety of clinical experience, both my own and that of colleagues.

Phil Mollon
July 2000

Acknowledgments

Chapter 6: a version of the section on Kohut, Klein and Bion was originally published in the British Journal of Psychotherapy (Mollon, 1986b).

Chapter 8: the account of Jo and the Outside People is based on a paper given to the International Society for the Psychological Treatment of Schizophrenia, Colchester, 16 September 1999. The section 'Depression: the thwarted self' is based on a talk given to the Taunton Association for Psychodynamics, Spring Conference, 13 March 1999.

Chapter 1
Rage, shame and presymbolic dread

> . . . the attempt to describe disintegration anxiety is the attempt to describe the indescribable.
>
> (Kohut, 1984: 16)

Psychoeconomic crises

A woman is admitted to a psychiatric unit, complaining of anxiety, depression, and a sense of being persecuted and controlled in various ways by a number of people. Her account is somewhat vague. She appears perplexed. Initially the clinician attempts to explore what events or experiences might have led to her becoming disturbed. Certainly there had been troubling areas of her life – a miscarriage, the break-up of her marriage, conflicts with her parents, her teenage son turning to drugs. However, the patient seems to become more agitated and angry as these aspects of her life are explored. Whether or not they form part of a relevant background to her current mental state, she clearly does not feel understood or relieved by the psychiatrist's effort to explore them. What does lead her to become calmer and to feel understood is when the doctor shifts tack and begins to tune in empathically to the patient's sense of her mind disintegrating. He begins to speak to her of how frightening this must be, and of the unspeakable agony of experiencing her mind – her very self – as having undergone some ominous change. The terror in her eyes begins to melt and she looks at him with just a hint of tentative trust and relief.

After identifying the most pressing anxiety and mental agony as the threat of disintegration of self, and communicating this understanding empathically, it becomes possible to put to the patient that she must have been experiencing stress or pain that had eventually become too much for her. She nods agreement and very cautiously begins to provide some clues as to the nuances of the distress in her life. These need not concern

1

us here. The important point is that an interpretive focus on *structure* of experience may at times have to precede the examination of *content*. When a patient is in the grip of disintegration anxiety, he or she is not concerned about what has led to that inner crisis – just as the inhabitants of a house on fire will have more pressing concerns than the initial cause of the flames.

This patient was not anxious (either consciously or unconsciously) about an impulse, an instinctual drive, a fantasy, or an object-relational need. The immediate cause of her anxiety was the disintegration of her experience of self (her self-structure). Allusions to such states are present in common words for madness, such as 'cracking up', 'crackers', 'crackpot', and 'potty'. The terror arises not from a presence (of an impulse or a feeling) but from an absence – a crack, a fissure in the mind. We may be reminded here of Balint's (1968) 'basic fault', a term suggestive of a structural metaphor of a building with a flaw within its foundations. Under stress, the fault gives way and a cleavage appears. It is this hole, this nothing, which creates panic and incommunicable agony. The deepest dread may be invisible and scarcely expressible in words.

Another patient speaks agitatedly of an experience the previous day. A man to whom she had expressed a sexual-romantic interest had rejected her rather brutally, telling her she was a fat and ugly cow whom he would not touch with a barge pole. Full of rage at the shame and humiliation of this, she shouts of her intention to visit him and stab him, or else stab herself in his presence. She recounts her despair that no man of the kind she likes ever seems to like her – and this leaves her feeling suicidal. In describing the episode she mentions that she went to a bar immediately afterwards and quickly consumed several strong drinks. Aware that there are many aspects of this communication that potentially could be explored, the psychotherapist attempts to address the patient's motivations behind her behaviour that led to her humiliation, a recurrent pattern in which she appears actively to elicit rejection. He also tries to examine the transference aspects – ways in which the patient has felt rejected and humiliated by him, both recently and in the past. None of these lines of enquiry makes any difference to the patient's obvious agitation and impulse to harm either herself or the man who had scorned her. However, what does lead to a marked calming of her mental state is the therapist's talking to her empathically of how she is feeling overwhelmed by her own emotions. He tells her that she had clearly been in a state of shock after her encounter with this man and that she had sought emergency relief by consuming alcohol. Moreover, he adds that everything she has been saying could be summarized as a communication of a state of mental *crisis*, in which she feels flooded with all kinds of emotions that she cannot manage. She nods in agreement and appears visibly calmer. In a markedly more reflective state of mind, she is then able to recognize, with more emotional conviction, that her personal worth and her potential for future relationships are not determined by the vicious response of the presumably rather disturbed man who insulted her.

In this example, the patient is calmed – her state of mind altered in a benign direction – by an interpretation that addresses not the *content* of her motivations, fantasies and affects, but instead empathically recognizes her state of being overwhelmed by her emotions. This is an interpretation of a *psychoeconomic* crisis (to do with the *quantity* of excitation). It is only after this has been addressed that she is able to be receptive to exploration of content (of motivations and fantasies, etc.). There is a paradox here. The patient's immediate anxiety is concerned with an *internal* state of psychoeconomic imbalance. Whilst precipitated by an experience with another person, the anxiety itself does not relate to a concern with a relationship. However, it is relieved by words given by another person (the psychotherapist).

Breakdown in the structure of experience

Content – especially that relating to conflicts with others – clearly is not always the most crucial and urgent aspect of a patient's presentation. This is emphasized in the following remarks by Kohut regarding a certain form of psychopathology:

> These patients initially create the impression of a classical neurosis. When their apparent psychopathology is approached by interpretations, however, the immediate result is nearly catastrophic: they act out wildly, overwhelm the analyst with oedipal love demands, threaten suicide – in short, although the content (of symptoms, fantasies, and manifest transference) is all triangular oedipal, the very openness of their infantile wishes, the lack of resistances to their being uncovered, are not in tune with the initial impression.
>
> (1972: 625–26)

Thus Kohut indicates that something else lies behind the apparent content – something that is driving the content but is distinct from it. He goes on to explain:

> The nuclear psychopathology of these individuals concerns the self. Being threatened in the maintenance of a cohesive self because in early life they were lacking in adequate confirming responses ('mirroring') from the environment, they turned to self-stimulation in order to retain the precarious cohesion of their experiencing and acting self. The oedipal phase, including its conflicts and anxieties, became, paradoxically, a remedial stimulant, its very intensity being used by the psyche to counteract the tendency toward the breakup of the self –

just as a small child may attempt to use self-inflicted pain (head banging, for
example) in order to retain a sense of aliveness and cohesion.

(1972: 626–27)

Kohut is arguing here that oedipal content – of conflicts and anxieties – is
intensified as a *psychic stimulant* to counter fears of disintegration. The
reaction to interpretation of this content may appear puzzling unless this
function is understood. He elaborates this point, as follows:

> Patients whose manifest psychopathology serves this defensive function will
> react to the analyst's interpretations concerning the object-instinctual aspects
> of their behaviour with the fear of losing the stimulation that prevents their
> fragmentation; and they will respond with an intensification of oedipal drama-
> tising so long as the analyst does not address himself to the defect of their self.
> Only when a shift in the focus of the analyst's interpretations indicates that he is
> now in empathic closeness to the patient's fragmenting self does the stimu-
> lation of the self through forced oedipal experiences (dramatising in the
> analytic situation, acting out) begin to diminish.
>
> (1972: 627)

Kohut is saying that in certain psychological conditions something has
happened to the *structure* on which experience is based – and that this
must be interpreted before content. By analogy, if a computer document
has become disrupted because of a fault in the computer, it is necessary
to attend to the malfunction in the software or hardware before
attempting to correct the deformations in the content of the document.

Fragmentation and rage

Kohut emphasizes rage – narcissistic rage – as one result of breakdowns
in the structure of experience and expectation. The encounter with
reality itself can be too much to bear, smashing as it does illusions of
control, predictability and knowledge:

> The enemy who calls forth the archaic rage of the narcissistically vulnerable… is
> seen by him not as an autonomous source of impulsions, but as a flaw in a
> narcissistically perceived reality. The enemy is a recalcitrant part of an
> expanded self over which the narcissistically vulnerable person had expected to
> exercise full control . . . narcissistic rage arises when self or object fail to live up
> to the expectations directed at their function . . .
>
> (1972: 644)

In Kohut's theorising, what threatens the individual when narcissistic
illusions of control are jeopardized is a return to the experience of disin-

tegration. Drawing on Freud's (1914) inference of an autoerotic stage –
suggestive of bodily incoherence – which precedes the coherence of the
stage of primary narcissism, as well as Glover's concept of 'ego nuclei'
(Glover, 1968), he postulated an early stage of the 'fragmented self'. The
possibility of regression to this stage is a source of profound fear – 'the
unspeakable anxieties accompanying . . . a prepsychological state'
(Kohut, 1984: 8). By 'prepsychological', Kohut meant a condition in
which there is no coherent and cohesive centre of experience. This is
clearly not an inevitable state, since Stern (1985) and others have
indicated that the newborn infant is in many ways an organized psychobiological being, but this benign state is dependent upon the appropriate
ministrations of the mothering one.

Writing from a very different perspective, Lacan too saw the aggression
inherent in the pursuit of the narcissistic image of coherence, driven by
the threat of a return to fragmentation – the stage of the 'fragmented
body-image' (Lacan, 1949; see also Muller, 1989). He inferred that the
earliest experiences of the baby are of fragmentation due to the prematurity of birth in the human species – 'a primordial Discord betrayed by
the signs of uneasiness and motor uncoordination of the neo-natal
months' (Lacan, 1949: 4). Lacan saw this as a state of infantile hell, represented most vividly through the paintings of Hieronymus Bosch. The
experience of fragmentation is displaced by the illusions of coherence
and completeness offered by an identification with the external *image*
found in a mirror or in the sight of another child – and later in the other
images offered by the pre-existing culture. For Lacan, the ego, the illusory
sense of a coherent self, is rooted in this alienating identification, yet
haunted by the ever-present threat of fragmentation, thereby giving rise
to a 'narcissistic passion' – 'the passionate desire peculiar to man to
impress his image in reality . . .' (Lacan, 1948: 22). It seems possible that
this passion and dread may lie behind the myriad ways in which human
beings seek to control one another and to impose their image and vision
on the social constructions of reality. When the rug is pulled from under
narcissistic illusions (of perfection, coherence, completeness and
control) the underlying fragmentation is exposed and rage is unleashed.

Shame

Shame is another affect that has been noted as a response to the
unexpected (Kohut, 1972; Mollon, 1993). Primitive forms of shame, self-
consciousness and embarrassment are shown by infants when their
expectations of a responsive maternal face are disrupted. Such narcissistic affects arise in the *gap*, the gaping crack between expectation and

the actual response of the other – a hole into which the shame-ridden person might wish to disappear. Shame and related affects are known to be peculiarly overwhelming, imbuing the whole sense of self with a desire to obliterate the excruciating moment of communicative incompetence. At such times, of misjudgement and misperception, the subject falters, stumbles out of the dance of human discourse – falling, no longer held by the illusory refuge of language and custom, the familiar and reassuring expectations that we have of one another. We are then reminded dimly of our original motor uncoordination and utter helplessness during our early life outside the womb.

Presymbolic dread

Perhaps more primitive, more fundamental than shame and rage, is the experience of dread in response to that which we cannot capture with our tools of representation and communication. We might call this 'presymbolic dread'.

This is the inarticulate agony felt by the patient whose structure of experience is fragmenting, whose sense of reality is receding, whose perception of self and other is warping, and yet whose access to words is ebbing away. Such a state of mind is pervaded by feelings of profound anxiety, unreality and perplexity. For example, a patient prone to this kind of fragmentation of experience would sometimes arrive at her session, looking bemused and frightened, and peering at the psychotherapist in apparent puzzlement. She might then ask, in all seriousness, 'Do you know who I am?' Whilst the question might have many meanings and implications, part of what it signified would be her uncertainty regarding her own identity, her existence in space and time, and her genuine doubts that the therapist could have been able to hold her in mind as a coherent entity. She could not take her own going-on-being (Winnicott, 1962) for granted. At the end of each session, she would jerkily pull her body and possessions together before juddering towards the door, as if uncertain of her capacity to remain in one mental and physical piece on leaving the external supporting frame of the therapy setting. Such states of fragmentation and perplexity can be a product of organic brain conditions, but they can also be a feature of more functional psychological disorders, stemming from childhood trauma or chronic failures of emotional containment by the environment (which fail to mitigate the inherent fragmentation of experience characteristic of the earliest period of life). Either way, the brain's normal capacities for making sense of the world and forming familiar and enduring patterns of representation are profoundly compromised.

A patient approached a clinic and asked to be referred to a psychoanalyst. The consultant asked him what was wrong that he should seek psychoanalysis. The patient replied that if he could answer such a question he would not need psychoanalysis. This was a perfectly apt answer. His experience of self tended to fragment and warp but he could not find words to identify, represent and describe this. The eye cannot see its own structure – without a mirror. Similarly a patient cannot identify, represent and think about the fragmentation in his own self without the mirror of psychoanalysis.

Our perceptual world is created by our brains. This created world is not identical with what Kant called the 'thing in itself', or what Bion (1970), from a psychoanalytic perspective, referred to as Ultimate Reality or 'O', and Lacan (1977) denoted as the 'Real'. In transactions with 'O', we form perceptions, meaningful organizations of patterns of sensory phenomena. We also create words and other symbols or signifiers as a means of representing phenomena, to ourselves and others. By means of signifiers we can manipulate 'reality' in our minds. But none of these representations is reality itself. There is always something beyond our symbols.

Grotstein (1997b: xv) comments:

> Bion's concept of 'O' and Lacan's concept of the Real each deal with the domain of the ineffable, which is Absolute Reality, Ultimate Truth, the domain that can never be embraced by imagination and symbolisation. When one is unprepared to experience it, it approximates the specular catastrophe of Sodom and Gomorrah.

Similarly, Hamburg refers to Lacan's presymbolic register of the Real as:

> moments of unmediated encounter with the world that are often traumatic and almost unbearable, as when the solidest ground beneath one's feet shakes violently during an earthquake.
>
> (Hamburg, 1991: 350)

According to Bion's (1962) theory of alpha function, sensory phenomena must be subject to a process that renders them meaningful. This 'alpha function' in the infant is helped by the 'alpha function' of the mother, involving her capacity to respond thoughtfully and appropriately to her baby's signals of distress or need. At one level, this can involve the development of primitive sensorimotor representations (Piaget's schemata and schemes) – familiar patterns of sensation as the world is grasped and manipulated. The mother's response of offering the nipple to the baby's mouth at the right time mates with the baby's inborn expectation, and produces a realization. Through this congruent meeting of expectation and mother's response, the sensation of nipple in mouth becomes meaningful. Bion states this as follows:

> The pre-conception. This corresponds to a state of expectation. It is a state of mind adapted to receive a restricted range of phenomena. An early occurrence might be an infant's expectation of the breast. The mating of pre-conception and realisation brings into being the conception.
>
> (Bion, 1963: 23)

This depends upon the mother's capacity for empathy – her willingness and ability to know what the baby needs, and when.

Without the process of alpha function, sensory phenomena do not become meaningful. They cannot be organized, represented and used for internal and external communication. Bion calls these unusable elements of the mind 'Beta elements'. They are outside the realm of symbolization – literally beyond the psychological. When alpha function fails, whether for constitutional or environmental reasons, the infant is bombarded by beta elements, nameless and meaningless particles of sensation and mental plasma. These are associated with the nameless dreads, the unthinkable agonies (Winnicott, 1962), the contentless anxieties of disintegration which cannot be articulated (although they can in principle be articulated by the analyst). This dread with no name and no thought forms a silent drive, unsensed and unknown. Bion captures the lurking yet invisible nature of this – 'the frightful fiend' – in his quote from Coleridge's poem:

> Like one that on a lonesome road
> Doth walk in fear and dread;
> And having once turned round walks on,
> And turns no more his head;
> Because he knows a frightful fiend
> Doth close behind him tread.
>
> (quoted in Bion, 1970: 46)

Presymbolic dread is normally unconscious, albeit a constant hidden persecutor-predator – *preying* on the mind. It becomes manifest in states of post-traumatic stress disorder. In this condition, after a person has experienced a severe trauma, such as an assault or an accident, the normal illusion of safety, the bubble of imagined security, is smashed, exposing raw terror (Ulman and Brothers, 1988) and death anxiety (Langs, 1997). This is usually understood as anxiety relating to the trauma, which has overwhelmed the person's capacities to adapt and cope, but it may also derive its devastating impact from the release into awareness of presymbolic dread – but no more expressible in words now (without psychotherapeutic help) than when it was unconscious.

Although presymbolic dread may be a particular feature of states of post-traumatic stress and also of psychosis, we may consider it to be in certain respects universal – a continual invisible persecution inherent in the human condition. For beyond what we can represent, whether at a sensory or more abstract conceptual level, lies Ultimate Reality – and a dread which, in its nature, cannot be grasped and represented directly. It can be given form only by images and narratives such as are to be found in horror films, or in accounts of the uncanny, or in religious imagery and symbolization of hell, the devil and the like.

The mother's empathic responsiveness as a bulwark against dread

Winnicott (1962), in his theory of early ego integration, suggests that dread without name or thought – the 'unthinkable anxieties' of going to pieces, falling for ever, having no relationship to the body, or having no orientation – form part of every human being's earliest 'experience'. He writes:

> At the stage which is being discussed, it is necessary not to think of the baby as a person who gets hungry, and whose instinctual drives may be met or frustrated, but to think of the baby as an immature being who is all the time on the brink of unthinkable anxiety. Unthinkable anxiety is kept away by this vitally important function of the mother at this stage, her capacity to put herself in the baby's place and to know what the baby needs . . .
>
> (Winnicott, 1962: 57)

All that stands between the baby and presymbolic dread is the mother's empathic response. Without this, the baby may look all right and may physically thrive, but in the hidden core of inner experience he or she is in pieces, but with no means of knowing, representing or communicating this psychic fact.

The presymbolic dimension and its terrifying bombardment of beta elements may be at the root of the many phenomena which Melanie Klein, throughout her writings, attributed to the death instinct. She considered that the infant was continually trying in phantasy to eject the terrifying force of death from within and to ally itself with the life instinct and the life-giving breast. The projection of the death instinct gave rise, in her view, to all the paraphernalia of persecutory figures of phantasy – of being devoured, torn to pieces, poisoned, burned, flooded, etc. However, Klein (1952), in a footnote, complements her views on the death instinct by quoting some remarks by Margaret Ribble (reporting on observations of 500 infants), on the way that the infant's experience of terror is moderated by the empathic responsiveness of the mother. Klein comments:

> Thus, regarding the relation to the mother from the beginning of life, [Ribble] stresses the infant's need to be 'mothered' which goes beyond the gratification by sucking.
>
> (1952: 89)

She goes on to quote further remarks by Ribble concerning the way in which the development of the child's personality and physiological integration are dependent on the attachment to the mother. She then quotes the following comments which suggest a primordial anxiety over chaos (and which echo Lacan's inferences regarding the 'fragmented body' deriving from the prematurity of the infant):

> The infant is, by its very incompleteness of brain and nervous system, continuously in potential danger of functional disorganisation. Outwardly the danger is of sudden separation from the mother who either intuitively or knowingly must sustain this functional balance . . . Inwardly the danger appears to be the mounting of tension from biological needs and the inability of the organism to maintain its inner energy or metabolic equilibrium and reflex excitability.
>
> (Ribble, 1944: 630; quoted in Klein, 1952: 89)

Ribble's clear implication here is that preservation or restoration of coherence and organization is brought about by the soothing responsiveness of the mother. Without this external assistance, the auxiliary ego, the infant lies continuously on the brink of chaos – the anarchic invasion of beta elements. Through the mother's receptivity and thoughtful responsiveness, the baby's world makes sense and order is established. When disorder threatens again, at whatever age, 'somebody must do something', the paradigmatic demand for the mother as transformational object (Bollas, 1987). The threat of disorganization – of entropy – will be experienced as a danger of annihilation and disintegration inherent in the baby's own psychobiology. Disorganization intrinsically lies outside the realm of symbolization and representation, since to represent (even at a sensory motor level) is to discover or impose organization. The dread of disorder derives from the presymbolic.

Perhaps, then, it is this presymbolic dimension which is the *ultimate* source of dread, terror and paranoia – indeed the source of the ubiquitous impulses to abuse and terrorize one's fellow human beings (Meloy, 1992). If the dread can be embodied in an other, made visible through the terror in the other's eyes, given form and focus through actual assault and injury to the other, then there can be a momentary sense of relief – mastery of the 'frightful fiend' that unceasingly pursues us, veiled in shadow behind our words and symbols.

Representation and illusion

The world that we apprehend through our senses is an illusion, created by the human brain. Our perceptual experience does not exist outside the activity of our brain. It is inherently a 'virtual reality'. What is beyond our senses and our capacity to represent and symbolize is unknowable – and this unknown includes our own selves and those of others. The terrible intuition of this haunts us – unspeakably. Perhaps this is part of what lies behind the anxiety and rage that has always been evoked by psychoanalysis – a discipline that threatens to enquire beneath the surface of phenomena.

It also follows that personal identity is in essence an illusion – a trick with mirrors – based on identifications with others, with images and roles that are socially created. As Wilshire (1982) persuasively argues, the evidence of mimetic identification is everywhere, in crowd behaviour, in fashions of all kinds, in body language, in opinions and so forth. By contrast, the evidence for individuality is rather slim. Identification with an available image creates an 'identity' – a representation of self – which gives birth to a sense of personal coherence. But such representations must fundamentally always be false – 'false selves'. They have no reality outside the images offered by the socio-cultural world. As Lacan puts it, '. . . they are constituted by a stagnation . . . similar in their strangeness to the faces of the actors when a film is suddenly stopped in mid-action' (Lacan, 1948: 17). Regarding this ubiquitous construction of 'self' out of an identification with alien images imported from others (or forcibly projected and imposed by others), Lacan comments starkly '. . . it might be said that at every moment he constitutes his world by his suicide . . .' (1948: 28).

A preoccupation with identity, the freezing of the image of the self (the creation of a 'false self'), appears to come about particularly when there is a threat of disorganization – a descent into Lacan's 'primordial discord'. In this respect it is no different from the delusional certainties of a psychotic person, arising as desperate attempts to create organization out of mental chaos. The alternative is the responsiveness of the empathizing partner (originally the mother) who is able to restore coherence and organization to the experience of self, thereby allowing life its flow and spontaneity, without the need to freeze the self in an alienating identity. Indeed the empathic connection to an other may be inversely associated with a preoccupation with identity. Those individuals who appear most concerned to promote and maintain a particular identity and to assert its superiority (one might think of Hitler, or a bigoted member of a northern Irish tribe, for example) often appear most lacking in empathy for others as well as in their own peace of mind. The merger with the larger group identity takes the place of *empathic* connection with others.

Our words, our beliefs, our customs and our theories, all work to offer an illusion of knowing – of knowing reality both psychological and physical. And yet our knowing of self and other can be only partial and imperfect. Ogden (1989) has drawn attention to the myriad ways in which we may attempt to defend against the persecutory awareness of not knowing. He comments:

> The mother's efforts at understanding, comforting, and in other ways providing for and interacting with her infant are inevitably narcissistically wounding to the mother since she will often feel at a loss to know what it is her baby needs and whether it is within the power of her personality to provide it even if she could somehow discover what he 'wants'. Winnicott's . . . use of the word *agonies* to refer to infantile anxieties applies equally to the pain of the mother's experience of not knowing.
>
> (Ogden, 1989: 202–3)

In defence against these agonies, the mother may substitute a false knowing, an illusory certainty. For example, there may be a resort to an external order, the clock, in place of a search for empathic knowing or intuiting of the baby's need. Ogden comments again:

> Such misnaming generates confusion in the infant as well as a sense that hunger is an externally generated event. In the extreme this mode of defence against not knowing becomes a persecutory authoritarian substitution of the mother's absolute knowledge for the infant's potential to generate his own thoughts, feelings, and sensations.
>
> (Ogden, 1989: 204)

Indeed all forms of certainty, of dogmatic knowing, and the imposition of one's beliefs on others, can be viewed as attempts to counter the persecution of not knowing. This can be as much true within the world of psychoanalysis as in other realms of human enquiry – but at least we have some rudimentary tools of understanding to help us bear our ignorance.

In order for the mother to begin empathically to 'know' her baby, or the analyst her patient, she must accept the imperfection of her knowing and thus be open to receive emotional communications – even if these are initially quite rudimentary. By applying her alpha function, thinking her way into the baby's (or the patient's) experience, she gropes towards empathy and 'making sense' of what otherwise are mere phenomena (such as a baby's 'noise') devoid of emotional meaning. This provision of alpha function – a kind of empathy arising from reverie – acts powerfully on the child's or the patient's mental and biological state. For making sense of experience and regulating affect are closely related. Talking about experience is calming. The alpha functioning mother or analyst assists in enabling emotional experience to be named, 'narratized', 'mentalized' (Fonagy, 1991; Fonagy, Target, Gergely and Jurist, 2000) and thereby 'digested' by the mind.

Kohut's healing legacy

In considering these realms of breaks, gaps and cracks in experience, the shame, rage and dread that arises in the collisions, misunderstandings and misconnections of human discourse, and the alienating identifications that cover these 'primordial discords', Kohut's novel perspectives present an innovative clinical instrument. Like Lacan, Kohut intuited that the experience of fragmentation of the mind-body self – 'the deepest anxiety man can experience' (1984: 16) – underlies the more specific anxiety of castration. However, he also recognized that fragmentation arises in the baby and child whose mental and physiological state is not regulated adequately by the caregiving environment. By understanding this, it becomes possible to focus on the process of regulation itself. A startling simplicity then becomes apparent. The antidote to fragmentation, shame, rage, dread and alienation – and the midwife to individuality and autonomy – is the experience of empathy from an other. This recognition is Kohut's healing legacy.

Summary

In the case of some states of mind, empathic recognition of disruptions in the structure of experience may be of more immediate importance than interpretations of content. Kohut recognized that intensification of drive-like impulses may arise as a result of breakdowns in the structure of experience. Shame and rage may erupt from the shattering of experience and expectation. The early psycho-biological state of the baby may be one of hovering on the edge of chaos, protected from this only by the appropriate ministrations of the mother. Kohut's idea of the 'fragmented self' and Lacan's account of the 'primordial discord' arising from the prematurity of the human infant both point to this aspect of early life. Those whose structure of experience is fragmenting may be overwhelmed by an inarticulate agony, being overwhelmed by phenomena which cannot be captured and communicated in words or other tools of representation – a state that could be termed 'presymbolic dread'. This may be linked with Bion's concept of 'Beta elements', Winnicott's 'unthinkable agonies', Kohut's 'disintegration anxiety', and Klein's 'death instinct'. Representation of the world experienced through the senses is an illusion created by the brain, which must be distinguished from what Bion called 'Ultimate Reality', or 'O', and Lacan called the 'Real'. Similarly, representations of 'self' – the sense of identity – are illusory. All 'selves' are in that sense 'false' selves. The threat of presymbolic dread may lie behind ubiquitious human strivings towards false knowing and false certainty, and the imposition of false identities on self and other.

Chapter 2
Discerning invisible structures

Nothing interferes more dramatically with acquiring a deep understanding than premature closure. If you think you know, then you cut yourself off from taking in more and more details with that pleasurable expectant puzzlement, until finally you see a totally unexpected configuration.

(Kohut, 1985b: 267)

Kohut's clinical discoveries and resulting theories provided a kind of photographic negative of psychopathology and of the relationship between patient and analyst. Instead of focusing on the overt content of the words and behaviour of the patient in analysis, he presented a picture of *what was not there* and how this absence was driving the patient's reactions. This searching behind the surface went beyond the usual analytic stance of seeing the manifest content as a disguised expression of something more hidden. Kohut looked for the *missing psychic structure*, whose absence resulted in desperate attempts to fill the gap with disintegrated and degenerative parodies of human need.

His concern with what is missing might be compared to the themes of 'blankness' in the writings of André Green (Kohon, 1999: 3) – blank psychosis, blank mourning, blank anxiety, psychic holes, etc. – who gave particular emphasis to the early childhood situation in which a mother becomes depressed and emotionally absent – the 'dead mother complex' (Green, 1983). In such circumstances, the child has not lost the mother per se, but has lost her emotional responsiveness. Modell (1999) has indicated how chronic childhood trauma deriving from the mother's emotional insensitivity may lead the child to develop a compensatory hypersensitivity to the inner life of others, as well as other outcomes:

To compensate for the fear of inner deadness, those suffering from a dead mother complex may be compelled to practice what can be described as a kind of emotional pump-priming, where they ensure their psychic aliveness by artificial means. For example, the fear of the deadness of the self may be negated through a hypersexuality or an addiction to thrills or induced crises.

(Modell, 1999: 84)

It is in this area – the study of the trauma of *blank* states, and the attempts to compensate for these – that Kohut's work has unfolded.

A perverse fantasy expressing missing psychic structure

Kohut writes of a patient (Mr A) who, at times of feeling disappointed in Kohut's empathic understanding of him, would experience an intensification of a particular perverse fantasy. In the fantasy, Mr A subdues a muscular man by means of some clever manoeuvre, then has the man tied up to a post; he then masturbates the helpless man and at the moment of his captive's ejaculation he would feel great sexual gratification combined with a sense of triumph and strength. Kohut explained this fantasy as an expression of something that the patient felt to be *missing* in his psychic structure as a result of the analyst's failure of empathy. The muscular man was a concretized and sexualized version of the idealized omnipotent father image. Mr A was attempting to counter his state of depletion by, in fantasy, acquiring strength and power through masturbating the muscular man, thereby draining him of his vigour, and magically incorporating the semen. However, Kohut emphasised that in essence this whole fantasy was merely a sexualized symbol of Mr A's need to participate in the strength of the idealized father. The fantasy would emerge when there was a collapse in Mr A's idealization of the analyst. Thus, the point of the fantasy was not that the patient's oral incorporative desires towards the analyst were in any way primary; rather, it was that their emergence was an indication of a disruption of the patient's sense of basking in the warm glow of feeling understood by the analyst. The fantasy did not *disguise* the patient's needs or desires; it expressed them vividly, but in a concretized and sexualized form. In a formulation frequently used by Kohut, the fantasy could be said to be a sexualized statement about a narcissistic need – a need for a response from the analyst that would maintain a sense of psychic cohesion and well-being.

Crucially, Kohut advised that on the whole the analyst should not interpret to the patient the details of the sexual fantasy. As he put it '. . . such fantasies are not made for insight; they are made for enjoyment' (1996: 9). He found that focusing on the sexual fantasy can tend to encourage the wish for sexual gratification. Instead, he would pose the question of why the fantasy has emerged at this particular point. He would then aim to show how the fantasy relates to the transference, in its total context of what the patient was seeking from the analyst and how the analyst was experienced as failing to provide this. In this way, the patient would be provided with the *non-sexual* meaning of the trans-ference desires – and how the fantasy revealed the experience of these not being met. Moreover, the patient would be helped to understand the effect of this thwarting on his experience of self – the sense of depletion and weakness.

Quite consistently, Kohut would focus on what was experienced as *missing* in the relationship with the analyst, and upon the patient's reactions to this absence. This may be part of the reason his work can be experienced by some as difficult to grasp and why his perspective is so often misunderstood. For example, because Kohut wrote extensively about the patient's needs for mirroring from the analyst, it is commonly assumed that he intended the analyst to offer mirroring or even overt admiration as some kind of legitimate gratification of the patient's narcissism. Here is what Kohut said about this in his Chicago lectures:

> . . . you don't have to mirror the patient to be effective as his analyst. *That really is a total mistake.* The meaning of mirroring, the essence of that concept, is not that you have to play act with your patient and praise him and respond to him and say that he is wonderful. No such nonsense. But you do have to show the patient over and over again how he defensively retreats because he expects that he will not get what he wants and that he doesn't dare to let himself know what he wants . . . Any patient who gets an unrealistic overdose of praise, who gets more than just an honestly empathic understanding of what his aspirations are, will be affronted. He will very soon be very angry at you.
>
> (Kohut, 1996: 373)

The truly radical core of Kohut's perspective was his recognition that primitive fantasies and archaic self and object images, and the wishes or drives associated with these – all the common currency of psychoanalytic investigation, whether Freudian, Kleinian or object relational – are often best understood as *derivatives* of experiences of fragmentation or depletion and as expressions of the longings for empathic (selfobject) responsiveness. Through Kohut's insights we are enabled to see beyond the mental *contents* of the disintegrating self, and discern the invisible structures behind these.

The selfobject – weaving the self from the fabric of the other

Kohut's radical perspective began with his observations that certain patients in analysis would show particular patterns of transference-like reactions. If the analyst were experienced as empathically understanding, in tune with the patient's emotional experience, and if breaks in the analysis were not imminent, then the patient would appear to benefit in two ways: (1) he or she would experience a sense of relative well-being; (2) he or she would show relatively good mental functioning, in terms of quality of thinking, and absence of signs of psychosis or other severe disturbance. However, at other times the patient might appear much more disturbed, fragmented in thought and feeling, in the grip of perverse sexual fantasies and compulsions, perhaps hypochondriacal, somewhat haughty and paranoid, possibly overtly grandiose, or preoccupied with mystical feelings. Kohut began to recognize that these reactions occurred when the patient experienced a failure in the analyst's empathy – this including an empathic attunement to the kind of response that the patient needed from the analyst at any particular moment.

Narcissistic injuries

This failure could be quite subtle. For example, Kohut described a patient (1996: 28) who had a particular hobby which his previous analyst had apparently belittled because he spent enormous amounts of time and money on it rather than attending to his job, and, as a result, had lost one job after another. Eventually the analysis with Kohut had evolved to a point where the patient could be more open about his hobby, no longer hiding it in shame, and began to talk to the analyst about it, sharing what it meant to him and how enjoyable it was. Kohut listened for about 40 minutes, speaking only when the patient asked if he understood some technical detail. Then Kohut asked when the hobby had originally started. The patient told him, but was then silent for many sessions afterwards. Kohut's later understanding of this sequence was that the patient had arrived at a point when he could share his interest and excitement with the analyst, looking for a mirroring response of interest in return. However, after 40 minutes, Kohut could not stand being placed in that position and felt compelled to be an 'analyst' by enquiring about the origin of the hobby. The implicit message of this was that the patient should undertake analytic work rather than just enjoy talking about the hobby. Whilst it is unrealistic to expect that an analyst will not inflict 'narcissistic injuries' of this kind, in the form of subtle rebuffs and imperfections of attunement, the insights Kohut presented were regarding the links between these and the patient's subsequent reactions. He emphasized that it was not until late in his professional life that he began to develop an appreciation of these vicissitudes of the patient's narcissistic economy.

In another example, Kohut described the reactions of a severely disturbed man (Mr G) when he announced he would be away for a week.

Mr G shifted to a near delusionally grandiose state of mind, coldly isolated, paranoid and hypochondriacal. Interpretations focused on the meaning of the separation in terms of object love and aggression were ineffective. Eventually Kohut stumbled on the crucial point that had provoked the patient's withdrawal and regression. Mr G had withdrawn not in response to the forthcoming break per se. Rather, it was in response to the tone of voice in which the analyst had announced it. Mr G had experienced this as unempathic and defensive. On reflection, Kohut concluded that when he made the announcement he had not been in an appropriately receptive and empathic state of mind, ready to explore the patient's feelings, but instead had been thinking of *himself*, in terms of fearing a stormy response and phone calls in the middle of the night. Mr G experienced this attitude and resulting tone of voice as a traumatic disappointment in the analyst's empathic capacities which he had previously idealized. After this sequence had been interpreted and explored, Mr G returned to a less disturbed state of mind, with a restored emotional connection to the analyst.

In an example of a more healthy patient, at a later stage of analysis (1971: 160), Kohut describes Mr I, who brought some childhood diaries to an analytic session and read them to the analyst. Following this, the patient had a two-part dream: he had been fishing and had caught a big fish which he brought proudly to his father; however, the father was not admiring but was critical; in the second part, he saw Christ on the cross, suddenly slumping, his muscles relaxing as he died. From this reaction, Kohut deduced that the patient must have experienced some lack of enthusiasm on the part of the analyst when he brought the diaries. The analyst had not been particularly aware of any emotional reserve and indeed had reacted with interest to the content of the diaries. Nevertheless, it seemed likely that the analyst may have perceived the reading of the diaries as an impediment to the more direct and spontaneous production of analytic material. As a result, the patient's mood slumped, he felt deflated, and had recourse to a masochistic merger fantasy, represented by the dream's allusion to the biblical account of Christ's reunion with God the Father. Kohut considered that the analyst had not appreciated fully the emotional meaning of the bringing of the diaries, which was not a resistance, but an analytic gift. The historical link was with the patient's experience of a narcissistic father who had tended to respond negatively to the child's progress in whatever area.

These three examples may be compared in terms of the nature and degree of the patient's reaction to the subtle narcissistic injuries experienced from the analyst. The first reacted with prolonged silence and withdrawal when the analyst interrupted his enthusiastic discourse about his hobby. A near psychotic regression was displayed by the second patient, with haughty grandiosity, paranoia and hypochondria, in response to the analyst's unempathic tone of voice. By contrast the third patient responded to feeling subtly rebuffed by creating a dream – this being a more contained and symbolic expression of a deflated mood resulting from narcissistic injury, as well as the efforts to compensate for this by resort to a fantasy of merger with an idealized father imago.

Kohut saw that in these and similar cases, the patient's state of mental well-being rested upon certain background transference-like configurations. Two features of these configurations were apparent. First, they were discernible primarily when they were disrupted; prior to this they were relatively silent and invisible. Second, they did not necessarily correspond to transferences of infantile relationships, although they might contain aspects of these; rather they seemed to express the patient's attempt to find a particular kind of sustaining or development-enhancing response from the analyst. In these transference-like configurations, the patient's mind and the analyst's empathic attentiveness would form a system. It would be as if the patient's mind rested upon functions provided by the analyst; self and object formed a functional system. Kohut captured the idea of the responsiveness required from the other in order to sustain the functioning of the self, in his new concept of the selfobject (a term which in earlier writings was hyphenated). It is important to distinguish this idea of the self drawing upon functions provided by the other, from the quite different concept of fusion of the images or representations of self and other. A person could have a clear differentiation of self and other whilst being deeply dependent on the selfobject functions provided by the other.

Definition of the selfobject

In his last book, Kohut defined the selfobject as 'that dimension of our experience of another person that relates to this person's functions in shoring up our self . . .' (1984: 49). A somewhat more obscure definition was given in his 1971 book where he was attempting to distinguish how the other can be experienced either in terms of narcissistic or object-loving dimensions: 'The small child, for example, invests other people with narcissistic cathexes and thus experiences them narcissistically, i.e. as self-objects. The expected control over such (self-object) others is then closer to the concept of the control which a grownup expects to have over his own body and mind than to the concept of control which he expects to have over others' (1971: 26–27). Thus the term 'selfobject' refers not to another person, but to an aspect of a person's *experience* of the other person. In his contribution to a symposium in 1980, Kohut

(1983) defined the concept as follows: 'In its strict sense the term "selfobject" denotes an inner experience, especially, though by no means exclusively, an inner experience of childhood that occurs when the child's self is firming' (1983: 392). Kohut then goes on to compare the developmental continuities of early and later selfobject experiences: 'Our mother lifted us up and held us close when we were babies and thus enabled us to merge with her calmness and strength; she was an archaic idealised selfobject. A friend puts his arm around us or understandingly touches our shoulder, and we regain composure and strength; he is a mature selfobject for us now' (397).

Differentiating object and selfobject

Kohut cautioned that the dependence on selfobjects can superficially appear to be an intense form of object hunger. However, he explained: 'The intensity of the search for and of the dependency on these objects is due to the fact that they are striven for as a substitute for the missing segments of the psychic structure . . . They are not longed for but are needed in order to replace the functions of a segment of the mental apparatus which had not been established in childhood' (1971: 45–46).

It is important to recognize that we can experience other people both as separate individuals ('objects', in the psychoanalytic sense) and also as selfobjects – a point which Grotstein (1983) calls the 'dual track' perspective. Often these two dimensions of experiencing the other may occur together. However, because the psychoanalyst is relatively unknown to the patient, in his or her reality as an individual person, the selfobject dimension is often particularly important. It may be paramount in the case of patients whose self structure is particularly fragile. When the selfobject dimension predominates, the analyst may be relegated to a role of supplying functions, and treated as if a part of the patient's psyche rather than a separate person.

The dream of the disintegrating ship

Kohut (1993) gives an example of this in criticizing a clinical presentation by one of his colleagues, Anna Ornstein. The patient and the analyst had recently been discussing the prospect of eventually terminating the analysis. The patient then had a dream: there was a ship, at sea, and although the hull seemed firmly held together, in fact it was in great danger because all the nuts and bolts had gone and the ship might fall apart or turn over. The analyst took this as a 'self-state dream' – i.e. a dream which expressed in visual metaphor the state of the self. She interpreted that the dream represented the patient's anxiety about the end of the analysis when the safe shore of the treatment setting would no longer be available. Kohut considered that whilst this interpretation was broadly along the right lines, it was incorrect in one particular detail. He pointed out that the dream contained no reference to a shore or not reaching a shore. The two anxieties depicted in the dream were (1) that the connecting links that held the structure together were missing, and (2) that the structure was in danger of turning over. Therefore, Kohut argued, the dream was *not* portraying the loss of the supportive figure of the analyst, but instead concerned the fragmentation of the self and its lack of equilibrium and orientation. Whilst the analyst's actual interpretation approximated an accurate empathic description, it incorrectly assumed that the patient was worried about the loss of the analyst and was experiencing a wish to refind a safe analytic shore; in fact the patient's dream appeared to be entirely concerned with the danger of disintegration. The analyst was not, at that moment, being perceived as an individual person, but as a function within the patient's self, represented by the nuts and bolts.

Kohut argued that the provision of accurate empathic understanding is important because only then can the patient feel sufficiently secure to proceed further. He speculated that, had the analyst correctly interpreted the manifest dream imagery of the disintegrating ship, the patient might have disclosed further, previously unarticulated, fears of disintegration of his body–mind self. Moreover, he might have recalled childhood fears about his health and sanity, perhaps evoked when his mother was physically or emotionally absent. He might even have recalled traumatic childhood experiences when tentative attempts at separation or independent movement were met with subtle parental withdrawal.

Self-state dreams

Kohut (1971) gives other examples of self-state dreams in which the patient portrays the experience of being supported by an impersonal function provided by the analyst in the role of selfobject. In one dream, the patient is in a rocket, circling the earth, but protected from shooting off into space – i.e. psychosis – by the invisible security of the potent pull of gravity. In the second dream, the patient is on a swing, swinging higher and higher, and yet is not in danger of flying off, or of getting out of control. Such dreams can occur, Kohut suggests, when the patient's infantile grandiosity or exhibitionism (aspects of narcissism) are mobilized through analytic work, threatening loss of self or dangerous overstimulation and hypomania. These dangers are countered by the sense of safety provided by the relationship with the analyst, experienced as a selfobject.

Varieties of selfobject

Kohut described three main varieties of selfobject needs and selfobject transferences: the mirroring selfobject – associated with the need to elicit confirming and approving responses; the idealizing selfobject – associated with the need to feel linked to a selfobject who can be idealized; the twinship selfobject – associated with the need to feel in contact with an other who is felt to be essentially similar. However, Kohut acknowledged the likelihood of other selfobject needs that could be found to be important in particular circumstances or stages of development. For example, Wolf (1994), one of Kohut's closest collaborators, describes three others: the *adversarial selfobject*, who is experienced as a 'benignly opposing other who continues to be supportive and responsive while allowing or even encouraging the self to be in active opposition and thus confirming an at least partial autonomy' (1994: 73); *efficacy experiences* involving 'the awareness of having an initiating and causal role in bringing about states of needed responsiveness from others . . . ' (see also Mollon, 1986c, 1993); *vitalizing selfobject* experiences, in which the child feels that the caregiver is 'affectively attuned to the dynamic shifts or patterned changes in its inner state, that is, across the specific categories of affects to the crescendos and decrescendos, to the surges and fades of the intensity, timing, and shape of its experiences (Stern 1985)' (Wolf, 1994: 74).

Kohut saw the three main selfobject needs as corresponding to what he saw as the three constituents of the self: the pole of ambitions (the grandiose self and the mirroring selfobject), the pole of ideals (the idealized selfobject), and the intermediate area of skills and talents (the selfobject of twinship).

Selfobject transferences

In his final book (1984), Kohut divided the selfobject transferences into three groups:

> (1) those in which the damaged pole of ambitions attempts to elicit the confirming-approving responses of the selfobject (mirror transference); (2) those in which the damaged pole of ideals searches for a selfobject that will accept its idealisation (idealising transference); and (3) those in which the damaged intermediate area of talents and skills seeks a selfobject that will make itself available for the reassuring experience of essential alikeness (twinship or alter ego transference).
>
> (1984: 192–93)

Kohut did not advocate that the analyst *do* anything to evoke a selfobject transference. Like other transference phenomena, he saw these as developing spontaneously provided the analyst did not interfere with their emergence. He contrasted this psychoanalytic view with the stance of those such as Aichhorn (1936), in work with delinquents, and Alexander and French (1946), in their exploration of brief psychotherapy, who advocated the analyst deliberately adopt a particular stance designed to foster or manipulate a transference image. Moreover, although it is not always immediately apparent from some of Kohut's theoretical accounts, it is evident in his clinical discussions that he viewed the selfobject transference as always interwoven with the historical transference as classically understood.

Kohut gave the following clear example of the spontaneous establishment of the mirror transference, in the case of Mr B (Kohut, 1971: 126–27). The patient was said to suffer a widespread but vague personality disturbance, suffering feelings of tension, alternating with emptiness, as well as intense rage at times, and also sexual and relationship difficulties. After a few weeks of work with a female analyst, Mr B began to experience the analysis as very soothing, 'like a warm bath'. During each week, he reported a marked lessening of his tensions, an improved sense of well-being and increased productivity at work. However, at weekends the tension increased, with hypochondriacal worries, irritability and rage. He began to realize that these weekend reactions were related to separations from the analyst. Mr B's reaction during one particular session was very illustrative of mirror transference soothing. He experienced a sudden intense sense of well-being, self-confidence and lessening of tension and feelings of emptiness after a remark by the analyst which contained the phrase, 'As you told me about a week ago.' What this meant to Mr B was that the analyst was listening to him, thinking about him, remembering him, and responding to him empathically.

This example demonstrates both the enhanced sense of well-being which the patient may experience in the mirror transference, but also the disintegration of this coherence and pleasurable tone at times of separation from the selfobject, such as the recurrent weekend breaks.

Another interesting example provided by Kohut is that of Mr E (1971: 130–32). During an early period of his analysis, Mr E tended to respond to tension states and feelings of emptiness, experienced during the weekend breaks in the analysis, by resort to exhibitionistic and voyeuristic perverse pursuits, including gazing at men's penises in public lavatories. However, he gradually became able to recognize the link between his compulsion to pursue these dangerous activities and the painful states of mind resulting from separation from the selfobject analyst. During one particular weekend, Mr E was able to reduce the need for these cruder methods of sustaining his self structure, by means of an artistic solution. He painted a picture of the analyst – but the analyst's eyes and nose were missing; in their place was a picture of the analysand. This image demonstrated with startling clarity the mirroring function of the selfobject. Mr E could feel that when he looked at the analyst he saw himself held in mind and reflected empathically. The selfobject analyst's perception of him seemed to be like the 'glue' that held the patient's self-image together. Moreover, the image of the patient and that of the analyst were incorporated into the same *structure*.

These two are examples of what Kohut termed the mirror transference – where the analysand's sense of well-being is dependent on the mirroring responsiveness of the analyst. However, Kohut also described the idealizing transference, where the analysand sees the analyst as the embodiment of such qualities of idealization as wisdom, knowledge, skill, perfection of understanding, etc. This idealization is relatively silent and invisible. It is revealed mainly by its disruption and the analysand's subsequent reactions. Perhaps because the idealizing transference is even more covert than the mirror transference, Kohut did not describe clear examples of this. Instead he tended to emphasize the analysand's response to breaches in the idealizing transference – the retreat to a haughty grandiosity or the search for more primitive or sexualized forms of idealization. The prior existence of the idealizing transference seems to be an *inference* based on such reactions.

Kohut's example of the idealizing transference (Mr A) – a defect in internal regulatory functions

One of the interesting features of this account is that although it is presented as an example of the idealizing transference, there is very little detailed description of the transference itself. Instead the focus is upon a reconstruction of the patient's childhood disappointments in relation to both his mother and his father – and, in particular, the derailments in his attempts to idealize his father.

Mr A, an unmarried man in his mid-20s, presented with worries about occasional homosexual preoccupations. However, Kohut also noted his tendencies to feel vaguely depressed and lacking energy, and to become enraged and then withdrawn, in response to criticism, lack of interest being shown in him, or the absence of praise from those he perceived as authorities. All that Kohut says about the transference itself is:

> In the cohesive therapeutic transference which established itself in the analysis,
> all these reaction propensities were clearly in evidence and permitted the
> gradual reconstruction of a certain genetically decisive pattern which had
> occurred repeatedly and had led to the specific personality defects of the

patient. Over and over again, throughout his childhood, the patient . . . had felt abruptly and traumatically disappointed in the power and efficacy of his father just when he had (re)-established him as a figure of protective strength and efficiency.

(1971: 58)

Idealization and disappointment

The father had been a prosperous businessman in Europe and when Mr A was aged 9, the family had emigrated to the USA. However, despite repeatedly telling Mr A of his exciting plans, the father was unable to establish himself successfully in America and would sell his businesses in panic when unforeseen events blocked his plans. Moreover, he would react with depression and hypochondriacal withdrawal in response to these failures.

During the analysis Mr A began to recall earlier examples of the idealization-disappointment sequence in relation to his father. From an early age, he and his father enjoyed a close relationship, and his father would sometimes take him to his factory and even playfully ask his advice about business matters. The relationship was then interrupted by the threat of German invasion and the father was away a great deal working to establish his business in another European country. Although the father managed to achieve this, his success was shortlived because the German army invaded the country they had escaped to. The family, being Jewish, then had to flee again and this led them to the United States.

A primary narcissistic vulnerability

In addition to the traumatic disappointments and disruptions in the relationship to the father, Kohut postulated that Mr A had suffered deficiencies in the empathic responsiveness of his mother in the earliest period of his life. These were 'not remembered but broadly reinstated by the patient's diffuse sensitivity to the analyst; specifically, to even slight imperfections in the analyst's ability to achieve immediate empathic understanding for all shades and nuances of his current experiences and moods . . .' (1971: 61). Thus Kohut reconstructed the mother's empathic unreliability on the basis of Mr A's sensitivity as revealed in the transference. However, he also pointed to supportive evidence of this on the basis of reports of the mother's current behaviour and personality; she was described as deeply disturbed, prone to intense anxiety and unintelligible excitement when under stress. Kohut hypothesized that these features of the early relationship with the mother had given rise to a *diffuse narcissistic vulnerability*, the components of which were as follows: he was extremely sensitive to slights by others and also to setbacks by adverse circumstances; he would react to these as if they were deliberately inflicted on him by an animistically experienced world.

Inadequate idealization of the superego

On the ground of this diffuse narcissistic vulnerability, derived from the faulty responses of the mother, Kohut postulated that Mr A developed a more specific psychological defect, namely 'the insufficient idealization of his superego . . . ' (1971: 61). In optimum development, Kohut theorized, the child *gradually* withdraws idealization of the father through repeated impingements of reality which result in nontraumatic disappointments; the idealization, the investment of perfection in the other, is taken back and used to build up an internal structure, the 'ego ideal' aspect of the superego. This is one example of the process Kohut termed 'transmuting internalization'. Because of the traumatic disappointments, Mr A had not been able to achieve transmuting internalization of the idealized father. The result was that he lacked the ability to find any lasting satisfaction in living up to his standards or in achieving his goals. There was no *internal* source of self-esteem. Instead, Mr A could obtain self-esteem only by attaching himself to strong, admired (i.e. idealized) figures whose approval and support he craved. Although Mr A's *idealization* of his superego was deficient, he did not lack the guiding and prohibiting functions of the superego, which Freud described as heir to the resolution of the oedipus complex.

Sexualization of narcissistic disturbance

Mr A's homosexual fantasies usually involved a theme of enslaving a strong and virile man whom he would masturbate and thereby drain of his power. Kohut argued that these fantasies were 'sexualized statements about his narcissistic disturbance' (1971: 71). They expressed, in a sexualized form, Mr A's longing for an infusion of strength and perfection from an idealized man, originally the father. In place of the missing inner ideal, Mr A had created an external sexualized image; moreover, in place of the source of self-esteem that derives from living up to internalized idealized values, Mr A had substituted a sexualized sense of triumph in stealing the qualities of power and perfection from the external ideal. Intriguingly, Kohut adds that these 'sexualized statements' are analogous to the theoretical formulations of the analyst, the difference being that they are in *opposition* to insight since they are created in the service of pleasure and relief from narcissistic tensions. Kohut is making the point here that the content of sexual fantasies reveals the underlying narcissistic tensions – as if they were the patient's private masturbatory formulation.

Impaired capacity to 'neutralize'

Kohut also postulated that one reason for the sexualization of narcissistic disturbance, in Mr A and other patients, is an impairment in the neutralizing functions of the psyche. This concept, which may be relatively unfamiliar to British psychoanalytic practitioners, was proposed by Hartmann (1964) and colleagues to denote the transformation of instinctual (sexual and aggressive) energy into a more 'neutral' form, suitable for use by the higher psychic functions. Kohut reasoned that the capacity to neutralize sexual and aggressive impulses derives in part from transmuting internalization, the building up of internal structures that channel impulses into reality-adapted and socially acceptable forms – functions which originally were performed by the selfobject. Kohut also noted that some patients represented the need for these desexualizing and de-aggressifying functions by dreams of books or libraries, expressing the search for symbols of the secondary (as opposed to primary) process (i.e. psychological expression which is reality based and culturally recognized). He gives the example (1971: 173) of a patient reported by Tolpin (1969), who represented mounting sexual tension during sleep by means of a dream of riding on a fast moving train; the dreamer got up from his seat and began to move from carriage to carriage; he realized he had left his books on his seat and went back to collect them; however, he discovered with horror that the part of the train containing his books had become disconnected from the part where he was now riding. Kohut saw this dream as portraying the anxious recognition that the patient's ego had been taken over by the sexual excitement and had lost its access to the drive-regulating and drive-elaborating functions of the secondary process, represented by the books. This particular patient suffered from premature ejaculation – and Kohut suggested that deficiencies in drive-regulating functions may often play a role in this condition.

Thus Kohut argued that defective regulatory functions give rise to sexualization of narcissistic tensions and also that these may be represented in the *content* of sexual fantasies.

Kohut's example of the twinship transference

In his 1971 book, Kohut regarded the twinship transference as a variant of the mirror transference. However, by the time of his last book (1984), he postulated twinship as a distinct selfobject need in its own right. He gives the following clinical example as one that contributed to his change of mind.

A woman patient began to develop 'quasi-fetishistic and quasi-obsessional preoccupations' during a period prior to Kohut's summer break. Her dreams and daydreams became focused on things rather than people, with a particular theme of placing a covering over objects – e.g. lids on jars and vases, corks in bottles, a plate over an aquarium, etc. When Kohut commented on this change in the content of her material, pointing out that it followed his announcement of his summer vacation, she responded with associations to lonely periods of her childhood when she was aged 6 or 7 and her family had moved to a new area, resulting in loss of the previous closeness to her grandparents, who had offset the emotionally distant quality of her parents. She recalled that she used to keep a bottle with a stopper on her desk, imagining that it contained a person – 'my genie' – with whom she would have endless conversations. This memory was associated with some shame because, so it emerged, she had continued a version of the conversations with the 'genie' into her adult life. Kohut offered the interpretation that since the associations to the genie had been evoked by his announcement of his absence from her for several weeks, the captive in the bottle probably represented him, this being a transference revival of her childhood attempts to cope with the loss of the grandparents. No doubt many analysts would have made just such an interpretation. However, the patient, with some embarrassment, gave an unequivocal rejection of this hypothesis. She insisted that it was not the analyst in the bottle and had not been either grandparent in childhood. In fact, Kohut explains 'Then as now the captive was a little girl, a twin, someone just like herself and yet not herself to whom she could talk, who kept her company and made it possible for her to survive the hours of loneliness when she felt that no one other than her companion in the bottle cared for her' (1984: 196).

Prior to this material, Kohut had been assuming that the patient was presenting a mirror transference. However, he came to realize that, unlike certain other patients, she did not need him to respond with empathic mirroring. Instead, she had felt sustained by his simple presence, allowing her to experience him as in essence just like her. She did not need him to speak to her. As with the original twin in the bottle, she would speak but would not expect any response. Silent communion with the twin was often her preferred experience.

From this patient Kohut also gained a clearer sense of a distinction between a pathological and a normal version of the twinship experience. Whilst the genie in the bottle fantasy represented the pathological variant, the patient also presented a memory describing a normal twinship selfobject experience. She recalled being in her grandmother's kitchen, aged about 4, her grandmother kneading dough on the table, while the patient too kneaded dough on a smaller table next to the grandmother's larger one. Kohut notes that such selfobject experiences, and similar ones such as a little boy working next to his daddy with daddy's tools in a basement, have inherently a rather quiet and undramatic quality. They provide silent nutrients for the developing self.

Narcissistic equilibrium in the primary matrix

Kohut theorized that at times, when well protected and nurtured, the infant experiences a primary narcissistic equilibrium – 'a psychological state whose perfection precedes even the most rudimentary differentiation into the later categories of perfection (i.e. perfection in the realm of power, of knowledge, of beauty, and of morality)' (1971: 63–64). If the mother's empathic responsiveness is sufficiently adequate to prevent intolerable delays in the restoration of equilibrium, when it has been disturbed by bodily and psychological needs, then the developing infant will gradually surrender the illusion of absolute perfection. The important factor, according to Kohut, is the principle of *optimal frustration*. This allows the process of transmuting internalization to take place. As the mother inevitably fails in minor ways, in her provision of soothing, empathic understanding, warmth and holding, relief from hunger, pain, tension etc., the infant gradually withdraws investment in the archaic image of absolute perfection and 'acquires in its stead, a particle of inner psychological structure which takes over the mother's functions in the service of the maintenance of narcissistic equilibrium . . .' (1971: 64). However, if the mother's responses are grossly unattuned or unreliable, then the process of *gradual* deinvestment in the image of perfection is disrupted. Then the building up of internal structure, the gradual taking over of the mother's functions through the process of transmuting internalization, does not take place. The resulting behavioural manifestations of this basic failure in narcissistic development consist of a general sensitivity to disturbances of physical and psychological equilibrium, and a tendency to react to these with a mixture of withdrawal and rage.

One point worth noting here is that a clinician who did not employ Kohut's framework might conclude that a patient who showed this kind of diffuse narcissistic vulnerability was probably suffering from an innate intolerance of frustration. Kohut emphasized how the capacity to manage emotions and psychological tensions develops out of the matrix of soothing functions originally provided by the selfobject mother.

Disturbances of equilibrium – self-state dreams

In the absence of the reliable and repeated availability of soothing from caregivers, the child will fail to establish healthy forms of self-soothing (and may resort to pathological forms, such as dissociation, self-stimulation, self-harm, substance misuse, etc.). At times of later stress involving injuries to self-esteem, such a person may appear overwhelmed and disorganized. This may be apparent in a hypersensitivity to sensory stimulation, or in a psychosomatic reaction. For example, the person may complain of noise or smell or sunlight or temperature, to an extent that might appear excessive, or he or she may report headache or other pains. At such times dreams may reflect this overwhelmed state where the cohesion of the self is threatened. Kohut comments in a 1974 lecture:

> . . . the dreams of the previous night . . . don't lend themselves to the ordinary kind of analysis of content. They are more chaotic . . . things are falling apart. They are disorganized . . . 'exploded' dreams like the disarticulated diagrams of mechanical contrivances that are purchased to be assembled at home – perhaps body parts . . . or rapid, apparently incomprehensible content shifts from one section of the dream to the next, and to the next . . . crumbling structures . . .
> (Kohut, 1996: 149–50)

Thus Kohut described how the disintegrating structure of the self may be portrayed in dreams – which he called 'self-state dreams'. Kohut's approach when faced with a patient in a *psychoeconomic crisis* would be to listen calmly, avoiding premature interpretation, before commenting empathically on this state of feeling narcissistically injured and overwhelmed, and then searching for its precipitants and their meaning.

The line of development of narcissism and the self

A crucial part of Kohut's novel theorizing was his postulating that narcissism was not in essence a primitive state of mind, to be gradually outgrown and replaced by object love (i.e. love for others), the position Freud had originally described. Instead, Kohut saw narcissism as pursuing its own developmental line, from archaic to more mature forms.

Following hints in Freud's 1914 paper *On Narcissism*, Kohut theorized that the disturbance of the infant's original narcissistic equilibrium, as a result of the inevitable shortcomings of maternal care, gave rise to two developmental lines of narcissism as the child attempted to replace the original experience of perfection: a grandiose and exhibitionistic image of the self – *the grandiose self*, and the *idealized parent imago*. In the first position, the child's illusion is 'I am perfect'; in the second position, the illusion is 'You are perfect – and I am part of you.' Both positions depend upon the empathic and responsive availability of the selfobject caregiver. Through gradual disillusionment and the process of transmuting internalization, the archaic grandiose self is transformed into mature, socially integrated ambitions, self-esteem and self-confidence, whilst the position of the idealized object is transformed into internal ideals, admiration for others and capacity for enthusiasm.

Commenting on his use of the term 'grandiose self', Kohut comments:

The terms 'grandiose' and 'exhibitionistic' refer to a broad spectrum of phenomena, ranging from the child's solipsistic world view and his undisguised pleasure in being admired, and from the gross delusions of the paranoiac and the crudely sexual acts of the adult pervert, to aspects of the mildest, most aim-inhibited, and nonerotic satisfaction of adults with themselves, their functioning, and their achievements.

(1971: 25)

Similarly, the phenomena of the idealized parent imago cover a spectrum, from vague mystical preoccupations and crude sexual voyeurism, to the mature capacity for admiration and the valuing of ideals.

The therapeutic mobilization of the grandiose self gives rise to a range of phenomena collectively called the *mirror transference*, whilst those that arise from the mobilization of the idealized parent imago are referred to as the *idealizing transference*. According to Kohut, these transferences consist of the 'amalgamation of unconscious narcissistic structures (the idealized parent imago and the grandiose self) with the psychic representation of the analyst which becomes drawn into these therapeutically activated, narcissistically cathected structures' (1971: 29).

By observing the movements of regression and progression in the analysis of patients with narcissistic disturbances, Kohut was able to discern the lines of development of narcissism. These concern the way the self is structured, experienced and represented.

The deepest regressions noted by Kohut were to the stage of the *fragmented self* – prior to the establishment of what he termed a *nuclear* or *cohesive* self. This corresponded to the earliest developmental stage which Freud (1914) had referred to as that of autoeroticism. Freud had viewed this period as characterized by an absence of the ego, a lack of integration of the drives, an absence of relatedness to others, and a seeking of instinctual satisfaction in the body – basically a state of fragmentation of the mind-body self (a view which may be also compared with a perspective offered by Lacan (1949) regarding a primary state of fragmentation prior to the 'mirror stage' of development). When a patient regresses to this state of fragmentation, he or she may attempt to explain or describe this experience by means of hypochondriacal brooding about the body or the mind. Kohut argued that nothing is gained psychotherapeutically by focusing on the experience of fragmentation per se. These experiences are beyond the reach of the healthy part of the psyche, as evidenced by the way the patient may describe parts of the body feeling 'strange', 'foreign', 'odd', 'unreal', etc. All such terms express the way that the experience of fragmentation is, inherently, outside the patient's psychological organization – and are therefore what Kohut would describe as 'prepsychological'. Kohut would not address or interpret the *content* of fragmentation directly, but instead would help the patient to identify the precipitants of the narcissistic regression (such as feelings of disappointment in the analyst, or of feeling misunderstood or slighted).

Kohut (1971) made some important observations regarding certain patients who, whilst not psychotic, do not have a firmly established cohesive self. Such people, who may often be described as having schizoid personalities, have learned to distance themselves from others because of a correct preconscious awareness that a narcissistic injury, resulting from emotional involvement, may have the potential to initiate an uncontrollable regression beyond the nuclear cohesive self. This emotional distancing may not reflect an inability to love, nor a paranoid perception of others, but an accurate assessment of their own narcissistic vulnerability and potential for regression to the fragmented self. Kohut considered that psychoanalysis, which involves a transference regression whereby the pathogenic nucleus of the patient's personality becomes activated in relation to the analyst, is not appropriate for those who have not established a cohesive self – i.e. patients who could be described as schizoid, borderline, or psychotic. For these patients, a psychoanalytically informed psychotherapy is the more appropriate, which focuses in a supportive way on the patient's regression potential and on identifying the triggers for this.

Most of Kohut's writings have focused upon the analysis of patients who have established a cohesive self, but nevertheless suffer disturbances in the realm of narcissism. These patients may display temporary or fleeting regressions to a partial state of the fragmented self, but there remains a sufficient area of psychic health to prevent a complete and irreversible descent into psychosis. The symptoms of such patients tend to be vague and ill defined, although he or she may be able to describe work inhibitions, perverse sexual activities, or pervasive but subtle feelings of emptiness or depression, or of unreality. These rather fluid states are often alleviated once the narcissistic transference is established, but become exacerbated when this is disrupted. The patient is unable to focus on or describe the central disturbance because of the 'nearness of the pathologically disturbed structures (the self) to the seat of the self-observing functions in the ego' (Kohut, 1971: 16).

Disruptions in the relationship to the selfobject analyst may evoke a regression along the developmental lines of narcissism, of the grandiose self and the idealized (or omnipotent) object. Thus the regression in the realm of the grandiose self might involve a retreat from mature forms of self-esteem and self-confidence, to solipsistic and imperious claims for attention and admiration (the stage of the grandiose self), and further to the stage of fragmentation with resulting hypochondriacal brooding. The regression in the realm of the idealized object might involve a retreat from mature forms of admiration for others and the ability for enthusiasm, to a compelling need for merger with powerful others (the stage of the idealized parent imago), to the stage of fragmentation, resulting in disjointed mystical feelings. If regression proceeds past the stage of fragmentation and into psychosis, there may be a *delusional reconstitution* of the grandiose self, resulting in cold paranoid grandiosity, or a delusional reconstitution of the omnipotent object, resulting in images of a powerful persecutor, or of influence by inanimate forces.

Thus the bulk of Kohut's work concerned psychoanalytic therapy with patients who had achieved a cohesive self, but who were prone to regress along the line of narcissism, in the realm of the grandiose self or the idealized object. However, he also made some valuable observations concerning those whose establishment of a cohesive self was sufficiently fragile that they lived with the danger of regression to the stage of fragmentation and the possibility of delusional reconstitution of the grandiose self or the idealized object. In Kohut's view, psychoanalysis – whose essential process he defined as one in which 'the pathogenic nucleus of the analysand's personality becomes activated in the treatment situation and itself enters a specific transference with the analyst before it is gradually dissolved in the working through process' (1971: 13) – is appropriate for the former group of patients, but not for the latter, in whom a transference regression could lead to a severe fragmentation of the self. For these more vulnerable patients, a psychoanalytically informed psychotherapy is the more appropriate.

The nuclear bipolar self – discerning a structure

Kohut seems not to have clearly differentiated between his use of the terms 'cohesive self', 'nuclear self' and 'bipolar self'. These all appear to have similar meanings. In *The Analysis of the Self*, he writes of the significance of the establishment of a cohesive self following an earlier stage of fragmentation. Although in the two subsequent books (1977 and 1984) he still writes about cohesion and fragmentation, he gives more emphasis to the terms 'nuclear self' and 'bipolar self', sometimes giving the impression that these are synonymous. These terms represent Kohut's attempt to discern the hidden core structures, in themselves invisible, that lie behind the manifest observable clinical phenomena of narcissistically disturbed patients. His inferences were not based on direct observation of children but upon psychoanalytic reconstruction of childhood development on the basis of the transference.

Here is how Kohut writes of his inferences regarding the origin of the self:

> In trying again and again, in analysis after analysis, to determine the genetic roots of the selves of my analysands, I obtained the impression that during early psychic development a process takes place in which some archaic mental contents that had been experienced as belonging to the self become obliterated or are assigned to the area of the nonself while others are retained within the self or are added to it. As a result of this process a core self – the 'nuclear self' – is established. This structure is the basis for our sense of being an independent center of initiative and perception, integrated with our most central ambitions and ideals and with our experience that our body and mind form a unit in space and a continuum in time. This cohesive and enduring psychic configuration, in connection with a correlated set of talents and skills that it attracts to itself or that develops in response to the demands of the ambitions and ideals of the nuclear self, forms the central sector of the personality.
>
> (1977: 177–78)

Note that Kohut is pointing to two aspects of the formation of the self here. First, the idea that a process takes place whereby certain mental contents are designated part of 'self' whilst others are designated 'not self'. Second, this process is linked with the establishment of a structure composed of the two poles of our central ambitions and ideals, which draw upon our skills and talents.

What did Kohut mean by this idea of the sorting of mental contents into 'self' and 'not self' and how and why would it take place? Part of what he had in mind is suggested by some remarks on the origin of the self in *The Restoration of the Self*. He points out (1977: 99) that although the infant cannot have any reflective self-awareness, he or she is from the beginning related to by an empathic environment which does regard him or her as possessing a self. The newborn may thus be described as having a *virtual self*. Moreover, this environment of the principal caregivers has expectations of the child's self, which channel it in specific directions. These expectations on the part of the environment have a sorting function, affirming some potentials whilst disregarding others. Kohut comments:

> At the moment when the mother sees her baby for the first time and is also in contact with him (through tactile, olfactory, and proprioceptive channels as she feeds, carries, bathes him), a process that lays down a person's self has its virtual beginning – it continues throughout childhood and to a lesser extent later in life. I have in mind the specific interactions of the child and his selfobjects through

which in countless repetitions, the selfobjects empathically respond to certain
potentialities of the child (aspects of the grandiose self he exhibits, aspects of the
idealized image he admires, different innate talents he employs to mediate
creatively between ambitions and ideals), but not to others. This is the most
important way by which the child's innate potentialities are selectively
nourished or thwarted.

(1977: 100)

Kohut goes on to say that this selection by the responsiveness of the
environment, which does not necessarily reflect the *conscious* attitudes
of the parents, gives rise to the *nuclear* self.

Why does Kohut link this environmental selection and shaping of the
infant's virtual self with the idea of a structure consisting of the poles of
ambitions and ideals, and associated talents and skills? This seems to be
because Kohut's clinical experience showed that patients whose selves
were vulnerable gave evidence of damage or deficit in these two areas of
the grandiose self (the natural exhibitionistic display) and idealization. He
perhaps concluded therefore that these were the two areas in which the
parents, or other principal selfobjects, could exert the main effect in determining the direction of the self; this would be in terms of what capacities
and talents the parent responded to with approval and affirmation
(mirroring) and what qualities the parent provided for the child to idealize.

In a paper entitled *On Courage* (from the early 1970s, but published
1985), Kohut makes a rather clear statement about the nuclear self. He
comments that there may be a simultaneous existence of several selves,
or even contradictory selves, with varying degrees of stability and importance, but there is normally one self that is most centrally located in the
psyche and which is the most stable and resistant to change. He states:

I like to call this the nuclear self. It is composed of derivatives of the grandiose
self (i.e. of the central self-assertive goals, purposes and ambitions) and of
derivatives of the idealized parent imago (i.e. of the central idealized values).
The nuclear self is thus that unconscious, preconscious and conscious sector in
id, ego, and superego which contains not only the individual's most enduring
values and ideals but also his most deeply anchored goals, purposes and
ambitions.

(1985a: 10–11)

Kohut also notes (1985b: 218) that as this nuclear self is formed,
'something clicks and we have a degree of autonomy . . . (which) we call the
self' and that this self is then a centre of initiative with its own goals and
ideals. Thus he argues that our autonomy comes about, paradoxic-ally,
through the shaping provided by the selfobject experiences offered by our
parents, which we then make our own, through using these experiences to

build the structure of our self. Kohut also emphasizes in the following passage the 'free will' arising from the establishment of the self and its inherent impetus to realize its inner developmental programme:

> While the environment has contributed to its formation, from a certain time on the self is a coiled spring, a wound clock . . . In other words, it is a structure that, though it has its limitations, is firmly formed and, from that moment on, has free will.
>
> (1996: 390)

However, another basis for Kohut's arguments regarding the selective inclusion and exclusion of mental contents in the formation of the self, comes more directly from the detail of his clinical experience – particularly the case of Mr M (described in *The Restoration of the Self*, Kohut, 1977). Kohut had observed that his patients sought selfobject experiences in relation to mirroring or idealization. However, he also began to appreciate that if a child had experienced deficits in relation to one dimension of narcissistic development (e.g. mirroring), then he or she could still form a coherent and viable self on the basis of the other dimension (i.e. idealization) – that the child had two chances, so to speak. Kohut found that in the analysis of Mr M the consolidation of the patient's self was achieved essentially in relation to the pole of idealization linked to his father and thus by means of the working through of an idealizing transference. Although some aspects of Mr M's earliest deprivations, relating to experiences with his unempathic mother and also linked to a stay in an orphanage, were addressed in the transference at an earlier stage of the work, Kohut believed that 'the deeper layers of his defective (depressive, lethargic, "dead") self (the self of his stay in the orphanage) were never exposed to full view in the transference' (1977: 52). He discerned a process during the analysis in which there came about an exclusion of the most defective areas of Mr M's personality from the nuclear bipolar self. The healing process appeared to be one in which the patient, spontaneously through the analytic work, gave up the pursuit of pathological solutions to the needs of the sickest part of the personality and instead focused upon building upon the areas of relative health. Kohut clearly believed that attempting to revisit in the transference the most damaging experiences of childhood could lead to an irreversible regression and disintegration of the self.

Comparison with Kernberg's formulation of narcissistic personality

Kohut and Kernberg began writing about narcissism around the same time. Somewhat confusingly, Kernberg adopted Kohut's term 'grandiose self', but used it somewhat differently. For Kohut, the grandiose self is a normal and inherent aspect of the line of development of narcissism, a polarity within the tripartite structure also encompassing twinship and the idealized other. However, for Kernberg (1975), the grandiose self is a pathological structure consisting of a fusion of the images of the actual self, the ideal self and the ideal object. He equates this with what Rosenfeld (1964) referred to as 'the omnipotent mad self'. For Kernberg, this pathological grandiose self functions to deny dependency and is 'a rigid defense against more primitive, pathological object relations centered around narcissistic rage and envy, fear and guilt because of this rage, and yet a desperate longing for a loving relationship that will not be destroyed by hatred' (1975: 274). In Kernberg's clinical descriptions, this pathological grandiosity appears rather overt – a conscious grandiosity – whereas Kohut's patients with narcissistic pathology tend to be characterized by low self-esteem, depression, and feelings of loneliness and depression – resulting from the repression of the natural (invisible) grandiose self. Thus they may have been writing about somewhat different groups of patients – possibly corresponding to the distinction between 'thick and thin-skinned' narcissists, described by Rosenfeld (1987) and Bateman (1998). Probably Kernberg's clinical and theoretical account corresponds more closely to the popular image of a 'narcissistic' character. Certainly, the malignant narcissism of criminal psychopaths, manifest in profound egocentricity, attitudes of entitlement and arrogance, often seems to reflect the grossly pathological grandiose self described by Kernberg. Discussion of a range of perspectives on narcissistic disturbance is provided in Mollon (1993).

Summary

Kohut's novel contribution was to focus not so much on the overt content of the patient's discourse, but upon the invisible absences of psychic structure that were driving the search for compensatory experiences. Some comparison may be made with André Green's theme of 'blank' states. Compulsive and abnormal sexual pursuits can be an attempt to shore up weakened narcissistic functions of the psyche. Kohut began to recognize that, in the case of some patients, his or her psychological functioning depends on the empathic attunement of the analyst. He called such mental systems selfobject transferences. This led to an appreciation that the child's 'self' was built up out of experiences with caregivers functioning as selfobjects – the self is woven from the fabric of the other. Kohut proposed that narcissism is not converted into object love during maturation, but follows its own line of development, through the positions of the grandiose self, twinship, and the idealized other. The deepest regression along this line of development would be to the stage of the fragmented self. Kohut wrote of a 'nuclear self' which he saw as the most centrally located self, which contains the person's deepest and most enduring goals and values. This nuclear self is a 'centre of initiative'. In the course of analysis, patients suffering from pathology of the self may spontaneously (but non-consciously) give up the pursuit of solutions to the needs of the most damaged pole of the self (e.g. the grandiose self) and instead seek to build upon areas of potential health (e.g. through the pole of the idealized other). Revisiting in the transference the most damaging experiences of childhood could lead to an irreversible regression.

Chapter 3

Perversion[1], the vertical split and the psychoeconomic dimension

> . . . to my mind, all worthwhile theorizing is tentative, probing, provisional – contains an element of playfulness . . . The world of creative science . . . is inhabited by playful people who understand that the reality that surrounds them is essentially unknowable.
>
> (Kohut, 1977: 206–7)

The vertical split

Another of Kohut's crucial contributions was his development of the idea that certain clinical presentations involve a split in the ego, a concept first proposed by Freud (1940b), based on his observations of fetishism. Freud had described how the fetishist may, in one part of his mind, accept the reality that a woman does not have a penis, whilst in another part, separated by a split in the ego, may maintain the belief that she does possess a penis, represented by the fetish. Kohut termed this a *vertical split*, since it allows coexistent attitudes or beliefs to exist side by side, which could be contrasted with the *horizontal split* of repression, whereby a content of the mind is denied access to consciousness. Freud's idea of the split originated in his study of a particular sexual perversion, but Kohut went further, to argue that in all perversions 'we find that there is a part of the personality intensely involved in a certain kind of pursuit, a pursuit driven by irresistible wishes for some kind of a fulfilment that seems totally out of keeping with the patient's personality' (Kohut, 1996: 48). He contrasted this with other conditions in which symptoms are not found acceptable, even by part of the personality, but are experienced as like a foreign body lodged in the personality. In the case of perversions,

[1] Some have argued that in order to remove the pejorative and judgmental connotations of the term 'perversion', some other word should be substituted, such as 'paraphilia' or 'neosexualities'. Others have argued that the term 'perversion' has continuing value, especially since it can refer to broader and deeper dimensions of personality, in addition to manifest sexuality. See Leigh, 1998.

one part of the personality is totally involved in the pursuit of these goals, even though they are at odds with other goals and values held by the patient. Kohut gives the example of a common situation during the analysis of narcissistic disorders, in which a man who is somewhat depressed, and whose analyst has gone away temporarily, may develop an intense urge to view pornography and may visit a seedy cinema or shop. Such activity may be quite incongruent with the man's other pursuits and his status in society. In one way the perverse activity is foreign to the rest of the personality, but on deeper examination, Kohut argues, the symptomatic behaviour has a long history and has coexisted with other quite different attitudes.

The present writer has observed related phenomena in certain patients who have created serious trouble for themselves by generating an elaborate web of lies involving their professional activities or financial situation. After the truth of the situation has come to light, it is sometimes possible to reconstruct the state of mind of the patient when he or she was wildly confabulating the fictitious events. The impression is that in one part of the mind the patient has believed his or her own lies and fantasies, whilst another part maintained an orientation to reality but turned a blind eye to the corrupt activities of the generator of lies.

In a similar way, the patient with a perversion maintains coexisting or alternating attitudes. Kohut describes a voyeur who would at times become utterly preoccupied with looking at male genitals. This would be quite at odds with his activities and preoccupations at other times. Kohut comments: 'Either he was this particular kind of a person, who could focus on nothing else but trying to look at male genitals, or he was the person who could not in the least understand what this urge was all about, who had no interest in it at all and was just going on with his usual life' (Kohut, 1996: 50). Contrasting with the position of a patient who is concerned about a symptom, where the analytic work can be undertaken 'with the aid, more or less, of a co-operative ego that has experienced this anxiety as something foreign that has interfered with its functions', in the case of a vertical split 'you have a total personality index that is side by side with another personality index, and the one is not connected with the other' (1996: 50). Therefore, the initial stage of the analytic work must be concerned with diminishing the vertical split between the divergent personalities.

What causes the vertical split? Kohut believed that it comes about when the mother rewards a particular aspect of the child's personality that conforms to her desires and expectations, but neglects crucial aspects of the child's own aspirations and needs for recognition. The child's needs for mirroring are hijacked and then turned against the developmental potential of the rest of the personality. In this way, mirroring becomes a developmental prison. The child's needs for mirroring of his (Kohut's examples of perversion are all male) own initiatives, his natural grandiose self, as well as his needs to idealize his father, are denied normal expression and fulfilment, but may emerge in the form of perverse or degraded sexual activities, especially voyeurism, exhibitionism and non-intimate homosexuality. All of these sexual variants, torn from the context of a relationship, are what Kohut termed *disintegration products* when the cohesion of the self is undermined. He also saw them as *sexualized expressions of narcissistic injury* and narcissistic need.

Mr E – the boy on a swing

The emergence of the sexualized expression of narcissistic need is illustrated clearly in Kohut's account of Mr E (1971: 158–59; 1996: 80–82). The patient would often revert to dangerous voyeuristic pursuits, particularly gazing at other men's genitals in public toilets, during separations from the analyst, or when he felt misunderstood by the analyst. Kohut regarded these as sexualized enactments of regressive wishes for visual merger with an idealized father. As the analysis progressed, Mr E began to recall relevant, affectively associated memories from childhood. He recalled the first episode of voyeurism in a public toilet as occurring at a country fair after he had asked his mother to admire his skill on a swing. His mother, ill with hypertension, showed little interest. Mr E, deflated and drained of all joy, then turned away from her and visited the toilet. As Kohut then describes, 'Driven by a force which he understood only now, but for which he could now, also, recall the appropriate feeling tone, he looked at a man's genital and, merging into it, felt at one with the power and strength that it symbolized' (1971: 159). Kohut saw this as a regression from the position of seeking from his mother a mirroring of his grandiosity (flying fantasies) to one of desiring merger with the idealized father imago.

Kohut provides further information about the origin of Mr E's preoccupation with looking and being looked at. Mr E had been an incubator baby for some months and he had been deprived of touch. Therefore, Kohut speculated, Mr E's needs for contact and security probably were channelled through the eyes; he could look at his mother even though she could not pick him up. Mr E's conflicts about looking were also apparent in the way that he would not look at the analyst. He feared that to look would overburden and embarrass the analyst. Kohut considered that Mr E felt that so much demand and neediness was implicitly contained in his need to look that the analyst would be made ill or might even die, as he felt had been the case with his mother. However, as Kohut notes, 'All he really wanted was the gleam in the mother's eye' (1996: 82).

Mr E's perversion was wholesomely transformed during the analysis. He became increasingly able to understand how his voyeuristic acting out related to rejections, separations, or failures of empathy experienced in the transference, and how these linked to his early rejections and deprivations. His regressions and perverse impulses did not immediately go, but Mr E became able to ask himself why these were occurring. He became more aware of this area of his personality as the vertical split lessened. Most significantly, Mr E began to use his visual gifts and preoccupations in an adaptive and creative way. He developed an artistic occupation and some of his visual creations were published. Kohut saw the image on one of his books. It was of a boy jumping with joy, but almost appearing to be flying – a clear allusion to the early episode of wishing to be admired by his mother for 'flying' on the swing.

Mr X, the stolen inheritance, and the lost can of gasoline

Mr X was twenty-two years old when he presented for analysis, complaining of loneliness, social isolation and shame about his sexual activities (described in Kohut, 1977: 199–219; 1996: 309–17). The latter consisted of frequent compulsive masturbation several times a day, accompanied by homosexual fantasies.

Mr X's mother had idealized him, but only so long as he stayed within her orbit. By contrast she had denigrated his father. The bond between them was close, an intimacy which excluded the father. She used to read Bible stories to Mr X, placing particular emphasis upon the connection between the boy Jesus and the Virgin. A favourite story was of Jesus in the temple, where he is portrayed as superior to all the older teachers. In this story (Luke 2, 48–49), Jesus is rebuked by his parents for being away from home without telling them where he was: 'Son, why hast thou thus dealt with us? Behold, thy father and I have sought thee sorrowing.' And Jesus replies: 'How is it that ye sought me? Wist ye not that I must be about my Father's business?' Kohut explains that this story represents the idealization of the son, whose greatness is linked to the mother (the Virgin), whilst the real father is denigrated. There is nevertheless a great father (God the Father), but it is not the mother's husband. The image of the idealized father is perhaps that of the mother's unconscious image of her own father.

From an early age Mr X felt a strong desire to enter the church ministry, but he did not actually do so. Kohut explains that although Mr X had entertained a grandiose identification with Christ, he had been unable to direct this into the vocation of a clergyman because his relation to religion had become sexualized. In particular, Mr X had a core masturbatory fantasy of crossing his penis with that of the officiating priest at the moment of receiving Holy Communion. As Kohut puts it: 'Thus at the moment of climactic ejaculation, the patient's preoccupation with a powerful man's penis, with oral incorporation, and with the acquisition of idealized strength found an almost artistically perfect expression in his sexualized imagery about the consummation of the most profoundly significant symbolic act of the Christian ritual' (1977: 201). Kohut also notes that this core theme was elaborated with all kinds of subsidiary fantasies and suffused with 'a fleeting sense of great strength, triumph and holiness' (1996: 313).

Mr X displayed an overt grandiosity and haughtiness, clearly derived from his having been a boy who was persistently aggrandized by his mother. However, this grandiosity related only to his experience of a self existing as an appendage to his mother. When he had tried to move away from his mother's orbit and pursue an independent initiative she would become coldly withdrawn. Thus the grandiosity based on the idealization by his mother and the denigration of his father actually left him still in need of an idealized father image, with which he could merge and draw strength for his independent masculinity. This was the need expressed in a sexualized form in the masturbation fantasy of crossing his penis with the naked priest whilst receiving communion (the body and blood of Christ).

A crucial clue to these deeper dynamics was present in some of Mr X's earliest communications in the diagnostic interview with the analyst. He complained that his mother and younger sister had deprived him of his inheritance from his father who had died some years previously. Initially this had been presented with a somewhat paranoid flavour and had raised questions about his analysability. However, Kohut concluded that this complaint by Mr X was a disguised statement that he felt deprived not so much of the financial inheritance, but of the far more important emotional legacy of identification with an idealized masculine father. This was the nurturance and emotional birthright which the mother's denigration, and his own oedipal collusion with this, had prevented him from receiving. All of this was obviously quite unconscious at the beginning of the analysis.

The early part of the analysis, prior to Kohut's supervision of the case, was not informed by an understanding of self psychology. Instead, during the first two and a half years, the analyst's focus had been upon Mr X's overt grandiosity, including his arrogance, isolation and his unrealistic goals. The interpretation of these was in terms of the developmental consequences of an 'oedipal victory', combined with an attempt by Mr X to deny that although his mother had appeared to prefer him to his father, the latter was nevertheless her real possessor who could 'castrate' the little boy. Such an interpretation combined a theme of oedipal victory with that of oedipal defeat, and saw the overt grandiosity as a defensive denial of the depression of defeat.

Kohut disagreed with this formulation, arguing that the overt grandiosity was not defensive but more directly the 'agent of his mother's ambitions' (1977: 203). Another way of putting this would be to say that what appeared as *Mr X's* grandiosity was in fact his *mother's* grandiosity, which had hijacked his development and was parasitically expressed through his personality. Kohut contrasted this with Mr X's own latent grandiosity: 'the boy's repressed grandiose-exhibitionistic self – an independent boyish self that had first yearned in vain for confirmation from the side of the mother and had then attempted to gain strength by merging with an idealizable, admired father' (1977: 203). This was a most original insight, that behind the overt grandiosity, which actually belonged to his mother, lay Mr X's own repressed and hidden latent grandiose self, which had failed to obtain the necessary support for its development. Failing to obtain mirroring responsiveness from his mother for his own grandiose-exhibitionistic initiatives, Mr X had turned unsuccessfully towards his father, attempting to merge with an idealized paternal image embodying strength and masculinity. It was this yearning, expressed in sexualized terms, which was enacted in the masturbation fantasy of crossing his penis with that of the priest.

A turning point in the analysis occurred after the second summer break. Mr X recalled that at the beginning of the vacation he had driven alone into the mountains and whilst driving he had daydreamed a lot. Although the analyst initially assumed that Mr X was communicating something about missing her during the break, he went on to convey quite a different meaning. He had had a particularly vivid daydream, in which he imagined that the car was running irregularly and eventually stopped. On looking at the fuel gauge he realized he had run out of petrol and pulled his car over to the side. He imagined himself trying to signal to request help from passing cars, but in his fantasy they all ignored him and his anxiety grew, as he saw himself alone and helpless. Then he had the thought that in the boot of his car, many years ago, he had stashed a can of petrol. He imagined looking in the boot, rummaging through all kinds of luggage, tools and other objects, and then finding the old can, battered and rusty, but still full of petrol. Thus, in the daydream, he was able to replenish his petrol tank and drive off.

Following the daydream, Mr X had wandered through the woodlands in the area to which he had driven. He found himself reminiscing about rare occasions when he and his father had taken walks through the woods. At these times he had felt a closeness to his father which had not been present at other times. Moreover, his father had on these walks impressed Mr X with his remarkable knowledge and skill regarding wildlife and hunting. The fact that these occasions were rare had meant that they were not integrated with the rest of Mr X's personality but had remained as enclaves in his experience. They were not talked about afterwards, as if both father and son knew that the mother would not approve. The point about this daydream, from Kohut's perspective, was that it indicated there had been some degree of relationship between Mr X and his father, and the rudiments of an experience of idealization of masculine attributes. These experiences were represented as the old petrol can stored in the boot.

Kohut explains that Mr X's personality was divided into two sectors by a vertical split. In one sector, he retained a grandiose identification with Christ, characterized by feelings of superiority and attitudes of arrogance, but this was based upon being an appendage to his mother. He had been aggrandized by his mother, but not for himself; she aggrandized him as an extension of herself, turning the little boy into her phallus. His true grandiose self was not mirrored by his mother and therefore was subject to repression. This second sector consisted of the repressed needs for mirroring and the yearnings for merger with an idealized father. Above this horizontal split of repression lay feelings of depression and emptiness. The repressed yearnings for merger found disguised and symbolic expression in the masturbation fantasies – along the same lines as the classic Freudian model of repressed impulses finding expression in displaced and derivative form through symptoms, dreams and daydreams. Kohut emphasized that grandiosity did not lie *on top* of the feelings of inferiority and emptiness. The patient would alternate between the experience of grandiosity and that of the depressed and empty self, these contrasting states of experience existing side by side, vertically split.

It was the overtly grandiose sector of Mr X's personality that was the most prominent. Although this invited interpretations – for example, that the grandiosity was a defence against underlying feelings of inferiority – these were of no value. Instead, the analytic work had to focus first on undoing the vertical split, so that the empty sense of yearning could move into the centre of awareness. It had been this empty yearning which Mr X had been speaking of unconsciously at the initial assessment when he had referred to having been deprived of his father's inheritance. Kohut explains this as follows:

The removal of this barrier has the result that the patient will gradually realize that the self-experience in the horizontally-split sector of his personality – a self-experience of being empty and deprived which, although underemphasized, had always been present and conscious – constitutes his authentic self, and that the up to now predominant self-experience in the nondichotomized sector – the self-experience of overt grandiosity and arrogance – did not emanate from an independent self but from a self that was an appendage to his mother.

(1977: 210–11)

The second phase of analytic work with Mr X focused upon the horizontal split, the repression barrier, so as to make conscious the hitherto *unconscious* structures of the nuclear self. Kohut puts this in terms of the metaphor of Mr X's daydream:

. . . the analysis should uncover the hidden supply of gasoline that can get him going again on the road of his life. Mr X, in other words, is helped to discover the presence of a nuclear self that had been formed on the basis of his relation with the idealized self-object, his father.

(1977: 211)

Kohut emphasized that although he was describing schematically two phases of analysis, and the enabling of the patient to turn his attention from one sector of his personality to another, he did not mean that the actual sequence of the work is as clearly separated as this.

Thus, for Kohut, the analyst's task is not to gratify the patient's narcissistic demands, nor to educate the grandiose sector of the psyche, nor yet to exhort the patient to give up his/her narcissism. Instead, the stance is one of 'acceptance which stresses the phase-appropriateness of these demands within the context of the transference revival of an archaic state' (1971: 179).

As a result of this accepting stance, in the case of those disturbances where there is a combination of vertical and horizontal splitting, the patient begins to encounter the repressed narcissistic needs:

The patient will then come face to face with formerly unrecognized defences which had protected him against the discovery that, despite the seemingly self-assured assertion of narcissistic claims by one sector of his psyche, the most centrally significant sector of his personality is deprived of the influx of self-esteem-sustaining narcissistic libido.

(1971: 179)

A significant sentence in Kohut's explanation of a diagram of the vertical and horizontal splits suggests a point not particularly explicit in the rest of his writings. He refers to the results of the analytic work undoing the vertical split: 'The narcissistic energies which are thus prevented from finding expression in the vertically split-off sector . . . now reinforce the narcissistic pressure against the repression barrier . . .' (1971: 185). It is as if Kohut is saying here that the narcissistic energies *leak away* through the vertical split leaving the main personality depleted; he implies that the mother's narcissistic use of the child hijacks (rather than nurtures) the child's narcissistic energies, leaving a rupture in the psyche through which there is continual leakage. Analytic work at the vertical split heals the rupture and stems the leak. Work can then take place at the horizontal split, where the now enhanced energic pressure pushes the repressed true narcissistic wishes through the repression barrier.

Kohut believed that the specific course of analysis is to a large extent predetermined by the patient's psychopathology. Thus, in the case of Mr X, the 'essential transference related to the reactivation of the needs of the unconscious nuclear self . . . the reactivation of a specific incompleted developmental task' (1977: 217). These needs were specifically focused on the pole of idealization directed at the father. As the associated developmental sequence was played out in the transference, the long-delayed tasks could be undertaken: first, merging with the paternal ideal, then transmuting internalization through gradual disillusionment, and finally integration of the ideals with the other constituents of the self.

Mr J and his fastidious shaving

Kohut (1971) gives another example of a patient with a personality structure combining a horizontal and a vertical split. For some time into the analysis, Mr J displayed only a flagrant grandiosity and exhibitionism. During one session he mentioned casually that after shaving in the mornings he would carefully rinse his razor and clean the sink before washing and drying his face. Kohut noted that although the account itself seemed irrelevant, it was presented in a slightly arrogant and tense fashion. In retrospect this was seen as the first indication of the presence of a hidden area of the patient's personality. Gradually they came to understand that the patient's overt vanity and arrogance was linked to his mother's acclaim for various performances in which he was shown off for the enhancement of her self-esteem:

> This noisily displayed grandiose-exhibitionistic sector of his personality had occupied throughout his life the conscious centre of the psychic stage. Yet it was not fully real to him, provided no lasting satisfaction, and remained split off from the coexisting, more centrally located sector of his psyche in which he experienced those vague depressions coupled with shame and hypochondria that had motivated him to seek psychoanalytic help.
> (1971: 180–81)

The shaving habit, in which performance of fastidious washing of his razor and the basin took precedence over attendance to his face, was an endopsychic replica of his need for his mother's acceptance of his displayed body-self and her rejection of this. Kohut notes:

> Gradually, and against strong resistances (motivated by deep shame, fear of overstimulation, fear of traumatic disappointment), the narcissistic transference began to centre around his need to have his body-mind-self confirmed by the analyst's admiring acceptance.
>
> (1971: 182)

Kohut and the patient came to understand that a crucial fear was that the analyst would value the patient only as a vehicle for his (the analyst's) own aggrandizement and would reject him if he displayed his own initiative in relation to his body and mind. The patient gradually became more aware of his hitherto repressed yearning for acceptance of his 'archaic unmodified grandiose-exhibitionistic body self', a yearning which had been hidden by the noisy display of narcissistic demands expressed through a vertically split-off sector of his personality. As these wishes were worked through and integrated the patient was able to arrive at a position where, as he humorously put it, he could 'prefer my face to the razor'.

What drives a perversion?

What gives a perversion its drive-like intensity? Kohut comments:

> When you talk to a person engaged in one or another form of perversion, he will assure you most of the time that the intensity of the pleasure surpasses anything that is otherwise imaginable . . . there is something much more irresistible in the urge toward the exercise of a perversion than there seems to be in the drive toward genital satisfaction.
>
> (1996: 2)

Why is there this quality in perversions which is like an irresistible addiction? And why does the ego appear so much more helpless and less able to tolerate delay in the case of perversions than is the case with genital drives? Kohut argues that this overwhelming quality of the motivation behind the perversion derives partly from the way that it is an attempt to fill a structural deficit; it is driven by a need rather than an instinct. The deficit is a hole in psychic structure, a missing area of psychic functioning that can be supplied only by another person. Failing the provision for this need by a caregiver, there may be an attempt to find a sexualized alternative to what was originally a non-sexual need.

Why does the need become sexualized? Kohut argues that early needs are closer to sexual experience than are later ones because the younger the child the more he or she is under the sway of basic pleasure–pain experience. He further argues that the intensity of the perverse urge is not explained by the pregenital fixation alone, nor by the search to fill the structural deficit alone, but by the convergence of the two:

> It is the convergence of the sexual pleasure-gain of the pregenital part-instinct, added to the irresistible quality of the need to fill a structural defect, that makes the urge so intense and so irresistible.
>
> (1996: 4)

Kohut gave examples of how the structural deficit and associated need could be concretized and expressed in terms of bodily desires entwined with sexual pleasure. One case he describes is that of Mr A (1971; 1996), previously discussed in Chapter 2, who had developed a core sexual fantasy in which he would subdue a muscular man and then tie him up and masturbate him. At the moment of the man's ejaculation Mr A would experience a mixture of sexual gratification and feelings of triumph and strength. Kohut's view was that the muscular man was a representative of the idealized omnipotent father imago, and that in the fantasy Mr A was obtaining his strength through masturbating him. This was thus a concrete bodily expression of a non-bodily need for the attention and responsiveness of a father who could be idealized and admired. Since the structural deficit could not *really* be filled by sexual fantasy and masturbatory activity, the perverse solution had to be repeated again and again addictively. During the course of the analysis Mr A's need for the fantasy lessened. However, it would be revived with renewed intensity at times when he felt misunderstood by the analyst or in response to analytic breaks.

Kohut describes the reconcretization of Mr A's selfobject needs in the terminal phase of analysis. For example, he had a dream in which he swallowed a clarinet and it continued to play inside him; an X ray was taken and a tiny analyst was sitting in his bowels. As Kohut puts it:

> And then, at the end of the analysis, with the loss of the analyst about to occur, the old archaically sexualized needs for the idealized father were revived, and the sexualized imagery of internalizing the father analyst were revived. Reflecting the stress of ending the analysis, the analyst became in his dream a part of him, somewhat unmetabolized at that point, but part of him nevertheless.
>
> (1996: 11)

Mr A had a further dream: he was tied to some kind of orthopaedic frame and somebody was pointing a finger closer and closer to his anus. Kohut comments:

In other words, what had gradually been internalized in a manageable, small, bit by bit process of internalization over the years of analysis had again become temporarily concretized in terms of anal penetration, anal incorporation, oral incorporation, or what have you – swallowing the analyst whole again. He wanted the analyst to penetrate him.

(1996: 11)

One interesting point here is that a psychological need can be expressed in concrete (bodily) or non-concrete terms. The earliest versions of selfobject need are obviously experienced bodily, and are met through the physical care given to the child. For example, soothing is given to the baby through physical holding, rocking and so on, whereas the same function can be provided later through empathic verbal responses employing symbols (words). When a selfobject need is not met at a psychological (non-concrete) level, there may be a regression to an earlier bodily version of the need. This may combine with psychosexual regression so that the selfobject need is grafted on to pregenital pleasure, thus creating the addictive intensity of a perversion.

The psychoeconomic dimension

The economic dimension of mental life, so important in Freud's perspective, has tended to fade from prominence in the contributions of many psychoanalytic theorists. However, it remained central for Kohut. Indeed, it could be viewed as the most fundamental dimension that runs through all of Kohut's concepts of development, of psychopathology, and of psychoanalytic cure (Rubovits-Seitz, 1999). It is there, for example, in his concepts of optimal and traumatic frustration, traumatic neurosis, and the development of tension-regulating structures through transmuting internalization. Just as Freud continued to postulate an 'actual' neurotic core to psychodynamic defence neuropsychoses, a psychic situation of excessive tension, so Kohut considered that the failure of selfobject availability in childhood led to narcissistic tensions which had an economic reality. For Kohut, narcissistic tensions, including the needs for soothing and merger with images of strength, were real in an absolute, quasi-physical sense, and could not be eliminated and repudiated but only transmuted through normal development or through psychoanalysis. Without this transmutation, the narcissistic tensions would result in inhibitions or in perversion (or both), as the instinct-like needs press against the repression barrier.

This perspective on the 'actual' neurotic basis of perversion, the tension of unmet selfobject needs, prevents Kohut's approach having the subtly moralistic tone found in some British and French psychoanalytic points of view, especially those influenced by Melanie Klein (e.g. Chasseguet-

Smirgel, 1985; Grunberger, 1971). For Kohut, the overcoming of a perversion was not a matter or insight, choice, acceptance of reality, or tolerance of depressive pain, etc. It could be genuinely overcome only through transmuting internalization, based on the gradual working through of innumerable microtraumas of selfobject failure, resulting in internal structures of tension-regulation.

In Kohut's view, the absence of adequate selfobject responses in the childhood of patients with narcissistic disorders, including those with perversions, results in a deficiency of structures of self-soothing. Such people are therefore 'thin-skinned', easily hurt and offended, prone to overwhelming shame, and their fears and worries tend to expand without limit, becoming boundless and catastrophic. Kohut notes that these patients are subject to recurrent traumatic states, both in analysis and in life in general. He comments:

> At such times the focus of the analysis shifts temporarily to a near-exclusive consideration of the overburdenedness of the psyche, i.e. to a consideration of the existing psychoeconomic imbalance.
>
> (1971: 230)

Patients with narcissistic disturbances are excessively shame-prone. Kohut gives the example of exaggerated shame reactions to the memory of committing a *faux pas*:

> His mind returns again and again to the painful moment, in the attempt to eradicate the reality of the incident by magical means, i.e. to undo it. Simultaneously the patient may angrily wish to do away with himself in order to wipe out the tormenting memory in this fashion.
>
> (1971: 231)

He emphasizes the importance of the analyst's tolerance of the patient's repeated recounting of the painful event:

> For long periods the analyst must participate empathically in the psychic imbalance from which the patient suffers; he must show understanding for the patient's painful embarrassment and for his anger that the act that has been committed cannot be undone.
>
> (1971 p 231)

Thus, for Kohut, this is not a matter of tolerating mental pain, surrendering illusions of omnipotence, or of reaching the 'depressive position', as it might be for many British Kleinian-influenced analysts. Instead it is a matter of building psychic structure in the context of a psychoanalytic relationship.

Kohut points out that often the traumatic states may be precipitated by events within the analysis. Paradoxically it may be correct and empathically given interpretations which give rise to psychoeconomic trauma. Although these effects might superficially look like a negative therapeutic reaction – due to unconscious guilt or envy, for example – this is not the case. Kohut gives an example of a patient who, in talking about his restless loneliness, mentioned that his mother had seemed to dislike her own body and would recoil from physical closeness; the analyst had commented that his restlessness seemed to relate to his never having experienced himself as 'loving, lovable and touchable'. The patient responded with excitement, declaring 'Crash! Bang! You hit it!', and shortly afterwards became tearful. The following day he arrived in a disheveled, excited and disturbed state, reporting that he had not been able to sleep; he also mentioned grossly sexual fantasies about the female analyst, dreams of eating breasts, and a variety of bizarre images and fantasies. Kohut explains this as follows:

> In essence the patient's traumatic state was due to the fact that he had reacted with overstimulation and excitement to the analyst's correct interpretation. His vulnerable psyche could not handle the satisfaction of a need (or the fulfilment of a wish) that had existed since childhood: the correct empathic response of an all-important figure in his environment.
>
> (1971: 234)

Kohut advises that the most helpful response to these traumatic states is for the analyst to explain to the patient that the understanding attained in the previous session, and the fulfilment of the wish for (empathic) understanding, had been overexciting.

Mr Z and the father bearing gifts

A further example of traumatic overstimulation as a result of selfobject needs being suddenly overwhelmingly met is given in Kohut's famous paper *The Two Analyses of Mr Z* (Kohut, 1979). Kohut describes how he treated the same patient twice, first from a perspective informed by classical psychoanalysis, and then (when he returned for a second analysis) on the basis of his new understandings of self psychology.

Mr Z reported a dream during the first analysis: the father arrived loaded with gifts; the patient was intensely frightened and attempted to close the door to keep the father out. During the first analysis, Kohut interpreted this in terms of the patient's ambivalence towards the father as an oedipal rival. The background was that when Mr Z was three and a half years old his father had become ill and was hospitalized; following this he left to live with another woman, a nurse, but returned to the patient and his mother when Mr Z was five years old. Mr Z remained close to his doting but dominating mother. His masturbation fantasies had masochistic content, involving being made to have sex by a strong, demanding and insatiable woman. Childhood versions of these fantasies involved being bought and sold by women and being treated like an object that had no will or initiative of its own. In his overt manner, Mr Z appeared grandiose.

Whilst Kohut's earlier understanding was of an oedipal situation in which Mr Z wished to retain exclusive possession of his mother and viewed the father as a hated and feared rival who would castrate him and repossess his mother, his later emphasis was upon Mr Z's need for a strong father who could help free him from the domination by his mother. From this perspective, the return of the father when Mr Z was age five, and perhaps also the revival of selfobject hopes within the transference, would have been traumatically overstimulating:

> Having been without his father during the period when the male self is phase appropriately acquired and strengthened via the male selfobject, the boy's need for his father for male psychological substance was enormous . . . so he had been exposed to . . . a traumatic state by being offered with overwhelming suddenness, all the psychological gifts for which he had secretly yearned, gifts which indeed he needed to get.
>
> (1979: 18)

Fears of primitive narcissism

Kohut's explanation of narcissistic anxieties is always set essentially in terms of psychoeconomic threat – the destabilizing potential of narcissistic energies, sensations and images that have not been moderated, harnessed, socialized and integrated into the ego through the transmuting crucible of selfobject experiences. He writes:

> . . . the danger against which the ego defends itself by keeping the archaic grandiose self dissociated and/or in repression is the dedifferentiating influx of unneutralized narcissistic libido (towards which the threatened ego reacts with anxious excitement) and the intrusion of archaic images of a fragmented body self (which the ego elaborates in the form of hypochondriacal preoccupations).
>
> (1971: 152)

Thus Kohut describes the central anxiety in the narcissistic disorders as the fear of the disorganizing intrusion of early forms of narcissism and their energies. Within this spectrum, he specifies four particular anxieties: (1) the fear of the loss of the reality self through ecstatic merger with the idealized parent imago – or quasi-religious regressions involving a sense of merger with God; (2) the fear of loss of contact with reality through grandiose excitements; (3) shame and self-consciousness (in response to the threatened intrusion of crude exhibitionism); (4) hypochondriacal anxieties (reflecting the sense of the break-up of the cohesive body–mind self).

One point that Kohut makes about the narcissistic anxieties is that they often have a vague quality, making them difficult to perceive with clarity. He contrasts these with oedipally based anxieties, where, for example, there is a fear of being killed or mutilated by an adversary of superior strength. Even when oedipal anxieties are expressed in regressive pre-oedipal imagery, the movement of the analytic material will be towards the elaboration of a specific fear. In the case of narcissistic anxieties, however, the longer the analytic work proceeds, the more vague the content may appear to become. Kohut observes:

> The patient may ultimately speak of vague physical pressures and tensions, or of fears of loss of contact, of contentless, stimulating anxious excitement, etc., and he may begin to talk of childhood moments of being alone, of not quite feeling alive, and the like.
>
> (1971: 154)

This inherent vagueness of narcissistic anxieties may have meant that prior to the provision of Kohut's conceptual lens, it was not possible for most analysts to perceive them.

Summary

Kohut described the coexistence of horizontal and vertical splits in the personality – the former corresponding to the idea of repression, and the latter forming a dissociation between incompatible goals and attitudes. In the case of perverse structures of mind, there may occur states in which a person engages in certain sexual pursuits that are at odds with attitudes and behaviours occurring in another mental state. Kohut believed these vertically split states arose when a mother selectively rewarded aspects of the child's personality that conformed to her desires and expectations, whilst ignoring or discouraging aspects that reflected more of the child's own initiative. The mother's 'mirroring' would thus act to 'hijack' the child's personality, creating a false self that is at odds with the more authentic developmental potential of the child. Narcissistic needs for mirroring and merger with an idealized selfobject would not be met in the relationship with the mother, and would be blocked by the combination of vertical and horizontal splits. However, these narcissistic needs would find expression through sexualized variants – such as overt sexual exhibitionism or voyeurism. These sexual compulsions have an intensity that derives from the fact that they are attempts to fill a structural deficit. Early structural needs are easily sexualized because the young child operates largely in accord with the dimension of sensory pleasure and pain. The build-up of narcissistic tensions gives rise to needs for soothing. Without soothing, there will emerge a psychoeconomic crisis of excessive tension. The absence of adequate structures of self-soothing mean that a person is emotionally 'thin-skinned' and shame-prone. Correct and empathic interpretations can in themselves lead to psychoeconomic trauma because they can be overstimulating. In Kohut's theorizing, the psychoeconomic dimension of mental life was always important. Narcissistic anxieties are based on psychoeconomic threat – of the destabilizing potential of raw narcissistic exhibitionism and idealization.

Chapter 4
The healing process in Kohut's psychoanalysis

> Clearly every explanation, however valid within the framework of our current knowledge, must not only be considered a gain, but also a barrier to further thought, a potential obstacle to seeing the new and appreciating the unexpected.
>
> (Kohut, 1984: 125)

The historical transference and the selfobject transference

There are two common misunderstandings of the clinical implications of Kohut's concept of the selfobject transferences. One is that the Kohutian analyst would actively 'mirror' the patient and in that way attempt to provide a 'corrective emotional experience' (Alexander and French, 1946). Referring to this idea in his 1972 Chicago Lectures, Kohut commented: 'That really is a total mistake . . . The meaning of mirroring . . . is not that you have to play act with your patient' (1996: 373). Kohut meant that the mirror transference (and the idealizing transference) was to be *analysed*. In *The Analysis of the Self*, Kohut describes the analytic task as follows:

> As in the analysis of the transference neurosis, the analyst's essential activity lies in the main in the cognitive field: he listens, he tries to comprehend, and he interprets. His evenly hovering attention must move with the flow of the analytic material as he participates in the slow, painstaking . . . task of analysing the manifestations of the activated grandiose self during the working through phase of the mirror transference in which the analysand assigns to him the performance of only one function: to reflect and echo his grandiosity and exhibitionism . . .
>
> If the analyst . . . truly comprehends the phase-appropriateness of the demands of the grandiose self . . . then the patient will gradually reveal the urges and fantasies of the grandiose self and the slow process is initiated . . .

which leads to the integration of the grandiose self into the structure of the
reality ego and to an adaptively useful transformation of its energies.

(Kohut, 1971: 175–76)

The second common misunderstanding is that a focus on the selfobject
transference somehow meant that the traditional idea of the historical
transference – the repetition in relation to the analyst of conflictual
wishes and fears from childhood – would somehow become less relevant
in relation to patients with narcissistic personality disorders. Some of
Kohut's theoretical accounts could give this impression. However, his
detailed clinical accounts illustrate that although the selfobject transference represents the patient's search for development-enhancing
responses that were not available in childhood, this is also interwoven
with the repetition, in relation to the analyst, of historical patterns from
childhood.

Kohut (1984) notes that certain patients will respond seemingly
favourably to the analyst's communications during an initial stage,
showing behavioural improvement, but may then suddenly appear to
deteriorate, this alarming development being accompanied by a barrage
of criticism and reproaches against the analyst. Why is there this period of
calm before the storm and why is the patient initially able to tolerate the
analyst's errors of empathy, only subsequently to become intolerant of
them? Kohut's answer is clear:

> What happens is nothing else but the transference clicking into place. Thus
> during the calm before the storm, the analyst and the patient have jointly
> explored the patient's traumatic past, allied in the shared pursuit of a goal;
> once the storm breaks loose, however, the analytic situation has *become* the
> traumatic past and the analyst has *become* the traumatizing selfobject of early
> life.

(1984: 178)

Here Kohut uses the term 'traumatizing selfobject'. He also, elsewhere,
refers to a 'pathogenic selfobject'. Does this introduce some confusion?
To state the conceptual problem crudely, mostly Kohut implies that a
selfobject is, almost by definition, a good thing, but here he is referring to
something bad – traumatizing or pathogenic. In the selfobject transferences the patient appears to be soothed and his or her functioning
enhanced until the selfobject experience is disrupted. The idea of a
selfobject that is itself pathogenic or traumatizing seems a contradiction
in terms. How does the idea of a pathogenic selfobject relate to Kohut's
definition of the selfobject as 'that dimension of our experience of
another person that relates to that person's function in shoring up our

self . . .' (1984: 49)? Kohut must have meant that a pathogenic selfobject is that aspect of our experience of another person where we are searching for the enhancing of our development and the sustenance of our self, but are actually experiencing the response as psychologically toxic. Perhaps a clearer term would be the 'anti-selfobject'. A caregiver could perform their selfobject functions well or poorly, but if their response to the child was actually damaging or restrictive of the child's development, then they are offering the reverse of a selfobject, which could be described as an 'anti-selfobject'.

One of Kohut's (1984) clinical examples illustrates these points.

Clinical example

The patient, a professional man in his 40s, approached Kohut after hearing him speak at a public lecture. He had seen a number of psychotherapists and analysts in the past but was extremely critical of all of them, describing them as grossly lacking in empathy. In addition he was very critical of his parents, blaming them for his severe emotional difficulties; he described his mother as having been totally involved with her church and its dogma, whilst his father had been withdrawn and uninvolved with the patient as a child. His presenting complaint was a chronic sense of unreality. Kohut commented that the analytic work with him developed along similar lines to the patient's previous attempts at therapy – with the significant difference that the treatment was not broken off.

Although initially uneasy about taking on this patient, in view of the relentless and monotonous criticism of previous therapists, and with some concern that there might be an underlying paranoid psychosis, Kohut did agree to proceed. The work began in an atmosphere of co-operation and the patient appeared to develop an essentially positive attitude towards the analyst. The patient seemed accepting of Kohut's interventions which linked his perceptions of his experiences in therapy with his experiences in childhood. However, he would become annoyed and impatient whenever he felt that Kohut was viewing the previous therapists as transference figures rather than as truly malevolent enemies. Another worrying symptom was that the patient would often develop severe headaches before his sessions.

However, an alarming deterioration took place after about a year of analysis, when Kohut was away for several weeks. On his return, over a period of weeks, the patient became increasingly dominated by his headaches, to the extent that he could talk of little else. The quality of the headaches also changed, from a more ordinary physical pain, to an unspeakable discomfort which appeared more psychological than physical. Kohut's initial approach was to link the patient's headaches to the break in the analysis and feelings of abandonment, loss of support, and hypochondriacal concerns about the body. The patient did not find this interpretation helpful, pointing out that he had not felt upset whilst Kohut had been away, nor initially on his return.

Then after the emergence of further material suggesting another interpretive possibility, Kohut offered an alternative explanation. He postulated that as a result of the analytic work the patient had opened himself more to emotional interactions with the world and that, as a consequence, he was now facing anxieties and tensions from which previously he had walled himself off; this was leaving him continually traumatized and overburdened by emotional impingements. At first the patient reacted favourably to this interpretation, providing some confirmatory evidence and his facial expression brightening considerably. Then, after a few sessions exploring this theme, he began again to criticize Kohut severely, accusing him of lacking all understanding and of ruining him. He also began to complain of people in his environment who upset him with their behaviour or manner, for example by the shrillness of their voices. At one point he even suspected that his television had become more shrill in its sound and took it to a repair shop, suspecting it had been tampered with.

Naturally Kohut became alarmed about the patient's deteriorating mental state. However, he managed to retain his awareness that such developments in selfobject transferences are less dangerous than they might appear, providing the analyst is able to retain an analytic stance and attempt to resonate empathically with the patient's communications. Kohut emphasized that this was not easy because the patient's complaints were always based around real flaws in his emotional response, even if these were exaggerated. He commented:

> The patient, as I finally grasped, insisted – and had a right to insist – that I learn to see things exclusively in his way and not at all in my way.
>
> (1984: 182)

Further understanding of the patient's experience of Kohut gradually emerged. The patient had felt that the content of the interpretations had been cognitively correct, both concerning the break and his increased sense of impingement resulting from greater emotional openness. However, he had felt additionally traumatized by perceiving Kohut's remarks as cognitively generated, without being based in feeling what the patient felt. In this way the patient felt that Kohut was repeating the essential trauma of his early life. Kohut notes that at such an impasse, the question of whether a 'borderline' condition will or will not become an analysable disorder depends upon the analyst's capacity and willingness for self-scrutiny – a point that relates to what he calls the 'principle of the relativity of diagnostic classification and specific prognosis' (a point also pursued by Brandchaft and Stolorow, 1984). Kohut comments:

> To hammer away at the analysand's transference distortions brings no results; it only confirms the analysand's conviction that the analyst is as dogmatic, as utterly sure of himself, as walled off in the self-righteousness of a distorted view as the pathogenic parents (or other selfobject) had been. Only the analyst's continuing sincere acceptance of the patient's reproaches as (psychologically) realistic, followed by a prolonged (and ultimately successful) attempt to look into himself and remove the inner barriers that stand in the way of his empathic grasp of the patient, ultimately have a chance to turn the tide.
>
> (1984: 182)

As these considerations continued to inform Kohut's stance, the patient began to present further material offering a new and initially not fully understood direction, relating to his father. His sensitivity towards noise began to subside. However, his reproaches against Kohut continued, but became more specific and focused. His complaints, against both his father and the analyst, were that each had wanted the patient to look up to them rather than responding to his own ideas and initiatives. Kohut saw this as another attempt at a mirror transference rather than an idealizing transference. He explains as follows:

> The archaic mirror transference in which the seriously disturbed, unresponsive maternal environment of early life had been revived psychosomatically in the diffuse noise-hypersensitivity-headache syndrome was now replaced by the more focused syndrome of transference reproaches directed at the nonmirroring father who was preoccupied with his own self enhancement and thus refused to respond to the son's originality and talents.
>
> (1984: 183)

Kohut does not give a full account of this case and we are not told in any detail how the analysis developed after the impasse subsided. However, the description of the case is embedded in the context of a discussion of the movement in analysis from an early phase in which the analyst may be required to provide only empathic understanding, to a phase in which explaining can take place. Kohut considered that the phase of explaining involves more objectivity, and invites the patient to be more objective about himself – and thus the patient's capacity to tolerate explanation as well as understanding indicates developmental progress.

Whilst different analysts may take different views regarding the understanding of this material, what does seem clear is that the patient was seeking a particular kind of response from the analyst but felt he was receiving another kind of response – one that duplicated damaging interactions from childhood. The selfobject dimension of transference, the search for mirroring, represented the *hope* of finding a development-enhancing response, whilst the historical or repetition dimension of transference represented the *fear* of encountering again the damaging environment of childhood. Kohut found that his own experience of the patient, as well as the evidence of the series of failed attempts at therapy, indicated that attempts to challenge or question the patient's point of view were fruitless – and, moreover, that such attempts would lead to an increasingly intransigent position and a worsening impasse. By contrast, if the patient's complaints were listened to and appreciated as having a core of validity, and if the analyst did not attempt to dispute the patient's perception, then gradually the analysis could move on and new understanding would emerge.

No doubt some analysts would argue that this example illustrates how certain patients attempt to control the analyst's mind and behaviour – and that Kohut's stance represents not good analysis but instead a collusion with the patient's pathology and fantasies of omnipotence. The only real argument against this is that Kohut's acquiescence, at least for a time, in seeing things only from the patient's point of view, did allow the treatment to continue, whereas a confrontation would almost certainly have led to another angry breaking off by the patient.

The lawyer and the three dreams: traditional and self psychological approaches to defence and resistance

Although Kohut continued to make use of psychoanalytic concepts of defence and, to some extent, resistance, his understanding of these changed radically as his self psychology developed. Basically he began to see that what might look like resistances, devoted to maintaining a pathological status quo, may actually be the patient's desperate strategies to preserve the bedrock of a nuclear self, especially if this is precariously established. He states this point as follows:

> Defense motivation in analysis will be understood in terms of activities undertaken in the service of psychological survival, that is, as the patient's attempt to save at least that sector of his nuclear self, however small and precariously established it may be, that he has been able to construct and maintain despite serious insufficiencies in the development-enhancing matrix of the selfobjects of childhood.

(1984: 115)

Kohut (1984) presents a lengthy case vignette illustrating the differences between more traditional psychoanalytic formulations and the newer perspectives offered by self psychology. He discusses the case first from a more traditional Freudian drive psychological point of view, and then from the point of view of self psychology.

The perspective of traditional (USA) Freudian ego psychology

The focus of Kohut's discussion is upon three dreams that occurred during a three-month period in the fourth year of analysis of a middle-aged male lawyer.

Dream 1

The dreamer is at a summer resort, either a hotel, motel or bungalow, but he is sleeping on the front lawn, feeling uncomfortable, thrashing around, resulting in his becoming uncovered. He is worried that people passing by might see him uncovered.

Dream 2

The dreamer was being honoured by a legal association and was to receive a prize; he was informed of this by the man sitting next to him, who also explained that there was to be a compromise whereby he shared the prize with someone else. On going to the podium, he was given the prize, which was a camera. To everyone's surprise he took a picture of the audience. Prior to telling this dream, the patient reported that he had behaved more maturely with his wife recently, cancelling an engagement of his own in order that she could attend a concert with her girl friend.

Dream 3

The dreamer's friend, John, was with him during his analytic session, lying next to him on the couch, but there were also other people in the room. Then an older man had a heart attack and the dreamer moved to help, performing mouth to mouth resuscitation as learned.

Kohut explores the dreams and related material in relation to four psychodynamic themes: sibling rivalry, exhibitionism-voyeurism, anality, and the oedipus complex.

Sibling rivalry

The patient's only sibling had been a brother two years younger, who had been his mother's favourite. The patient perceived the brother as having achieved this favoured position by being compliant and conforming to the mother's expectations. He himself responded by withdrawing into an attitude of superiority, particularly in relation to academic pursuits, where he was in reality intellectually the superior.

Kohut describes how this sibling rivalry could be seen as contributing to a form of *resistance* in the analysis. He explains that the patient had the impression that analysts are very interested in dreams, especially since his previous analyst had admonished him that dreams are the 'royal road to the unconscious'. Therefore, the patient would feel that to present dreams and submit to their being analysed was to be compliant and conforming like his hated sibling. Partly this attitude, of wanting and not wanting to offer dreams, was expressed by a pattern of telling Kohut a fragment of a dream but then veering off into intellectual discourse about the general meaning of dreams and so on. In addition, the patient would directly accuse Kohut of pressuring him to have dreams, remember them and analyse them, just like the previous analyst, as well as trying to make him conform generally to the rules of analysis. Kohut notes that this pattern would intensify at those times when the patient would in some way fantasize that the analyst was turning to a preferred sibling who was more conforming.

Kohut then indicates how dreams 2 and 3 both contained clear references to sibling rivalry. In dream 2 the patient shares a prize with a sibling figure, whilst in dream 3 the patient has to share the couch with a brother figure. However, the dreams also represent the patient's attempts to elicit the analyst's approval and to establish a special bond with him: in dream 2 he behaves in a mature way – of which the analyst might be expected to approve – sharing the prize with a sibling; in dream 3 he, rather than the brother, saves the analyst's life.

Exhibitionism-voyeurism

Kohut then turns to the themes of exhibitionism and voyeurism, again focusing on the dreams. Dream 1, which portrayed the patient's shame at being seen naked followed the frustration of his wish to have a light on whilst making love with his wife so that he could see her and be seen by her. In traditional terms, the exhibitionistic wish had intensified through frustration and was expressed in inhibited and censored form in the dream. The exhibitionistic desire was also clearly apparent in dream 2, where he is told by his neighbour (the analyst) that his performance is to be honoured in front of an audience. However, he turned this around so that it was he who looked at the onlookers by taking a photograph of *them*. This manoeuvre could be seen as an instance of the mechanism of turning passive into active. He visually embarrassed others when he felt the discomfort of being visually embarrassed himself. Whereas dream 1 represented the passive aspect of being looked at, dream 2 represents the turning of this into the activity of looking.

Kohut also discusses the patient's pattern of turning the tables in relation to shame in connection with some transference interactions that occurred during two sessions between dreams 1 and 2. In the first of these sessions, the patient spoke with great warmth of how he had recently become able to converse more freely and in a more human way with his colleagues in his office and also with his wife and children. He indicated that he felt this improvement was a result of the analytic work, but also that it derived from his experience of the analyst's general human and empathic attitude. The patient also noted that sometimes he would speak with elements of Kohut's own tone of voice and choice of words. He also was aware of fleeting thoughts that Kohut would be pleased with him. However, in the following sessions the patient launched a fierce verbal attack on psychoanalysis. He complained that analysts were dogmatic, forcing their views on patients and often were more sick than their patients. Kohut listened to this tirade for some time before remarking that it was in striking contrast to the positive view of analysis that he had expressed the previous day – and wondered aloud whether there was some link with his having spoken yesterday of his identification with the analyst and his expectation of the analyst's pleasure in hearing of his progress. In response the patient recounted a memory of an event when he was in law school. This had involved an exercise wherein some of the students participated in a mock trial, watched by other students and the faculty staff. Afterwards the partici- pants would be subject to scathing criticism of their performance and knowledge of the law. The patient had felt terrified but had cleverly turned the tables on the audience by appearing to pursue an erroneous line of legal defence, only to reveal suddenly, to their stunned surprise, that he had deliberately misled them and that his apparent error was in fact a brilliant stratagem leading to success. Kohut considered that this memory indicated that the patient's pattern of turning passive into active, of shaming and embarrassing others at the point when he felt he was in danger of being shamed and embarrassed was a deeply ingrained one. He does not at this point give any clear explanation of this sequence, although he returns to it when later discussing the view from the perspective of self psychology.

Anality

Kohut then discusses the theme of anality, which had apparently played a large role in the previous analysis. In fact this did not emerge as a signifi- cant theme in the analysis with Kohut, although the patient would often repeat, seemingly with pleasure, certain remarks and phrases the previous analyst had used in relation to this. However, a relevant historical point was that the patient's mother had been in the habit of giving him enemas regularly until he was ten or eleven years old. This seemed to be consistent with the outlook of the previous analyst, that the patient resisted the production of dreams and free-associations, just as he had earlier resisted and resented the parting with his faeces.

Oedipal aspects

Finally, Kohut considers the material in terms of evidence for an incompletely resolved oedipus complex and resistances derived from this. He points out that traditional analysis might consider all the preceding defence-resistances to be the result of a defensive retreat from the conflicts of the oedipal complex to those of the pre-oedipal period. Moreover, the competitiveness with the brother could be viewed as a regressive version of competitiveness with the father. His voyeuristic-exhibitionistic features and fears of passivity could derive from frightening primal scene observations or fantasies. The anal preoccupations with resistance to loss of faeces might be considered a displacement from castration anxiety. In addition, the patient may have combated castration anxiety by emphasizing a phallic image of the mother with the enema syringe, and by fantasizing himself as the passive woman (in the enema situation) whilst still retaining his penis.

The perspective of self psychology

Kohut begins by explaining that the self psychological approach gives less emphasis to individual defences and resistances, but focuses more on the patient's total personality. His own cognitive style, he says, is to construct first a tentative hypothesis concerning the patient's nuclear self and its central programme. This mode of thought leads Kohut to a consideration of the patient's childhood. He describes three vignettes of the patient's mother's behaviour.

The mother's behaviour

One of these episodes was termed 'the interrupted basement game'. The father once played hide and seek with his two sons in the basement. They were all having a good time when suddenly the mother appeared at the door, expressing wordless disapproval. The joy went out of their game and after continuing listlessly for a few minutes, the boys retired to their bedrooms and the father went to his club.

In the second memory, the patient, as a little boy of four, awoke one morning from a nightmare in which he fell off a high building. The mother immediately took him to the top of a skyscraper to demonstrate to him that there was nothing to be afraid of.

The third recollection of his mother's behaviour concerned her attitude to his bowel functions. She believed that regularity was important and that disturbances such as irritability and failure to concentrate at school were due to the presence of faeces in the body. Moreover, she considered that bowel movements should occur in the mornings. For these reasons she applied an enema every day.

Kohut concludes from these vignettes that the picture of the mother as remembered by the patient was of a woman who lacked warmth, was moralistic, duty-oriented, ritualistic, joyless, and suffering from a diffuse hypochondria displaced on to the patient.

There were initially relatively few memories of the patient's father, who seemed to have been experienced as somewhat distant, taking little interest in the children. He did, however, show some greater capacity for liveliness and joy, being successful in his career and having been an outstanding athlete as a college student.

Thus, Kohut notes that the problems of this patient showed a paradigmatic similarity to those of several others that he had written about. The patient was exposed to 'development-thwarting influences' from his mother, whilst his father, seeming to offer potentially a greater capacity for joyful living, withdrew both physically and emotionally.

Sources of health

Kohut asks the question of how it was that, despite this development-stifling early environment, the patient still managed to remain relatively healthy and capable of responding to new opportunities for psychological growth, such as were provided by the analysis. More specifically, he asks why and how the patient was able to preserve his nuclear self.

Kohut suggests that the patient's strength rested partly upon an innate capacity to maintain hope of finding a development-enhancing selfobject. Like other cases Kohut described, he appeared to have given up on the search for a *mirroring* selfobject and instead was focused (unconsciously) upon finding an *idealizable* one.

Kohut then asks what environmental supports there might have been for the patient's preservation of a nuclear self and of hope of finding a suitable selfobject. He points to the small contribution of the patient's father – there was at least the memory of the game in the basement and he did not appear to have actively interfered with the patient's development in the way that the mother did. A figure who may have been of more positive significance was the patient's maternal grandfather, who seems to have remained a figure of idealization for the patient's mother. Although this meant that the mother devalued both the patient's father and the patient himself, the positive aspect was that the child could see that the mother was at least *capable* of idealizing a man. The grandparents also provided relatively happy times for the patient and his brother during vacation visits. Although the patient did sometimes report positively tinged memories of his mother, Kohut was inclined partly to doubt their validity, because these tended to occur during a back and forth movement in which the patient would begin to gain some psychological distance from his mother and recognize her psychopathology, but then retreat from this perception and begin to doubt his own mental functioning. Moreover, these more positive memories of his mother usually related to times when the family had been on holiday with the grandparents when presumably she felt more supported by her own parents. Nevertheless the mother did regularly read stories to the two boys, boyish adventures, which Kohut believed may have contributed to the patient's enjoyment of adventurous trips as an adult. Overall Kohut concludes that the patient's selfobject transference indicated a developmental move away from the mother and to the paternal images of the grandfather and the father.

Self psychology perspectives on the dreams

Kohut then returns to considering the patient's defence resistances in relation to the three dreams. The patient believed that his brother had been preferred by his mother because of his superior physical grace and because of his compliance. In reaction to this perception, the patient had become withdrawn in an attitude of superiority. This was repeated in the analysis in the following way. Whenever he felt understood by Kohut he would withdraw. It was as if the patient's view was that other patients (his brother) might wish to be understood but he did not – as exemplified in his about-turn after telling the analyst of his improvements. Kohut comments:

> Thus, after proudly reporting to me that he had behaved maturely towards his wife and, in his dream, receiving recognition from me (albeit shared with a brother) of his progress, he suddenly turned the situation topsy-turvy and, raising the camera and exposing me to the painful limelight, denied ever having asked for a self-confirming mirroring response from the mother-analyst.
>
> (1984: 140)

Kohut also emphasizes that this kind of dynamic conflict and defence does not involve a desire to be loved but instead 'a need for self-enhancing reflection: to be looked at, approvingly and admiringly and, with this self-confirmation, to be able to go on with the further firming and development of this core of our being' (1984: 140).

Kohut now interprets the dream of stunning the audience by taking their picture as an indication of the patient's efforts to guard his self against the intrusions of his disturbed mother and her crazy preoccupations. He notes that the patient frequently saw analysis in similar terms as a crazy system in which analysts impose their fixed ideas upon compliant patients. It became possible for Kohut and the patient to begin to understand his attitude towards his brother in a different way. His withdrawal and attitude of superiority was not essentially based on an opting out of competition with his brother, but rather 'was the product of his early recognition, however dimly formed, that his brother was being irrevocably damaged by the mother because, unlike the patient, he could not maintain the integrity of his self against her oppressive demands and expectations' (1984: 142). Apparently the brother did indeed turn out to be more damaged, becoming a drifter, unsuccessful, with no stable relationships and unable or unwilling to obtain psychological help.

Exhibitionism-voyeurism from a self psychology perspective

Kohut then considers again the theme of exhibitionism-voyeurism from the point of view of self psychology. He argues that, like any child, the patient would have needed to be mirrored, 'to be looked upon with joy and basic approval by a delighted parental selfobject' (1984: 143). However, his mother's defective ability to provide this, combined with her needs to incorporate her sons into her own hypochondria and control not only their bodies and behaviour but also their thoughts, as well as the unavailability of a father who could take pride in his sons, meant that the patient did not receive sufficient of these developmental nutrients. Therefore, his needs for self-enhancement through mirroring would come to be associated with intense shame and embarrassment (because they would remain intense, infantile and unintegrated with the mature personality). However, unlike his brother, the patient had not surrendered totally to the control by his mother, but had preserved his self through the adaptive aggression of turning passive into active. Thus he became a sadistic voyeur, exposing the other to shame and embarrassment. This sequence is illustrated by the shift from the dream of being naked in public and experiencing the shame of exposure, to the dream of suddenly taking a picture of the analyst-audience.

Anality – the self psychology perspective.

Next Kohut turns to discussion of the theme of anality. Apparently this had been prominent in the previous analysis, the analyst assuming that the patient and his mother had enjoyed the enemas and that he had retained his faeces in order to prolong the pleasure, resulting in some kind of anal orgasm. According to the former analyst, the patient had been unwilling to reveal this forbidden pleasure to himself or the analyst, and it was this secret clinging to a regressive pleasure that caused his resistance to analysing these experiences. Whilst Kohut thought this was a theoretically coherent and plausible formulation, he noted one fact that was inconsistent with this. The patient did not appear to wish to hide this anal material but would sometimes refer with seeming pleasure to these interpretations of his previous analyst. What eventually emerged was that the patient's motivation in recalling the anal theme from the first analysis was not his own anality, nor a wish to play the first analyst against the second, but was to do with his pleasure in the *way* the first analyst had presented these interpretations. It was the warmth and vitality of the former analyst's tone of voice. He would say to the patient: 'First you are holding back for all you are worth, but then you are making a b-i-i-i-g production.' The patient had loved this playful use of words – and the lively interest that he had not found originally with his father.

Oedipal aspects – the self psychology perspective.

Finally, Kohut considered the oedipal theme, which classically would be viewed in terms of competition with the father and reactive passive homosexuality with defence-resistances against both of these. Kohut found that the theme of the father was not prominent until relatively late in the analysis, after the conflicts to do with his mother and his brother had been analysed. However, the patient's feelings about his father did emerge, both in the transference and in related memories about his father. The understanding that emerged was not to do with an oedipal death wish against the father and a defence against this, but a longing for a strong and vital father-analyst who could be idealized. Dream 3, which involved the revival of the father-analyst who had had a heart attack, expressed not a death wish but the desire to resuscitate and transform the analyst from a old sick and dying man into a vital and responsive ideal. Kohut says this interpretation was supported by associative material about the analyst, the father and the grandfather.

Kohut discusses one memory of the grandfather that emerged late in the analysis prior to the patient's discovery of his secret idealization of the analyst. Apparently, one of the ways the mother had interfered with the patient's capacity to idealize the grandfather had been to exaggerate the latter's physical frailty, implying that he was so ill with heart disease that he was likely to die at any moment. When the patient was about fourteen, the grandfather had invited him to dinner at his private club, an exclusive 'man to man' get together. What the patient emphasized in recalling this was an apparently insignificant detail. The cab had by mistake dropped them off a block away from the club. Although it was a cold, windy and snowy night the grandfather walked vigorously without any discomfort – a fact which was completely at odds with the picture presented by his mother.

The idealizing transference

Thus the healing process with this patient was by means of the establishment and analysis of an idealizing transference. Alongside the idealization of the analyst, the patient also recovered memories relating to embryonic idealization of the grandfather, and, to a lesser extent, the father. Kohut also notes that in the transference, one of the patient's fears was that the analyst would knuckle under when belittled just as his father had in relation to his mother. Moreover, he had wanted Kohut to display his strengths and achievements openly, in the same way that the maternal grandfather had built his house in a conspicuous place on a hilltop. Late in the analysis, he told Kohut he had always secretly admired him, although he had hidden this by belittling him – a pattern which had also been the case in childhood in relation to his father. The patient did make considerable gains in his capacity to relate and express his emotions and to laugh and generally to be more warmly human.

Kohut's general comments on defence and resistance.

As Kohut saw it, traditional Freudian analysis gave primacy to the idea of cure through insight, through cognitive and emotional understanding. Resistance would thereby be seen essentially as resistance to insight, to knowledge. This was different from Kohut's finding that although insight is achieved in a self psychologically informed analysis, this is not the essential vehicle of healing. The patient achieves health through the establishment and working through of a selfobject transference which strengthens the nuclear self. Kohut introduces a concept here which he terms the principle of the *primacy of self preservation* (1984: 143). He argues that 'it is the self and the survival of its nuclear program that is the basic force in everyone's personality and . . . , in the last resort and on the deepest level, every analyst will finally find himself face to face with these basic motivating forces in his patient' (1984: 147). Crucially, Kohut then concludes that what might appear to be resistances to analysis, such as the areas of sibling rivalry, voyeurism, anality and attachment to the mother, which he described with the lawyer patient, should all be understood as essentially healthy psychic activities 'because they safeguard the analysand's self for future growth' (1984: 148). Similarly, the analysand's 'resistance' to the unfolding of his selfobject needs in the transference is in the service of the self because such needs have to be met in a gradual and modulated way. Kohut emphasizes emphatically: 'All these so-called resistances serve the basic ends of the self; they never have to be "overcome"' (1984: 148).

Kohut gives another example of how an apparent 'resistance' may be reframed as a positive psychological strength, again from his discussion of his lawyer patient. The patient tended to intellectualize, often speaking of his own psychic life in terms of mechanisms and dynamics – and indeed regarding himself as a 'thinking machine'. For a long time he preferred the more 'scientific' interpretations of his previous analyst, framed in terms of wish, anxiety and defence, rather than the broader 'genetically based reconstructions of chronic attitudes to which I [Kohut] tended to turn in order to explain his behaviour, whether in treatment vis-à-vis me or elsewhere' (1984: 150). However, Kohut came to understand that the patient's intellectualizing had actually been a great achievement of his early life, a means whereby he could defend himself against the intrusive craziness and illogicality of his mother. The patient's tendency to intellectualize did recede during the analysis but this was not as a result of interpreting it as a resistance to treatment, but was part of the general developmental progress through the selfobject idealizing transference.

The significance of the two developmental opportunities

One of Kohut's most interesting findings was that a patient seems to have an inherent developmental agenda which he or she plays out in analysis, provided the opportunity is offered. This agenda does not necessarily involve revisiting and working through in the transference the areas of deepest damage and deprivation, nor those of the most intense and archaic need. He found that patients will often 'choose' not to enter those areas, perhaps for good reason. Commenting on the patient's unconscious awareness of what is needed developmentally and also what is best avoided for the purpose of psychic survival, Kohut remarked: ' . . . the analysand's capacity to assess his own psychological state is in certain situations potentially vastly more accurate than the analyst's' (1977: 20). He distinguishes this from the more ordinary situation in which a patient is, under the influence of a specific anxiety, avoiding a developmental task that could be beneficial if faced. What he noticed was that patients might spontaneously bring certain areas of early developmental conflict and need to the transference whilst giving much less emphasis to other areas, which nevertheless may have been highly important in giving rise to the present psychopathology. Of course these 'decisions' as to what to bring to the transference are not conscious, but appear to reflect an inherent healing agenda which seeks facilitation by the analyst.

Miss V

One of Kohut's simpler examples of this process is the case of Miss V (1977: 58–62). This concerns a forty-two-year-old single woman artist who sought help because of periods of empty depression when she felt lethargic, lifeless and unproductive. Kohut came to the view that these enfeebled self states related to childhood experiences when her mother was subject to periodic depressions against the background of a chronic emotional disconnection from others and possibly some borderline schizophrenic characteristics. This meant that Miss V suffered traumatic disappointments in relation to her needs for mirroring from her mother. Her mother's responses were either absent or bizarre because of psychotic misperceptions of the child's needs.

Kohut reconstructed from the qualities of Miss V's depressions, when triggered in the transference, that as a young child she would have felt burdened by demands she could not fulfil. In particular she appeared to have felt an obligation to relieve her mother's depression and to have experienced a deep sense of failure over her inability to do so. Her childhood conclusion was that before she could receive acceptance, approval and affirmation she first had to meet her mother's similar needs. In struggling to extricate herself from the pathogenic relationship with her mother Miss V had turned to her father and established a strong bond with him. He did respond much more to his daughter's needs. His frustrated artistic talents and ambitions formed the basis of Miss V's paternal ideal and a *potential* source of strength for her self. Although the father provided some psychological sustenance, this was not sufficient to compensate for the lack of appropriate response from the mother.

Kohut reports that the focus of working through in the analysis was not directed at the primary structural deficit relating to the mother's flawed responsiveness, but instead was concerned with an idealizing transference relating to the insufficiently established compensatory structure derived from interactions with the father. Miss V did improve through the analysis, her depressions becoming much less severe. Kohut saw this occurring not as a result of a healing of a primary defect (relating to the mother) but due to the rehabilitation of the compensatory structure (deriving from the father). He explains:

> Specifically, the crucial transference revivals concerned events when the father himself appeared to be so severely disappointed by his wife's frustrating emotional flatness and lack of empathy that he, too, seems to have become

temporarily depressed and thus emotionally unavailable to his daughter . . . at the very time when his daughter needed him most, when the mother was depressed and the daughter expected her idealized and admired father to be a bulwark against the pull of lethargy that emanated from the mother and threatened to engulf the child's personality.

(1977: 62)

Kohut's case of Mr M

Kohut provides a longer and more complex account of how a patient may choose unconsciously to build upon one of the two developmental opportunities, in his example of Mr M. The discussion of this case takes up the bulk of the opening chapter of Kohut's *Restoration of the Self* – an opening which, paradoxically, is concerned with termination. Perhaps the reason why issues to do with the termination of analysis are given such a prominent and theme-setting position is because they demonstrate that (a) psychoanalytic healing follows its own inherent agenda, and (b) this is not based essentially on the acquisition of insight, although (c) it does involve working through a transference.

Mr M was in his 30s, in analysis with a female analyst working under Kohut's supervision. His wife had left him, he suffered a serious and chronic disturbance of self-esteem, feelings of apathy and inner emptiness, and also experienced inhibition in his work as a writer. His feeling of being only 'half alive' was countered by intense sexual fantasies of achieving sadistic control over women; his enactment of these with his wife had contributed to his marital breakdown.

Kohut reports that certain transference phenomena, as well as direct memories, suggested that Mr M had experienced his mother's emotional responsiveness towards him as insufficient and faulty. Two particular memories appeared relevant here. One was of often trying to look at his mother suddenly in order to see her real facial expression before she had time to adopt what he feared was a false face of interest and friendliness covering her real indifference. The other was of an occasion when he injured himself and spilt some of his blood on his brother's clothes; without waiting to grasp the true situation, the mother rushed to take his brother to hospital, leaving Mr M behind. Kohut notes that these memories both suggest that his mother's empathic responses were faulty rather than completely absent. His compulsive looking to check her facial demeanour suggests that he had not entirely given up hope of finding empathy and attunement.

Rather late in the narrative, Kohut mentions the important point that Mr M had been abandoned by his natural mother and left in an orphanage until three months of age. Kohut concludes that 'Not only must he have been traumatized by the repeated failure of his adoptive mother to respond appropriately to his needs during the preverbal period, but behind these layers of frustration there hovered always a nameless preverbal depression, apathy, sense of deadness, and diffuse rage that related to the primordial trauma of his life' (1977: 25). He points out that this early deprivation and trauma would probably have compromised his reactions to his adoptive mother. These could have been in the direction of intensified oral greed and violent temper reactions to frustration, or perhaps along the lines of a residual apathy, discouraging the mother from persisting in her attempts to relate to her adopted baby. From the transference, Kohut was inclined to surmise that Mr M had tended to react with increased rage followed by withdrawal when faced with frustration by the mother.

Kohut believed that the failure of the maternal mirroring functions left Mr M with a *primary structural deficit*. By 'structure' Kohut meant a capacity to perform a function originally performed by a selfobject. In Mr M's case, he was unable to manage (to 'curb and neutralize') his grandiosity and exhibitionism that would be activated during his writing. He would become overexcited and anxious and as a result would inhibit his imagination or stop writing – hence his 'writer's block'. Kohut reconstructed that following the primary failure in relation to the mother's mirroring functions, Mr M had turned to the father as an idealized selfobject, in order to build a *compensatory structure* – especially relating to the father's skill with language. Thus:

> . . . it was by means of words that the patient, throughout his adolescence and as an adult tried to find, in an aim-inhibited, socially acceptable way, fulfilment for the derivatives of his grandiose and exhibitionistic strivings . . . In his writings, describing and criticizing various artistic productions, he could now, by using the father's idealized power, translate his yearning for an empathic mother's response into appropriate words and sentences; even his unrelieved primary desires for the texture of the responsive body of his mother could find symbolic expression in certain verbal descriptions he had to compose in the pursuit of his professional activities.
>
> (1977: 11–12)

Kohut hypothesized that the secondary compensatory structure, based on the relation to the father as an *idealized* selfobject, especially with regard to *skills and talents* with words, provided a channel for the expression of narcissistic needs in the realm of *grandiosity and exhibitionism*. To state this in terms of his model of the bipolar self, the weakened pole of grandiosity-exhibitionism (in relation to the mother), was buttressed by the stronger pole of idealization (in relation to the father), the two poles being linked through the domain of talents and skills (with words). The problem for Mr M was that although the father had functioned better as an idealized selfobject than the mother had as a mirroring selfobject, he had still failed his son in certain ways – resulting in a weakness in the compensatory structures that Mr M had tried to build up in the realm of language and creative writing. This meant that Mr M could not comfortably contain and channel his grandiose-exhibitionistic excitement and, more specifically, he often experienced difficulty in translating his imaginings, which took the form of visual imagery, into appropriate language. The difficulty in containing and channelling states of excitement is an example of the *psychoeconomic* dimension of mental life that Kohut particularly emphasized.

Action-thoughts

According to Kohut, the analytic cure took place on the basis of an initial period of work which focused on aspects of the maternal mirror trans- ference. Sufficient work was done here to enable the patient to activate crucial aspects of the paternal idealizing transference – and through the working through of this sector, the rehabilitation of the compensatory structures could take place. Kohut discusses the implications of three acts that related to the termination phase of Mr M's analysis: (1) he bought an expensive violin yet almost immediately lost interest in playing it; (2) he cultivated a relationship with an adolescent boy whom he allowed to idealize him; (3) he founded a 'writing school' to help people from a variety of backgrounds learn how to write by sorting their ideas into manageable portions and also by becoming more receptive to word imagery. Clearly the latter two acts involved helping others to establish the selfobject functions that Mr M himself had sought, whilst the first was more to do with his own exhibitionistic expression. Kohut distinguishes these activities – which he calls 'action-thoughts' – from acting out, in the usual sense of resistances or action substitutes for insight. He considers such action-thoughts to be creatively initiated steps, expressions of devel- opmental achievement – to be interpreted but not given up except insofar as they are replaced by other activities arising from further devel- opment. These are perhaps rather like certain functions of dreams.

Thus, Mr M's action of buying an expensive violin and then giving up his interest in playing it could be seen as an enactment of his relin- quishing his attempt to gratify his exhibitionism through direct sensual appeal. This occurred as he was moving from the (for him) cruder form of exhibitionism of music to the (for him) more aim-inhibited (neutralized) exhibitionism of writing. Mr M had in fact taken up playing the violin during the analysis, particularly during the working through of the mirror transference. In his fantasies accompanying his playing, he offered his grandiose self to an admiring and listening audience without the two fears, of maternal disinterest and hypomanic overstimulation. This activity and accompanying fantasies functioned to express the exhibitionism that was activated in the mirror transference but could not be fully contained within the psychoanalytic situation. Kohut saw this as unconsciously like 'a form of psychoanalytic homework through which he tried to learn to express his exhibitionistic strivings in realistic yet gratifying ways' (1977: 39). The giving up playing the violin expressed another developmental message – that of moving from the search for mirroring from the mother to the wish to identify with the idealized father in pursuit of skills in writing. As the idealized transference was worked through, particularly in relation to the childhood disappointments suffered as he had attempted to elicit his father's interest, then the secondary compensatory structures became sufficiently firm that they could act as a vehicle for the expression, through writing, of grandiose-exhibitionistic strivings. The move from playing the violin to writing represented the selfobject search from mother to father and the strengthening of Mr M's previously precariously established (bipolar) self. This was for Mr M a highly successful developmental solution. Kohut states: 'His work as a writer enabled him to gratify his grandiose-exhibitionistic strivings to display himself to his mother, satisfy his need to merge with his idealized father, and enjoy the employment of the genuine talents he possessed' (1977: 40).

The second action-thought that Kohut describes is the development of Mr M's friendship with an adolescent boy. Mr M reported to the analyst that he was fascinated by the father's attitude to the boy, which was described as respectful, close yet allowing independence and separateness. Moreover, the boy himself was seen as both pridefully independent, yet also warmly respectful of the father. One particular incident with the boy was of considerable significance. Mr M had taken the boy to a ball-game and noticed among the crowd an ex-girlfriend. He was initially worried about speaking to the woman in case the boy felt hurt by losing Mr M's full attention. However, on beginning to speak to the woman, whilst carefully monitoring his companion's reaction, he realized that the boy did not seem to mind at all. On discovering this, Mr M felt unaccountably joyful, feeling that something important had taken place within himself, but not understanding what. As this was explored in the analysis, what became clear was that Mr felt that this scene with the boy and the ex-girlfriend had enacted a crucial developmental step which he had not achieved originally in his adolescence – the establishment of a sense of independence from the idealized selfobject father, an achievement of self-sufficiency through transmuting internalization.

Mr M's third action-thought was his founding of a writing school, a project that had been germinating in his mind for some time. One factor that had previously inhibited him in doing so was a fear that he would lose interest in it and not bring the idea to fruition. Kohut notes that such fears often express a patient's worry that a significant structural defect still exists, and that insight alone would not resolve the problem. The fact that Mr M eventually became able to realize his ambition suggested that a genuine termination of the analysis was approaching. What Mr M offered his students was the opportunity to internalize a specific structure to do with the use of language – particularly concerned with the transmuting of formless imagery into words. The functions of this structure were to channel, organize and socialize (neutralize) archaic grandiose-exhibitionistic strivings. Or, as Kohut put it: 'Expressed in metapsychological terms, the structure Mr M offered to his alter egos (taught his students) were the aim-inhibiting, discharge-delaying, substitution-providing verbal patterns that transform primary-process imagery into secondary-process ideation' (1977: 47). In addition, Mr M, as an enthusiastic teacher, functioned as an inspiring paternal ideal for his students.

Defective nuclear self

According to Kohut's formulation, Mr M's pre-analytic personality was characterized by a defective nuclear self. The damage was widespread, affecting all three areas of this structure: the two poles of grandiosity-exhibitionism and idealization, and the intermediate area of skills and talents required to fulfil the demands of the ambitions and ideals. The damage was most severe in the pole of the grandiose self, which gave rise to defensive structures – the sadistic sexual fantasies. What became of these? Apparently they did appear at times in the early stages of the analysis, as the mirror transference (relating to the mother) was partially worked through, but receded into the background as the focus of analysis shifted to the idealizing transference and to working through disappoint-ments relating to the father. Kohut clearly considered that Mr M's case was an example of how a patient will, according to an unconscious agenda of healing, exclude those areas of early personality development that cannot be contained, managed and worked through in a psycho-analytic transference – 'the deeper layers of his defective (depressive, lethargic, "dead") self (the self of his stay in the orphanage) were never exposed to full view in the transference' (1977: 52). Although some aspects of the primary defect were worked through in the initial mirror transference, Kohut did not believe that this was sufficient to account for the improvement Mr M eventually showed. Instead of dealing with the 'dead' self, Mr M used the analysis to strengthen 'compensatory struc-tures designed to increase the activity of the healthy parts of the nuclear self and to *isolate and bypass the defective ones*' (1977: 49; italics added). Perhaps an implicit analogy is with heart bypass surgery; there is no attempt to heal the most severely damaged areas of the heart, but instead a new structure is created which compensates for – literally bypasses – the defective structures. For Kohut, the genuine point of termination of the analysis was reached 'when Mr M abandoned the fruitless attempt to strengthen his rejected and enfeebled self with the aid of fantasies of sadistically enforced acclaim and turned to the successful attempt to provide the healthy sector of his self with patterns for creative expression' (1977: 54).

The analytic work with Mr M was in the realm of narcissism – comprising, in Kohut's framework, the poles of grandiosity-exhibitionism and idealization. The developmental task was to strengthen Mr M's self through analysis of its two poles. Kohut emphasizes that the favourable development was not in terms of facilitating a move from narcissism to object love; rather it was that the rehabilitation of Mr M's self meant that he was more free to pursue object-related activities – a 'welcome bonus' (1977: 41) obtained secondarily from the work on the self.

So how *does* analysis cure?

Whilst Kohut considered that analytic work, whether classical or self psychological, was based on the establishment and working through of transferences, and that the analyst's task consisted essentially of interpretation, he did not believe that the cure was achieved through insight. This was his view long before he developed self psychology. Instead he believed that the healing and strengthening process of analysis proceeds through *transmuting internalization*. It is very important to understand that Kohut was *not* advocating the analyst do anything different from analysis as classically understood – the essential analytic task is to interpret the transference – but the understanding of the process and the content of interpretations might be rather different. For Kohut, insight might be the *vehicle* that delivers the psychoanalytic cure, but it is not the essential *means* of cure.

Kohut states this very clearly in the following passage:

> In contrast to those – including James Strachey (1934) – who believe, in harmony with the spirit of the Age of Enlightenment of which Freud was a true child, that it is the power of reason which cures, the self psychologically informed analyst holds that with regard to all forms of analysable psychopathology the basic therapeutic unit of the psychoanalytic cure does not rest on the expansion of cognition. (It does not rest, for example, on the analysand's becoming aware of the difference between his fantasy and reality,

especially with reference to transference distortions involving projected drives.) Rather it is the accretion of psychic structure via an optimal frustration of the analysand's needs or wishes that is provided for the analysand in the form of correct interpretations that constitutes the essence of the cure.

(1984: 108)

In understanding this passage it is necessary to bear in mind that by 'psychic structure', Kohut meant the capacity to carry out certain functions previously performed by a selfobject, such as a parent or the analyst – it could be described as 'internalized function'. This psychic structure is built up through transmuting internalization – the gradual internalization of function through the innumerable benign (growth-promoting) failures, frustrations and prohibitions emanating from the selfobject. A related concept is Kohut's idea of optimal frustration. Here is how Kohut describes the role of this in child development in an early paper (1963) predating his development of self psychology:

As a result of having introjected many experiences of optimal frustration in which his infantile drives were handled by a calming, soothing, loving attitude rather than by counter-aggression on the part of his parents, the child himself later acts in the same way toward the drive demands that arise in him.

(Reprinted in Kohut, 1978: 370)

Through these repeated experiences of optimal frustration, the process of transmuting internalization takes place whereby the child is able to take over the functions of modulating, transforming and socializing basic impulses and strivings. Ways are found for the analysand's needs to be integrated with reality. The innumerable 'microinternalizations' of trans-muting internalization should be distinguished from the more gross internalizations of 'objects' – such as the superego or the internal objects described by Fairbairn (1952). Transmuting internalization of parental and psychoanalytic function occurs, according to Kohut, in classical analysis as well as that informed by self psychology. It applies to the management and transmutation of narcissistic strivings as well as those that are object instinctual.

A further crucial process must take place in order for the psychoana-lytic cure through transmuting internalization to take place. A transference must be established, whereby the thwarted needs and desires of childhood are revived. The psychoanalyst's interpretations help to remove defences against the awareness of these. However, the continual frustration of these needs and desires, in their raw and archaic form, provides a persistent stimulus to growth and the development of mature solutions; Mr M's taking up playing the violin during the working through of the mirror transference is one example of this.

In the working through of the transference, the childhood frustrations, disappointments, deprivations and thwartings of developmental needs are relived in relation to the analyst. These are understood and interpreted by the analyst, both in terms of their current significance in the transference and also in relation to their historical precursors in childhood experience. Insight provides support to the curative process but 'the essential structural transformations . . . are brought about by the fact that the old experiences are repeatedly relived by the more mature psyche' (1977: 30).

For Kohut the analytic work of reconstruction of childhood, on the basis of the transference, was crucial. Why? Basically it is because the psychoanalytic reconstruction of childhood provides the patient with a deeper experience of empathy *and* thereby facilitates his or her own self-empathy. Kohut argued that whilst the analyst's accurate and empathic interpretations of the patient's here-and-now experience in the transference are helpful and do indeed promote a movement towards health, the results of these 'tend to be ephemeral' (1984: 106). By contrast, he argues that:

> Well-designed verbal interpretations, on the other hand – which explain the patient's psychological reactions (in particular and par excellence his transference experiences) in dynamic terms . . . and which, furthermore refer to the genetic precursors of his vulnerabilities and conflicts – will implant the wholesome but, heretofore, ephemeral experience of having been understood into a broader area of the upper layers of the analysand's mind . . . and will thus allow him to recall this experience during the subsequent all-important period of working through.
>
> (1984: 106)

What Kohut appears to be saying here is that here-and-now interpretations of the transference are indeed of some help – a 'wholesome but ephemeral experience' – but the empathic reconstruction of childhood development provides a broader perspective and framework within which the analysand can view his or her own reactions. This broader perspective facilitates the working through process in the transference.

Another recurrent feature of Kohut's emphasis is his consistent focus on subjective experience. On the whole he did not regard it as an essential part of the analyst's function to address the data of objective reality. His or her task is to understand the patient's *subjective* reality, both in the transference and in the childhood as reconstructed through the transference. Kohut did allow that occasionally it might be necessary, *in order to preserve the analysis*, to point out that certain expectations, demands or perceptions may belong to childhood and are unrealistic in the present (see 1977: 30). Nevertheless, he was clear that such clarifications of reality are not an essential component of the psychoanalytic cure.

Summary

Two common misunderstandings of Kohut's position are (a) that the analyst should 'mirror' the patient, and (b) that the traditional idea of the historical transference (of the repetition of conflictual relationship patterns from childhood) becomes less relevant in the case of patients with a narcissistic disturbance. In fact, Kohut advocated analysis (not gratification) of the transference, and he described the interweaving of the historical and the selfobject transferences. Kohut regarded as the essential vehicle of healing not insight per se, but the establishment and working through of a selfobject transference. He refers to the principle of the primacy of preservation of the (nuclear) self, to indicate one of the fundamental motivations confronted during psychoanalysis. Kohut discovered that patients seem to have inherent developmental agendas that are played out in analysis, provided the conditions allow this. Sometimes, the natural healing agenda will involve an avoidance of the areas of greatest psychic weakness and, instead, a strengthening of a compensatory structure. In practice, this would usually mean that a full establishment and working through of a mirror transference would not take place but instead the patient would establish and work through an idealizing transference. During the working through, the disappointments, deprivations and thwartings of developmental needs are relived in relation to the analyst. These are understood in terms of both their current significance and their historical precursors. Through transmuting internalization, the traumas of childhood are mastered by the more mature psyche. Reconstruction of childhood experiences is helpful because it facilitates the patient's empathy for him/herself.

Chapter 5
Empathy and the intersubjectivists

> . . . we are primarily . . . attempting to look at the psychological universe, as it were, *via* introspection and empathy and to bring order into the *inner* experience of man. . . By empathy, by the use of a variety of cues that we obtain, and on the basis of the essential similarity between people, we can, with some hope of correctness and accuracy grasp what another person feels, experiences, thinks.
>
> (Kohut, 1996: 350)

The empathic-introspective vantage point

A philosophical rigour is woven throughout the fabric of Kohut's theorizing. An early paper, *Introspection, Empathy and Psychoanalysis* (1959) set the conceptual and methodological scene for much of what followed in his later clinical and conceptual innovations. Basically, Kohut argued that the domain of psychoanalysis is defined by that which is available to introspection and empathy. The data of psychoanalysis – thoughts, wishes, feelings, fantasies, anxieties – cannot be observed in physical space. They are available to introspection, in ourselves, or through empathy with others. Crucially, Kohut defined empathy as *vicarious introspection*. He criticized the use within psychoanalysis of quasi-biological concepts which went beyond the domain available to introspection or empathy – for example, the idea of life and death instincts and the related concept of the repetition compulsion:

> The concepts of Eros and Thanatos do not belong to a psychological theory grounded on the observational methods of introspection and empathy but to a biological theory which must be based on different observational methods.
>
> (1959: 227)

Instead, for Kohut, the data gathering field of psychoanalysis was determined by the consistent use of the observational tool of introspection and empathy – 'this observational method defines the contents and limits of the observed field' (1959: 212). Whilst he did not argue that intro-spection and empathy are the only relevant methods of observation for the psychoanalyst, he did insist that these are the essential and most decisive modes of inquiry. Kohut believed that this emphasis distin-guished his perspective from that of other psychoanalysts whose frameworks he considered to be based on a more external vantage point – such as the separation-individuation theory of Mahler, or the attachment theory of Bowlby, or the 'identity' concept of Erikson. According to Kohut, the work of such theorists lies outside of the domain of psychoanalysis, as defined by the empathic-introspective framework. He states this very firmly in a letter to a colleague in 1978:

> The framework within which Spitz's and Mahler's theories belong and within which their statements find their meaning is the framework of sociology. In other words, however psychologically insightful and sophisticated these great contributors are, they deal in essence with social relationships and they must therefore, formulate their findings in sociological – interactional, trans-actional – terms . . . what is at stake here, as demonstrated by a comparison of the results obtained when the same data are seen from one point of view or from the other, is a decisive difference between the outlook of the child observer and the outlook of the introspective-empathic psychologist, which is mine.
>
> (1990: 571–72)

Kohut regarded his development of the methodological stance of reliance on the empathic-introspective vantage point as one of his most important contributions. It was from this position of examining phenomena consistently from within the patient's point of view, that Kohut's new clinical observations and insights proceeded – his recog-nition of the selfobject transferences and his formulation of the bipolar self. He firmly considered psychoanalysis to be a science, whose data were those provided by empathy and introspection. The observation of data gives rise to theory, as the analyst attempts to order and formulate phenomena, but theory then guides further observation – a circular process of mutual influence of observation and theory. However, Kohut frequently expressed his preference for what he termed 'experience-near theorizing', as opposed to 'experience-distant theorizing'. He believed that his empathic-introspective stance tended to give rise to more experience-near theorizing than had been typical of classical psychoanalysis, as developed in the USA by Hartman and colleagues. Kohut described the interaction between observation and theory as follows:

Anyone who has studied the conception of the bipolar self should realize that I alternate between direct clinical observation in the transference (concerning the child's turning from a disappointing selfobject to a less disappointing one) and experience-distant theorizing (the formulation of the clinical findings in dynamic-structural terms as a shift from the functional preponderance of one pole of the self to that of the other one, a formulation in turn, related to the concept of compensatory structures).

(1978: 269)

Kohut was also fond of emphasizing that the psychoanalyst should not only be open to new observation – should be prepared to be surprised – but also should be able to entertain a variety of hypotheses. By having a range of interpretive and theoretical perspectives in mind, the analyst-observer can suspend judgement until it is apparent which is the most satisfactory formulation. He describes the psychoanalytic method of science as follows:

I think that we should remain faithful to the approach that has been so rewarding to us up to now: prolonged empathic immersion into psychological material; the appreciation – analogous to the various images we 'see' in clouds or in Rorschach inkblots – of as many alternative configurations as we can derive from the data that our empathic immersion has provided for us; further observation to determine which of the closures, if any, will stand the test of time (e.g. which of the alternative clinical hypotheses is supported by subsequent material); and ultimately the formulation in theoretical terms of that particular product of empathic understanding which has proved to be the most correct and accurate, for the purpose of communication and with the aim of fitting the single experience-near finding into a pre-existing broader experience-distant context.

(1978: 271)

A thought experiment

In a relatively early contribution, Kohut describes a remarkable *thought experiment*, concerning the understanding of depression, to illustrate his view of the interplay of empathy and theory. His intention is to demonstrate

how empathy pervades the processes by which the explanation of the primary data, perceived via empathy, is ultimately achieved in our science, and how its use may bring about that mixture of subtlety of understanding, nuanced formulation, and faithfulness to actual human experience, while yet rigorously maintaining the high degree of theoretical clarity that has always characterized psychoanalysis at its best.

(1968a: 94)

Kohut starts from Freud's (1917) statement that in depression, aggression initially directed outwards has been turned inwards, resulting in self-hatred and self-belittlement. He argues that this formulation, stated thus, allows the observer only a grasp of a sequential process, without a more full empathic understanding of the process in its totality.

First, Kohut notes some preliminary points regarding the aggression encountered in depression. It is possible to recognize empathically that the aggression is primitive and that it has a nagging quality. The patient's dreams may lead to association with cannibalistic preoccupations. Thus the observer may grasp, via empathy, that the aggression belongs to an oral sadistic experiential world, and that it has roots in early experiences concerned with feeding and weaning, and rage at a frustrating mother-breast, and so on. All this is quite familiar and commonplace to the analyst. However, Kohut wishes to comprehend, on both an experience-near and experience-distant basis, how it comes about that the rage that was directed at the object is now directed at the self.

Kohut next argues that the mood characteristic for depression is 'most closely understood via empathy with a baby or small child that has suffered a severe frustration at a particular, clearly circumscribed stage of psychic development, i.e., at the very moment when its cognitive development has just tentatively allowed it to recognize that the breast-mother is separate, that it is not under the child's absolute control (not as much, that is, under the child's control as is the control which adults expect to exert over their own bodies and minds), but that the breast-mother has a greater degree of independence vis-à-vis its needs' (1968a: 98). Allowing empathy and theoretical knowledge concerning the development of self-object separation to co-operate, Kohut arrives at the conclusion that the baby's oral frustration has two results: an upsurge of oral-sadistic rage; and an undoing of the tentative recognition of the separateness of the object. If the response of the caregiver has not been such that the baby can master, through its predictability, the sequence of need followed by feeding, then the rage becomes intensified and more primitive, and there is a regression in the child's cognitive grasp of a distinction between self and object. As a result of this cognitive regression, the rage is directed diffusely against this primitive fused image of self and object. At this point, from the external observer's point of view, the rage now appears to be directed at the self.

Part of Kohut's rationale for presenting this thought experiment, combining empathic and non-empathic processes, was to demonstrate the scientific status of his earlier assertion that the data of psychoanalysis are those derived from introspection and empathy. He indicates that his 1959 paper on this epistemological topic had been, in his view quite mistakenly, criticized as promoting a mystical, philosophical, and essentially unscientific position. Kohut's methodology was consistently based on the two processes of (1) understanding, based on observations derived from introspection and empathy, and (2) explanation, in which the empathically observed and understood data are fitted into a more experience-distant formulation. Experience-near and experience-distant perspectives continually inform and modify each other. For Kohut this was the appropriate scientific method of psychoanalysis. In his final contributions (1984), he describes how this method is also the two-stage process whereby expanding psychoanalytic knowledge is conveyed to the patient.

Stolorow and the intersubjectivists

Some who were strongly supportive of Kohut's work have moved on to develop the ideas of self psychology in a somewhat new direction, which they have termed *intersubjectivity* (e.g. Atwood and Stolorow, 1984; Stolorow, Brandchaft and Atwood, 1987; Stolorow and Atwood, 1992; Stolorow, Atwood and Brandchaft, 1994; Orange, 1995; Orange, Atwood and Stolorow, 1997). This approach is based on the idea that the clinical phenomena observed by psychoanalysts always occur in the context of two people (patient and analyst) interacting, each with their own subjective patterns of organizing their experience. Atwood and Stolorow state their position as follows:

> In its most general form, our thesis . . . is that psychoanalysis seeks to illuminate phenomena that emerge within a specific psychological field constituted by the intersection of two subjectivities – that of the patient and that of the analyst . . .The observational stance is always one within, rather than outside, the inter-subjective field . . . a fact that guarantees the centrality of introspection and empathy as the methods of observation.
>
> (Atwood and Stolorow, 1984: 41–42)

Crucially, they add, in an echo of Winnicott's (1947) remark that there is no such thing as a baby, but only a baby in relation to the caregiver:

> [C]linical phenomena . . . cannot be understood apart from the intersubjective contexts in which they take form. Patient and analyst together form an indissoluble psychological system, and it is this system that constitutes the empirical domain of psychoanalytic inquiry.
>
> (1984: 64)

These authors have consistently explored the implications of a radically intersubjective position, both for understanding development and psychopathology, and also for guiding the work actually in the consulting room. Although closely associated with Kohut's innovations, especially through the latter's emphasis on the introspective-empathic observational stance, and his concept of the selfobject which is embedded in the recognition that self and other form a psychological system, it is important to understand that Stolorow and colleagues were developing their intersubjective position independently of Kohut (see Stolorow, 1994). Their insights into the intersubjective nature of mental life were first presented in 1979 in the book *Faces in a Cloud: Subjectivity in Personality Theory* (Stolorow and Atwood, 1979). Here they explored the personal and subjective origins of the psychological theories of Freud, Jung, Reich and Rank, showing how each constructed formal systems that reflected their own emotional experiences, preoccupations and conflicts. Thus it was apparent that theories themselves are subjective creations, reflecting the personal concerns of their creators. Stolorow and Atwood comment: '. . . what psychoanalysis needs is a theory of subjectivity itself – a unifying framework that can account not only for the phenomena that other theories address but also for these theories themselves' (1992: 2). These authors' later emphasis on the point that both patient and analyst organize their experience within the consulting room on the basis of their personal subjective patterns gave rise to their view of the intersubjective field as a system of *reciprocal mutual influence* (Beebe and Lachmann, 1988). This position, whilst based on the method of 'sustained empathic enquiry', led them in directions slightly different from those of Kohut.

Intersubjectivist criticisms of self psychology

Stolorow, Brandchaft and Atwood state their agreement with three aspects of Kohut's self psychology: (1) the empathic-introspective mode of observation; (2) the emphasis upon the centrality of self-experience (which they see as implying 'a theoretical shift from the motivational primacy of instinct to the motivational primacy of affect and affective experience' (1987: 16); (3) the concept of the selfobject, defined here as 'a dimension of experiencing an object . . . in which a specific bond is required for maintaining, restoring, or consolidating the organization of self-experience' (1987: 16–17).

However, they go on to criticize self psychology using one of its own fundamental tenets – that psychoanalysis should be defined and delimited by the empathic-introspective mode. Thus they argue that the concept of 'self', as employed by Kohut, is confused and reifying. They point out that the term 'self' is used within self psychology both to refer to a psychological structure – an organization of experience – and as an existential agent. These two meanings become conflated in sentences such as the following, which are typical of those found in the self psychology literature: 'The fragmented self strives to restore its cohesion.' This sentence implies that an organization of experience, called the 'self', has undergone fragmentation, and that an existential agent, also called the self, is attempting to restore cohesion to that organization. Instead, they suggest that the term 'self' should be restricted to descriptions of the organizations of experience (including the subjective sense of personal agency), and that the existential agent should be referred to as 'the person'. Thus the illustrative sentence becomes: 'The person whose self-experience is becoming fragmented strives to restore his sense of self-cohesion.'

Kohut's concept of the bipolar self is seen as particularly problematic. They see reification inherent in this model, such that 'the poles of the self become ossified entities that belie the organic fluidity of human experience' (1987: 20). Moreover, they consider Kohut's metaphor of a 'tension arc' between the two poles as 'a retrogression to mechanistic thinking, reminiscent of the libidinal hydraulics of classical drive theory' (1987: 20), introducing phenomena not accessible to introspection and empathy. However, they regard the most serious problem with a bipolar concept of the self as being that it 'unnecessarily narrows the vast array of selfobject experiences that can shape and colour the evolution of a person's self-organization' (1987: 20). They prefer to think of a 'multidimensional self'.

Stolorow and colleagues expand the concept of the selfobject by proposing that 'selfobject functions pertain most fundamentally to the integration of affect into the organization of self-experience, and that the need for selfobject ties pertains most centrally to the need for attuned responsiveness to affect states in all phases of the life cycle' (1987: 20). Clearly this goes far beyond Kohut's initial positing of selfobject functions as comprising mirroring and idealization – and takes the field of exploration far beyond its roots in the study of narcissism, just as had indeed Kohut's own later theorizing (Kohut, 1984).

Not surprisingly, in the light of this line of criticism, Stolorow and colleagues also object to Kohut's (1977) idea of the drive-like 'disintegration products' resulting from fragmentation of the bipolar self in response to selfobject failure. They view this metaphor too as having an inherently mechanistic connotation, which obscures the meaning and *purpose* of these reactive states. For example, they point to the way in which lustful feelings and strivings can be an attempt to find an eroticized replacement for a missing selfobject experience, as Kohut himself described; similarly, rage can be an attempt to restore a collapsing sense of power and personal agency. Furthermore, Stolorow and colleagues argue that by not giving sufficient emphasis to these meanings and purposes of the supposed 'disintegration products', an important clinical distinction is blurred. This is between *reactive* sexualized or aggressivized transference configurations, and *primary* transferences whereby the patient is attempting to present, albeit conflictually, newly emerging sexual or aggressive aspects to the analyst in the unconscious hope that these will be recognized as developmental achievements.

A further objection is to Kohut's idea of transmuting internalization arising from optimal frustration. Stolorow and colleagues argue that the use of the term 'internalization' to refer to the process whereby autonomous regulation replaces regulation by the environment (Hartmann, 1939) introduces misleading physicalistic and spatial reifications. Moreover, they argue that the idea of optimal frustration as the basis for structure formation is a remnant of drive theory, an obsolete vestige which has no place in an empathic-introspective framework. Instead, they believe that structure formation occurs primarily when the selfobject bond is intact, or at least in the process of being restored. Rather than emphasizing optimal frustration, they propose alternative concepts, such as 'optimal empathy' and 'affect attunement'. In particular, Stolorow and colleagues place importance on the process of 'structuralization of self-experience': 'The analyst's consistent acceptance and empathic understanding of the patient's affective states and needs regularly comes to be experienced by the patient as a facilitating medium reinstating developmental processes of self-articulation and self-demarcation that had been aborted and arrested during the formative years' (Stolorow et al., 1987: 23).

Finally, Stolorow and colleagues criticize what they see as a false dichotomy between selfobjects and true objects in Kohut's theorizing. They see this as an outgrowth of Kohut's original (1971) juxtaposition of narcissistic libido and object libido. Again they consider this kind of concept to involve unnecessary reification. Instead, they suggest that the term 'selfobject' be used to refer to a particular dimension of experiencing an object. The implication of this for conceptualizing transference is that at times the selfobject dimension may be in the foreground, whereas at other times it is more of a background support enabling the patient to face frightening feelings and painful dilemmas. In other transference conditions the selfobject dimension may be absent and the emphasis is upon fears of repetition of traumatic relationship patterns:

> Here the analyst is not experienced as a selfobject, but as a source of painful and conflictual affect states, in turn engendering resistance. When, in such instances, the patient is resisting the emergence of central selfobject needs, it

makes no theoretical sense to speak of the analytic relationship as a
self–selfobject unit, because the selfobject dimension of these transference has
been temporarily obliterated or obstructed by what the patient has perceived as
actual or impending selfobject failure from the side of the analyst, and the
analyst must focus on the patient's fears of a transference repetition of traumatically damaging childhood experiences.

(Stolorow et al, 1987: 26–27)

Stolorow and colleagues see a shifting figure–ground relationship
between the selfobject and the repetitive dimensions of transference.
Analysis of the fears of transference repetitions allows the disrupted bond
to the analyst to be restored, so that the selfobject dimension can then
resume its place either in the foreground, or as part of the silent
background.

The centrality of Kohut's concept of self – an evaluation of Stolorow's critique

Unfortunately Kohut himself was not alive to answer these criticisms.
However some of his published remarks do have a bearing on what has
been argued, and suggest the lines along which he might have
responded.

Some particularly pertinent comments are to be found in Kohut's
discussion of Mr R, which was not actually published during his lifetime.
Here he argues that psychological phenomena must be examined from
two contrasting perspectives or models. One is that of the psyche 'as an
information gathering, information processing, acting and reacting
apparatus, i.e., man's psyche conceived as a machine which reacts to
signals from the environment' (1990a: 208) The other is concerned with
the idea of the psyche as activated from within: 'the self, to the extent to
which it has become a central structure which is capable of making active
choices and decisions . . . to the extent to which it is endowed with a "free
will"' (1990a: 209).

Kohut probably would not have entirely agreed with the theoretical
stance of intersubjectivity, insofar as it emphasizes that the psyche can
always be understood only in relation to other psyches – the two (or
more) subjectivities interacting. He did not see his psychoanalytic theory
as a field theory. Such a position he viewed as a kind of social psychology,
useful in its own right but essentially different from the empathic-introspective stance that discerns the individual's experience of free will and
of the self as a centre of initiative. That Kohut would not have found
himself entirely in agreement with Stolorow et al. is suggested by the
following remarks:

The analyst is . . . fully aware of the broad explanatory scope of field theories which focus on the interactions of individuals. These models, however, which focus primarily on energic processes between psychobiological units, do not facilitate the analyst's thinking about the phenomena to be explained by him within his own field of observation.

(1990a: 210)

The nuclear self

The particular phenomena that Kohut felt could not be explained by field or intersubjective models of the psyche were those to do with the experience of free will and the autonomy of the self. He was struck by the way that some heroic individuals will remain true to their ideals, even when these are in conflict with both external social pressures, and internal urges to preserve life and comfort. One extreme example he gives is that of solitary martyrs in Nazi Germany who preserved the integrity of their inner self and its ideals even at the expense of loss of physical life. He described the case of Franz Jagerstatter, an Austrian peasant who refused to compromise his Christian ideals by serving in the German army. Jagerstatter rejected all the compromises that were offered and calmly went to the guillotine in 1943. Kohut presents Jagerstatter's account of a dream which prompted his decision not to serve in the army:

> Right at the beginning I want to describe a brief experience during a summer night in 1938. First I lay awake almost until midnight even though I was not ill; but then I must have fallen asleep for a while because I was shown a beautiful railroad train which circled around a mountain. Not only the grownups but even the children streamed toward this train and it was almost impossible to hold them back. I hate to tell how very few of the grownups there were who resisted being carried along by this occasion. But then I heard a voice which spoke to me and said: This train is going to hell.

(1990b: 138–39)

Kohut explains:

> Jagerstatter reflected on the meaning of this dream. Ultimately he came to the conclusion that it depicted the Nazi invasion. It showed how everybody was jumping on the bandwagon, but that the movement which everybody joined was evil and that they would all be led to their utter destruction.

(1990b: 139)

Kohut describes a similar dream of Sophie Scholl, a 19-year-old girl, who, along with a group of others, formed a movement called the White Rose which actively opposed the Nazi regime in 1941 by distributing leaflets and posting notices on walls. After she was caught and knew she was to be executed by beheading on a particular day, she had the following dream the night before, which she told to her cell mate:

> I carried a child, dressed in a long white garment, to be baptised. The path to the church led up a steep mountain; but I held the child firmly and securely. Suddenly there was a crevasse gaping in front of me. I had barely enough time to deposit the child on the far side of it, which I managed to do safely – then I fell into the depths.
>
> (1990b: 148)

Sophie Scholl herself interpreted her dream to her cell mate – that the child was 'our leading idea – it will live on and make its way to fulfilment despite obstacles' (1990b: 148).

Commenting further on this dream in his Chicago Lectures, Kohut explained that the falling represented 'the loss of her total psychological body self, the ultimate dropping of self-esteem. Her own youthful, beautiful body was going to be horribly done away with' (1996: 253). However, the baby represented the preservation of her ideals which would live on after her, kept safe by her remaining true to them even in the face of death by mutilation. If she had opted to preserve her physical life, which she probably could have done by recanting or turning informer, her ideals would have been destroyed.

Kohut argues that this awareness of a capacity to choose, even when it conflicts with the natural inclinations to seek pleasure and avoid pain, indicates an autonomy of self which psychoanalytic theory must accommodate:

> The more deeply an analysis penetrates, the more clearly the analysand recognizes the essence of those deepest of his ambitions and ideals which make up his nuclear self . . . the more vivid and real becomes the analysand's experience of being able to choose and to decide, the more certain he feels of possessing access to the capacity of exercising his 'free will' – whether he chooses to live in accordance with the reality-pleasure principle . . . or whether he chooses to transcend the reality-pleasure principle . . . and disregarding even his cherished body self . . . strives towards that fulfilment of his nuclear self which, in the symbolism of religion, is celebrated as saintliness and as eternal life.
>
> (1990b: 212)

Thus Kohut indicates there is something important in the human psyche, which, whilst *derived* from relationships and experiences with others, becomes *independent of* relationships and pursues its own agenda. He comments:

> The conclusion is, therefore, inescapable that certain qualities and functions of the self, once this structure has been fully formed, cannot be comprehended unless the self is conceptualized as an independent, autonomous unit, despite

the fact that there are other, broad areas of the personality, outside the
(nuclear) self, which must be coerced as interacting with the environment, in a
give-and-take relationship that is governed by the signals of the pleasure
principle, and despite the fact that the early environment of the child (the
child's selfobjects) makes decisive contributions to the forms and contents of
the self. Once the nuclear self has been laid down, however, it strives . . . to fulfil
its life curve. It moves . . . towards the realization of its ambitions and ideals . . .
And if an individual succeeds in realizing the aims of his nuclear self, he can die
without regret.

(1990b: 213)

One crucial but little recognized implication of comments such as these,
is that the nuclear self is not the same as the conscious sense of 'I'.
Indeed, a person can experience his or her nuclear self as a powerful
other within, as indicated in the following passage:

An individual's deepest ambitions and ideals, once congealed to form the
nucleus of his self, will drive and lead him with a force which, though in most of
us hidden by conflict, fear, and guilt, is in its essence independent of fear and
guilt, of expiation and reform. Man's need, therefore, to move toward the
realization of his deepest ambitions and ideals will, as I mentioned earlier,
allow him even to tolerate torture and to accept death . . .

(1990b: 214)

Kohut argued, on the basis of his clinical observations, that the nuclear
self can be in conflict with other more superficial selves. Many
individuals, he suggests, may adapt superficially to the external social
world, in such a way that the nuclear self is progressively isolated and
repressed:

The psychological outcome which is unfortunately more or less characteristic of
the psychological makeup of the majority of adults, is not an individual striving
toward a creative solution of his conflicts concerning the redefinition of his
basic ambitions and values, but a person who, despite his smoothly adaptive
surface behaviour, experiences a sense of inner shallowness and who gives to
others an impression of artificiality.

(1990b: 136)

By contrast, those who are in touch with and guided by their nuclear self
experience a sense of depth and joy in the pursuit of their goals and the
preservation of their values. Analysis can help the individual to restore
and have access to their nuclear self.

These various comments concerning the way an individual is directed
by a deep source of goals and ideals, even when this is in conflict with
more superficial motivations for pleasure, approval of others and
avoidance of pain, suggests that Kohut did indeed consider the nuclear

self to be an *autonomous* structure, not reducible merely to the conscious sense of agency. His view of the bipolar nature of the nuclear self, comprising the poles of ambitions and ideals, was derived not from philosophical reasoning but from the empathic-introspective stance in clinical psychoanalysis. Thus, the arguments by Stolorow and his colleagues for discarding the concept of the self as a bipolar structure would appear to ignore some of what Kohut himself felt to be most crucial to his observations and formulations. Kohut accounted for the heroic in man, the dedication to ideals even at the expense of surrendering the physical body, and overriding the pleasure-pain principle. The nuclear self, in his heroes, transcended the pressures of the immediate social environment. This is part of what makes his writings often very moving.

The argument by Stolorow et al. that the concept of the bipolar structure of the self 'unnecessarily narrows the vast array of selfobject experiences that can shape and color the evolution of a person's self-organization' (1987: 20) suggests that their focus is upon the relationship between patient and analyst – indeed upon the selfobject dimension of the relationship – whereas Kohut's focus was upon the patient's experience. Although it was through the consistent application of the empathic-introspective stance that the selfobject phenomenon was identified, it was by remaining focused upon the patient's experience – and not upon the field between patient and analyst – that Kohut located the bipolar self. Kohut did not see his self psychology as a form of relational psychoanalysis (Bacal and Newman, 1990).

That Stolorow and colleagues sharply diverge from Kohut over the importance of the self as a structure is demonstrated starkly by the following comment arguing against what they call the 'myth of the isolated mind':

> A second remnant of the myth of the isolated mind that persists in self psychology can be seen in the idea that the self possesses an innate nuclear program or inherent design . . . awaiting a responsive milieu that will enable it to unfold . . . Unlike ego psychology, which postulates the autonomous mind as the ideal endpoint of development, self psychology seems here to locate this ideal in the prenatal or genetic prehistory of the individual, as a pre-existing potential requiring only the opportunity to become actualized. Such an idea contrasts sharply with our view that the trajectory of self experience is shaped at every point in development by the intersubjective system in which it crystallizes.
>
> (Stolorow and Atwood, 1992: 17–18)

It will be readily apparent from the above examples of Kohut's views that this is not at all an accurate representation of his concept of the nuclear self and its origin. Kohut saw the nuclear self structure as developing within the early selfobject milieu, but once developed it then takes on its own autonomy and becomes a directing and leading force within the psyche.

However, Stolorow and colleagues present extensive and sophisticated arguments against what they see as the pervasive assumptions, implicit in much psychoanalytic theorizing, that the psyche can be considered in isolation from its relationship with others. Thus they point to how the patient is often portrayed as the 'chief director of the analytic stage' (Stolorow and Atwood, 1992: 22) who attempts to draw the analyst into old relational patterns or to make the analyst the target of projective identifications, or to maintain psychic retreats from relatedness to the analyst – and here they no doubt are thinking particularly of British Kleinians (e.g. Spillius, 1988b; Steiner, 1993). They argue that often insufficient attention is given to ways in which the patient becomes a co-actor in the analyst's drama – how the patient is subtly coerced into responding in accord with the analyst's assimilation of him or her to the analyst's preexisting categories and beliefs. Many variants of contemporary psychoanalysis do not fully take on board the point that it is the child-caregiver system and the patient-analyst system of mutual regulation that should be the unit of study. They ask why it is that these assumptions, that one psyche can be observed without *fully* taking account of the influence of the other (observing) psyche, appear so pervasive and difficult to eradicate, and suggest that they serve as shared defences against existential anxiety:

> . . . it is our view that this pervasive, reified image in its many guises serves to disavow the exquisite vulnerability that is inherent to an unalienated awareness of the continual intersubjective context. The impersonal machine, the autonomous ego, the omnipotent agent, the inviolable pristine self – all such images of the mind insulated from the constitutive impact of the surround counteract . . . what might be termed the 'unbearable embeddedness of being'.
> (Stolorow and Atwood, 1992: 22)

This may be so. Nevertheless, it is a misrepresentation of Kohut to suggest that he presented an image of autonomy and independence as the outcome of healthy development. His view of mental life, like so much in psychoanalysis, was more complex and acknowledging of paradox. For Kohut, the healthy individual is one who has become able to fulfil the potential of the nuclear self, and yet he saw human beings as forever dependent on the availability of selfobjects and vulnerable to disorders of the self in their absence. The nuclear self is dependent on the availability of selfobjects early in life, and upon the selfobject functions of the analyst, but once formed the nuclear self acquires its own autonomy.

Thus, Kohut's vision of development embraces both dependence and autonomy.

Stolorow's formulation of transference and the unconscious

Stolorow and colleagues have presented some interesting reformulations of both transference and the unconscious.

They point to the various ways in which transference is considered. One traditional view is of transference as *regression* to earlier stages of development and organization. A second is that of *displacement* – whereby emotions or impulses relating to an unconscious representation of an object from the past are transferred to a representation of a current figure in the external world. A third view of transference is that it involves *projection* of internal objects or parts of the self on to (or into) the analyst; this usage is particularly characteristic of analysts influenced by Melanie Klein. Yet another traditional view of transference is that of *distortion* – a distortion of reality as the analyst is mistakenly perceived in terms of images from the past or from the patient's internal world.

Stolorow and colleagues argue that transference may be better conceptualized as referring to the variety of ways in which the patient's experience of the analyst and the analytic situation are shaped by the patient's own psychological structures, the characteristic configurations of self and other that unconsciously organize his or her perceptions and expectations of relationships:

> Thus transference, at the most general level of abstraction, is an instance of organizing activity – the patient assimilates . . . the analytic relationship into the thematic structures of his personal subjective world.
>
> (Stolorow et al., 1987: 36)

This means that transference is not seen as a regression to or displacement from the past, nor essentially as projection (although projection may indeed occur for defensive purposes), but instead is viewed as an expression of the 'continuing influence of the organizing principles and imagery that crystallized out of the patient's early formative experiences' (1987: 36). This view is actually very compatible with the Sandlers' (1997) model of the 'present unconscious' which is organized by the templates derived from the experiences and phantasies of childhood – the past unconscious. Conceptualized thus, it is quite easy to include fully the contributions of the analyst to the patient's experience; the analyst's activity, including that of interpreting, is assimilated to the patient's recurrent configurations of expectation regarding relationships. Looked at in this way, the patient is not making a 'false connection' or 'distorting' what would otherwise be an objective perception of the analyst; it is inevitable that the patient will assimilate the experience of the analyst to his or her recurrent structures of organization of the subjective world. The analytic work can then be freed from the awkward position in which either the patient's or the analyst's perception is endowed with 'truth' or 'reality'. Nor does there then have to be an excessive concern with 'abstinence' based on a fear of 'contaminating' the transference, since the analyst's behaviour (including 'abstinence') is seen as inevitably and continually providing emotional material which the patient will assimilate to the recurrent internal configurations. Stolorow et al. conclude:

> When transference is conceptualized as an organizing activity, it is assumed that the patient's experience of the therapeutic relationship is always shaped *both* by inputs from the analyst and by the structures of meaning into which these are assimilated by the patient. We would therefore do away with the rule of abstinence and its corresponding concept of neutrality and replace them with an attitude of sustained empathic inquiry, which seeks understanding of the patient's expressions from within the perspective of the patient's subjective frame of reference. From this vantage point, the reality of the patient's perceptions of the analyst is neither debated nor confirmed. Instead, these perceptions serve as points of departure for an exploration of the meanings and organizing principles that structure the patient's psychic reality.
>
> (Stolorow et al., 1987: 43)

Stolorow and his colleagues' additional reformulation of the concept of the unconscious is based on their view that affect, rather than instinctual drives, should now be seen as the central motivational construct for psychoanalysis – a view that would be consistent with the influential emphasis of Sandler (e.g. Joffe and Sandler, 1968), for example. They point out that the work of developmentalists, such as Stern (1985) and Emde (1983; 1988a; 1988b), indicates that affectivity is grounded in the mutual attunement of the early infant–caregiver system. A purely intrapsychic origin of affect is untenable. From this point of view, the dynamic unconscious – the repression of feelings, memories, fantasies and perceptions which are feared will give rise to emotional conflict and danger – is always a product of the early intersubjective context. Most crucially, the dynamic unconscious is seen as containing those experiences that had to be denied expression because they were *perceived to threaten a needed tie to a caregiver* (an idea very similar to the theory proposed by J.J. Freyd, 1996).

Two further forms of unconsciousness are described by Stolorow and his colleagues. The *prereflective unconscious* consists of the organizing principles that unconsciously shape and thematize a person's experiences, these being derived from recurrent patterns of intersubjective experience with the early caregivers, along the lines of Stern's (1985) concept of repeated interactions that have become generalized (RIGs) or Bowlby's (1980) internal working models. This view is also compatible with that of Sandler, in the concept of the representational world (Sandler and Rosenblatt, 1962), and the later concept of the past unconscious, which provides the dynamic *templates*, but not the *content*, for the present unconscious (Sandler and Sandler, 1997). Thus the prereflective unconscious, like the Sandlers' past unconscious, contains organizing principles but not repressed content banished from consciousness. It might be regarded as a form of *implicit* memory (Mollon, 1998).

The unvalidated unconscious contains experiences that could not be given conscious expression because they had not evoked validating responsiveness from the early caregivers. Stolorow and colleagues argue that the child's developing sense of the world and self as real depends upon the validating attunements of the caregiving surround. The earliest preverbal validations occur in the affective attunements whereby the caregiver, through touch, facial expression, movement, vocal rhythm and so on, mirrors the child's emotional state. Later validations occur through verbal and other symbolic modalities. However, certain areas of experience or perception may be actively invalidated by the caregiver:

> Derailments of this developmental process can occur in any phase when validating attunement is profoundly absent. Under these circumstances, the child, in order to maintain ties vital to well-being, must accommodate the organization of his experience to the caregiver's. With the advent of symbolic communication and awareness of others as centers of subjectivity, such accommodation can result in a subjective world constituted in large part by an alien reality imposed from outside.
>
> (Stolorow and Atwood, 1992: 28)

This view is compatible with that of the cognitive psychologist J.J. Freyd (1996) in her 'betrayal trauma' theory of the forgetting of childhood abuse. She argues that a child will perceive and remember child abuse provided that the experience is met with validation and does not threaten a needed primary relationship. However, if the abuse is at the hands of a primary caregiver, then it is a form of 'betrayal trauma'; recognition of betrayal would threaten the relationship and so the awareness is blocked.

Stolorow and colleagues emphasize that all three of these realms of the unconscious – the prereflective, the dynamic, and the unvalidated – arise within the specific, formative intersubjective contexts of infancy and childhood. Thus repression, dissociation, or other forms of banishment from awareness, are intersubjective, rather than purely intrapsychic, processes.

Stolorow and Atwood (1992) argue that the reformulation of the three forms of unconscious and their intersubjective origins provides a clear response to critics such as Kernberg (1982), who has suggested that an empathic-introspective stance can lead only to a psychology of conscious experience.

Three forms of unconsciousness – clinical illustrations

Stolorow and Atwood (1992) illustrate their reformulation of the uncon-sciousness by reference to the dream of a 19-year-old woman, which occurred just prior to a psychotic episode. The dream was as follows:

> The dreamer stood in a country setting before a small structure that she said resembled an outhouse. Looking inside, she found a toilet. As she peered into the bowl, the water began gurgling, foaming, and then rising and overflowing. The flow became more and more agitated until an explosive geyser of uniden-tified glowing material erupted from the toilet, increasing in violence without apparent limit. At this point the dreamer awoke in terror.
> (Stolorow and Atwood, 1992: 36)

A crucial aspect of the patient's childhood had been severe sexual abuse by her father, from age 2, mainly involving oral sex. However, these activ-ities took place only late at night and were kept entirely secret from the rest of the family which maintained an image of great respectability in the community. Her father instructed her not to speak of the abuse and told her that their relationship was special and that their sexual activities were similar to those of royal families. On one occasion she did tell her mother about what was going on but she was screamed at and beaten for telling lies. Thus her experiences of abuse were dissociated from her experi-ences during the day, and indeed she did well in school and had many friends.

Despite this apparent good adjustment, two recurrent nightmares from her early and middle childhood gave some indication of the emotions that she was warding off. In one dream she observes dark spots on the floor, and above each spot any object would vanish and was annihilated; the spots were expanding, leaving less and less clear space, and she became increasingly desperate as she tried to avert her own annihilation. In the second recurrent dream she is lying on the floor whilst her body is pulled in opposite directions by elf-like creatures with strings attached to hooks which are embedded in her skin. Stolorow and Atwood explain the first of these dreams in terms of an expression of her sense of increasing threat to her psychological survival within the family. The second was seen as expressing concretely her sense of contradictory pulls on her sense of self exerted by the two versions of her father: the loving and responsible father of the daytime and the sexual abuser of the night-time. If she were conscious of the contradictory aspects of her experience in the family she would indeed feel pulled apart and torn into pieces.

Regarding the dream from age 19, Stolorow and Atwood argue that the dynamic unconscious consisted of areas of experience that had to be banished from awareness in order to maintain the needed tie to the caregivers – and this was represented by the underground material beneath the outhouse which bubbles up through the toilet. What the dream portrays is the breakdown of repression whereby overwhelming affects, previously disposed of, invade the upper space of consciousness. The prereflective unconscious is represented in the geometry of the imagery, whereby the public daylight world is separated from the underground area from which the frightening material emerges. The idea of an 'outhouse' is also suited to symbolize a place where unacceptable emotional material is placed. The unvalidated unconscious is demonstrated by the undifferentiated and unidentifiable glowing material that emerges from the toilet. This quality of being overwhelming whilst lacking specific objects that could be identified and given words, is characteristic of the unvalidated unconscious, since it consists of that which cannot be articulated because it has not received validation from others.

Stolorow and Atwood describe how gradually the patient's experience was explored and validated in a lengthy process of analytic therapy. They point out that in this case the dynamic unconscious and unvalidated unconscious coincided, but that at the beginning of the therapy the repressed material emerged in an undifferentiated form typical of the unvalidated unconscious. Only gradually were clear memories and feelings articulated.

Although Stolorow and Atwood's formulation of the three dimensions of the unconscious is conceptually helpful, Carveth (1995) points out that in their application to the patient's dream and other clinical material, they take for granted the primary process language which Freud (1900) originally elucidated as a feature of the dynamic unconscious. In this and other ways too, self psychology and intersubjectivity draw upon the fundamental insights first presented by Freud.

Stolorow's concept of 'sustained empathic inquiry'

Whereas Kohut wrote of the necessity for 'prolonged empathic immersion' in the patient's subjective world, Stolorow and colleagues prefer the term 'sustained empathic inquiry'. This is defined 'as a method for investigating the principles unconsciously organizing experience' (Stolorow and Atwood, 1992: 33), which they clearly distinguish, as would Kohut, from any attempt to fulfil literally and concretely a patient's selfobject longings.

Whilst the notion of sustained empathic inquiry, which focuses the analyst's attention on the elucidation of the prereflective unconscious principles that organize the patient's subjective world, is clearly felicitous and in line with other contemporary psychoanalytic theoretical and technical positions, such as that of the Sandlers (1997) and Fonagy (1991), some have pointed out that it seems inherently to restrict the scope of empathy. For example, Ornstein (1995) comments that this position appears to differ significantly from Kohut's characterization of empathy as 'the capacity to think and feel oneself into the inner life of another person' (Kohut, 1984: 82). In his commentary on a paper by Trop (1995a) which purports to demonstrate the superiority of intersubject-ivity theory by comparison with self psychology, Ornstein (1995) argues that this new view of empathy as focusing on the patient's organizing principles can lead to an interpretive process that is somewhat different from that advocated by Kohut – one that in some ways seems less empathic.

A discussion between Trop and Ornstein

Trop (1995b), in arguing the case for a post-Kohutian stance of inter-subjectivity, gives an example of witnessing a woman and small child in a pushchair in an elevator. The child looked excited by the changing lights on the display but the mother appeared apprehensive. She said to her daughter, 'Don't worry. The elevator ride will be over in a minute.' The child remained excited and then the mother pushed her back in her seat and repeated that the ride would be over soon. The child became subdued and leaned back with a blank look. When the elevator reached the ground floor, Trop said to the mother that her daughter had actually seemed excited by the lights and not worried. The mother turned away and continued on her way with her daughter.

Trop sees this as an example of unconscious organizing principles. He speculates that if the mother is afraid of elevators she requires her child to share this experience; the child will probably grow up with a fear of elevators but will not recognize that this has arisen on the basis of a message conveyed by her mother.

Ornstein (1995) in his commentary on the account, accepts Trop's description of the incident, but sees his remark to the mother, offering a correction of her distorted perception, as likely to be experienced as intrusive and unwelcome – as evidenced by the mother's turning away. He suggests that if a comment had to be made to the mother, a more genuinely empathic one might have been something like 'You tried to calm your daughter's worries, but it wasn't easy – you both made it down the elevator successfully at the end.' (British readers might find any such comment, Trop's or Ornstein's, culturally alien!) Ornstein speculates that the mother might have smiled in response to this empathic affirmation of her experience and might even have said, 'I don't know which of us was more anxious' – a remark that could have formed the beginning of a reflection on her own anxiety in response to feeling understood.

Ornstein's concern is that if the mother had been a patient in analysis and the elevator experience had been presented then Trop might again have focused his enquiry upon the mother's distortion of her daughter's experience – he wonders how on earth that could be considered an empathic enquiry. Ornstein applies similar criticisms to a longer clinical account in Trop's paper.

In Trop's (1995b) reply to Ornstein's criticism, he reveals an interesting stance. This is what he says:

> My subjective experience was the opposite of what Ornstein recommends be articulated. I did not experience the mother as trying to calm her daughter's worries, but rather as trying to calm herself by using her daughter to provide a twinship experience. My subjective experience was that she was using her daughter, but Ornstein recommends that I not use my subjective experience but rather ignore it. In my opinion, presenting his comments to the mother would serve to reinforce an archaic and embedded meaning pertaining to the mother's own sense of subjective danger.
>
> (1995b: 83)

What is remarkable about this response is how it does indeed reveal an assumption that the analyst knows best and should present his version of reality as a correction to the patient's distorting organizing principles. This is particularly surprising since Trop claims to be drawing directly upon the work of Stolorow and colleagues who give so much emphasis to the importance of avoiding a stance in which the analyst claims to arbitrate concerning the truth. It appears that Ornstein's worries may be warranted – that despite the careful meanings and clinical recommendations of Stolorow and colleagues, their reformulation of empathic inquiry as a focus on discerning the recurrent unconscious organizing principles that shape a patient's subjective experience can lead to a stance which is unempathic by more ordinary criteria.

Intersubjective, relational or intrapsychic psychoanalysis – where do we situate Kohut?

Kohut himself did not consider his self psychology to be a form of relational psychoanalysis. Indeed, as described above, he was concerned to distinguish his empathic-introspective position from that of those analysts and researchers who study the interactions between babies and caregivers or who view the analytic process as interpersonal. The field of study of such investigators he – possibly rather disparagingly – called a form of social psychology. Instead, Kohut wanted to examine empathically the patient's own experience, from the patient's own perspective, in the context of the transference relationship. He would have viewed his stance as one of focusing on the intrapsychic in the context of the self–selfobject relationship.

However, the relational tradition in psychoanalysis (Mitchell and Aron, 1999) – with its roots originally in the interpersonal framework of Sullivan, but now embracing intersubjectivity and a number of other influences, including British object relations theories – has become increasingly sophisticated and subtle in recent years. Consider the following comment by Ghent:

> Relational theories have in common an interest in the intrapsychic as well as interpersonal, but the intrapsychic is seen as constituted largely by the internalization of interpersonal experience mediated by the constraints imposed by biologically organized templates and delimiters. Relational theorists tend also to share a view in which both reality and fantasy, both outer world and inner world, both the interpersonal and the intrapsychic, play immensely important and interactive roles in human life.
>
> (Ghent, 1992: xviii)

Kohut may well have found himself comfortable with the trend described in this quote. After all, it seems clear that Kohut emphasized his empathic-introspective stance because he believed that although Freud's psychoanalysis was essentially based on this observational position, it had not sufficiently and consistently followed the discipline of observing and theorizing in experience-near terms. His concept of the selfobject gave vivid expression to his recognition that the child's and the analysand's subjective experience is profoundly embedded in the responsiveness of the other. He would probably not have disagreed with the aspirations of Stolorow and Atwood, articulated as follows:

> We hope it is clear that we seek not to eliminate psychoanalysis's traditional focus on the intrapsychic, but to *contextualize* the intrapsychic. The problem

with classical theory was not its focus on the intrapsychic, but its inability to recognize that the intrapsychic world, as it forms and evolves within a nexus of living systems, is profoundly context dependent and context sensitive.

(Stolorow and Atwood, 1999: 377)

Radical intersubjectivity

However, Kohut may have parted company with some of the more radical of those who have driven or leapt on the intersubjectivity train. For example, Renik (1993; 1996; 1999), in writing of the 'analyst's irreducible subjectivity', argues that since every person's perception of the other is determined by their own personal emotions and experiences, then it is actually an illusion to suppose that the analyst can accurately or objectively focus on the other's inner reality:

> I would say that it is impossible for an analyst to be in that position even for an instant: since we are constantly acting in the analytic situation on the basis of personal motivations of which we cannot be aware until after the fact, our technique, listening included, is inescapably subjective.
>
> (Renik, 1993: 414)

He sees the claims for analytic neutrality as fundamentally flawed, since countertransference awareness is usually retrospective, following some degree of enactment by the analyst (an assertion which some would find questionable (see Baker, 2000)). In place of the metaphor of the surgeon or the mirror, Renik proposes the metaphor of a skier or surfer, who must allow himself to be pulled this way and that by powerful forces which have to be managed rather than overcome. From this point of view, Renik argues against the emphasis of Kohut, as well as that of Stolorow and colleagues, that the analyst should focus consistently on the patient's vantage point. By drawing out some of the implications of considering the analyst's 'irreducible subjectivity', Renik helpfully focuses attention in a radical way upon questions of truth, subjectivity, objectivity, neutrality, and the aims of analysis.

Renik disagrees explicitly with the position of Schwaber, an analyst who, whilst not directly aligning herself with the self psychologists, has in a remarkably sensitive series of papers described the importance and the difficulty of staying focused empathically on the patient's vantage point (Schwaber, 1981; 1983a; 1983b; 1983c; 1986; 1990; 1992a; 1992b; 1995a; 1995b; 1996a; 1996b; 1997a; 1997b; 1998). Drawing on many clinical illustrations of how she fails fully to appreciate the patient's experience of the analysis but then later manages to grasp this with more accurate empathy, Schwaber speaks to the continual danger of the analyst unwittingly mistaking his or her implicit theories for the objective truth. For example, she comments:

> As clinicians we are enjoined to be agenda-free; we may have our preferred models of the mind, but they are not to be superimposed on the patient's material. Yet often our agendas, which may reflect our values or goals, are unknown to us and can be well rationalized, hidden behind our models of the mind, so as to keep them outside our awareness. We may feel we have no preferred agenda, but the patient may feel we do.
>
> (1990: 237)

However, responding to Grossman's (1996) and Gabbard's (1997) attempt to redress the balance and argue for the importance of the analyst's different, external, or 'objective' point of view, Schwaber adds:

> It is not that the analyst 'goes along' with the patient's view nor simply accepts it as such; rather she uses her own view to enable her to locate the subtleties of the inner logic of the patient's, which have not yet been clear to her. We must surely employ our view, or experience, *even vigorously so*, as an avenue to find the patient's, as long as we acknowledge ours for what it is – how it seems from within our vantage point – and listen with this realization.
>
> (Schwaber, 1997b: 1220)

By contrast, Renik believes the analyst should be free to state his or her own point of view, including self-disclosure, discarding any pretence that the analyst can achieve objectivity. In this way the analytic exploration proceeds through the interaction of the analyst's and patient's point of view. He argues that in place of a concern with 'truth' in an objective sense, the real goal of psychoanalysis should be that of helping the patient to feel better and achieve symptom relief: 'As I see it, in clinical psychoanalysis, as in the rest of science, what is true is what works.' (Renik, 1998: 492).

However, his position regarding objective truth and reality has been criticized on both philosophical and clinical grounds by Cavell (1998a; 1998b), who cautions that 'one slips from the idea that evidence can never be conclusive to the idea that evidence itself is unavailable . . . or from the idea that each of us sees things from his own point of view to the idea that what each of us sees is his own (subjective) point of view' (Cavell 1998a: 1200 – with a reply by Renik, 1999). Moreover, the danger of this point of view – certainly from the perspective of many British analysts – may be that all effort to monitor and contain countertransference could be surrendered. Some may feel that a more balanced position is offered by Carpy (1989), who argues that although complete control of countertransference is neither possible nor desirable, the patient's perception of the analyst's *struggle* to contain and understand evoked feelings has an important therapeutic effect – showing the patient that the analyst is receptive to, and is affected by, his or her communications and yet is willing and able to tolerate these; the patient can then identify with the analyst's capacity to bear painful feelings, which can thereby be given meaning and rendered less toxic – a theory derived from Bion's (1962; 1970) model of the mother's function of containing and thinking about the anxiety and other disturbing feelings projectively evoked in her by her baby.

Baker comments on the implications for psychoanalysis of views such as Renik's:

> I do not doubt that enactments are inevitable. What concerns me is the value currently being attached to their inevitability. The implicit permission for nonrestraint, together with the abandonment of basic concepts such as neutrality, abstinence, and anonymity, is a radical departure from classical psychoanalytic technique as hitherto practiced and understood.
>
> (2000: 150)

Perhaps there is value in the provocations to thought presented by Renik's arguments. However, it is ironic that the concept of intersubjectivity, which in part grew out of the empathic-introspective stance of Kohut, and the highly disciplined attention to the patient's subjective vantage point, should have now become associated with a position that, by emphasizing *inter*subjectivity, appears to promote countertransference enactments and denies the possibility of objective empathy! Perhaps this illustrates the way that any position, if taken to an extreme, may circle back to its opposite, just as the extreme left and right in politics will often resemble each other. The history of psychoanalysis is full of examples of individuals taking one element of theory and giving it undue priority, balance being found again several generations later. Freud's own theorizing was always characterized by balance, such that complexity was not sacrificed for the sake of an easy argument or slogan. Kohut was, I think, of similar mind.

The multiplicity of meanings of 'intersubjectivity'

It will be apparent, even from the range of authors discussed above, that the term 'intersubjectivity' is used in a somewhat confusing variety of ways. No doubt this is because in some way it expresses the concern of many analysts, of diverse schools, to be free of the constraints of a classic Freudian or ego-psychological intrapsychic model of the mind and of psychoanalytic technique – and to embrace a view that takes account of there being two people interacting and influencing one another in the consulting room. An earlier assumption that one person, designated the patient, free-associates, whilst the other, called the analyst, more or less objectively interprets, seems less and less tenable (Goldberg, 1994). Today we are much more aware of systems of interaction. We know that an observer influences what is observed. Moreover, developmental research increasingly tells us that babies are born into a relationship of mutual influence and regulation – and that the 'self' (and indeed the functioning of the brain itself) is relationally constructed.

Some analysts have always intuited these points. An obvious early example was Sandor Ferenczi and his experiments with the healing elements of the relationship – as indicated in his Clinical Diary (1988). The interpersonalists – such as Erich Fromm (1965), Harry Stack Sullivan (1956) and Clara Thompson (1950) – as well as object relations theorists, such as Ronald Fairbairn (1952), Harry Guntrip (1961) and later Otto Kernberg (1976), all gave explicit emphasis to the relational construction of the psyche. Winnicott saw the infant as developing within a facilitating environment of responsive maternal care, and formulated the import-ance of the opportunity to be alone in the presence of the other – the mother or the analyst (Winnicott, 1958). Robert Langs, with his concept of the bipersonal field, has, since the 1970s, argued strongly for the signifi-cance of the analyst's contribution to the patient's presentations of psychopathology in the consulting room (e.g. Langs, 1976). Greenberg and Mitchell (1983) gathered many such strands and identified a variety of relational models in psychoanalysis, which could be contrasted with drive models, as well as those that could be described as mixed. During the 1980s, psychoanalytic theorizing with a strongly feminist perspective began to emerge, developed by women analysts such as Jessica Benjamin (1988; 1990) and Nancy Chodorow (1986). These various tributaries have now become a broad and strong current, especially within North American psychoanalysis – as evidenced by the appearance of a book entitled *Relational Psychoanalysis: The Emergence of a Tradition* (Mitchell and Aron, 1999). Kohut's own contribution during the 1970s can be seen as just one (albeit important) element within this developing tradition – part of his significance being that Kohut was very much part of the mainstream of American psychoanalysis and would not have identified himself as a relational psychoanalyst (Rubovits-Seitz, 1999).

The accommodation of a relational perspective sometimes involves some stretching of concepts. For example, the original theoretical position of Melanie Klein – a profoundly important influence in British psychoanalysis – could not really be described as 'object relations' or 'relational' since it rested upon assumptions of the inherent conflicts between the life and death instincts and saw the personal environment as making only a secondary contribution to evolving psychopathology. It was not until Bion's groundbreaking, and deceptively simple innovation of expanding the concept of projective identification (from its original meaning of an intrapsychic phantasy) to include an interpersonal dimension that the Kleinian tradition was rescued fully from the solipsism of a closed world of instincts, although earlier leads had been offered by Heimann (1950) and Money-Kyrle (1956) in relation to countertransference (Hinshelwood, 1999). Basically, Bion (1962) suggested that projective identification involves more than just a phantasy – of projecting part of the self into the other – but actually has a real effect on the analyst's or mother's psyche, forming a crucial basis for emotional communication. More recently, Steiner (1993), again working within the Kleinian tradition, has distinguished between patient-centred interpretations (focusing on what the patient is doing defensively) and analyst-centred interpretations (focusing on how the analyst is being experienced); the latter allow much more concern with the analyst's contribution to the patient's experience, whereas the former tend to address the patient as if his or her psychopathology were essentially intrapsychically generated. As an example of how far some Kleinian thinking has evolved from the original emphasis upon instinctually driven and bodily-based phantasy, to an interest in a person's need to be understood empathically, consider the following remarks by Brenman Pick, one of the foremost of the London Kleinians:

> If there is a mouth that seeks a breast as an inborn potential, there is, I believe, a psychological equivalent, i.e. a state of mind which seeks another state of mind . . .

> Consider a patient bringing particularly good or particularly bad news; say, the birth of a new baby or a death in the family. Whilst such an event may raise complex issues requiring careful analysis, in the first instance the patient may not want an interpretation, but a response; the sharing of pleasure or of grief. And this may be what the analyst intuitively wishes for too. Unless we can properly acknowledge this in our interpretation, interpretation itself becomes a frozen rejection, or is abandoned and we feel compelled to act non-interpretively and be 'human'.
>
> (1985:157, 160)

Clearly this could be taken as a comment about intersubjectivity – the relationship of two people in the consulting room such that one state of mind seeks another state of mind. The proposed interpretation articulates what the patient is seeking from the analyst – an empathic sharing.

Many concepts originally derived from a purely intrapsychic model come under strain as relational dimensions are embraced. Grotstein (1994a) comments:

> Intersubjectivity has recently become a new flash word for many analysts of different schools for attempting to transcend the limitations of the concept of countertransference, which itself derives from the one-person model.

As a 'flash word', the term 'intersubjectivity' is rich in connotational meaning, to do with the relational, the personal and the systemic aspects of mental life, but it lacks definitional precision. However, we can perhaps identify some of the main ways in which the term is used – as summarized below.

Kohut did not use the term 'intersubjective'. However, he did draw attention to the way in which the mental state of certain kinds of patients is exquisitely responsive to the quality of the analyst's empathic attunement – thus indicating that the patient's mind is not a separate entity but combines with the mind of the analyst, functioning as a selfobject. Atwood and Stolorow took this perspective further, to develop the view that 'psychoanalysis is pictured here as a science of the intersubjective, focused on the interplay between the differently organized subjective worlds of the observer and the observed' (1984: 41–42) and that clinical phenomena cannot properly be understood other than in terms of their intersubjective contexts. They began to explore ways in which the organization of the two subjective worlds, that of the patient *and that of the analyst*, might interact, sometimes contributing to therapeutic impasse – a clinical paradigm which incorporates the idea of countertransference, but embraces much more in terms of the analyst's inevitable contribution to the emerging form and content of the analysis (Stolorow and Atwood, 1997). This point of view would be an example of what Poland (2000) refers to as a 'unified field' version of intersubjectivity. He links this to Heidegger's (1927) view of 'persons as beings-in-the-world, living in an experientially unified universe that does not contain the intervening spaces our dichotomizing minds create' (Poland, 2000: 29), an insight that reveals the inescapable embeddedness of the individual in a systemic context of interacting others. Taking such ideas to an even more radical extreme, Renik gives such emphasis to the 'irreducible subjectivity of the analyst' and of the illusory nature of neutrality that the possibility of objectivity appears obliterated. Yet another meaning of intersubjectivity is given by those such as Beebe and Lachman (1994), Stern (1985) and Benjamin (1990), who refer to developmental aspects of the child's need *for* recognition from the mother and capacity *to* recognize that the mother also is a person with her own mind and experience – a point of view that could also be linked to Fonagy's (1991; Fonagy and Target, 1996a; 1996b) discussions of 'mentalization' and 'theory of mind', the ability to recognize that another person too has a mind like oneself. Indeed the theme of recognition – being recognized or mirrored by the other and finding our self in the other's response (Winnicott, 1967; Kohut, 1971; Benjamin, 1988) is woven as a key thread through much of the recent discourse concerning intersubjectivity. Some related ideas are those of 'witnessing' (Poland, 2000) and 'acknow-ledgment tokens' (the analyst's grunts: Gerhardt and Beyerle, 1997), which refer to the therapeutic task, at times, of simply being empathically alongside the patient, bearing witness to important emotional experience, without the need for interpretation or verbal reflection beyond an encouraging grunt to indicate attention and involvement.

Most of the explicit discussions of intersubjectivity have been North American, but an excellent British contribution, which draws also on European thinkers, such as Derrida and Lacan, is that of Kennedy (1998) who explores the beginnings of a psychoanalytic theory of subject relations. Another interesting approach is that of the Spanish analyst Hugo Bleichmar (2000), who provides an integration of intrapsychic and intersubjective perspectives within a framework of motivational systems.

The dark side of intersubjectivity

On the whole, intersubjectivity – the finding of the self in recognition by and of the other – has tended to be regarded positively, as one of the foundations of healthy development in childhood and in analysis. However, it does have its dark side. The mirror offered by the other, by the family, or by society and culture, may be profoundly alienating. Mirrors can distort and can substitute a false image. This aspect is most explicit in Lacan (1949), but others, including Kohut and Winnicott (1967), have also pointed to ways in which the mother, in her desire for a particular kind of child, or in her depression or preoccupation with a dead child (Kohon, 1999; Lewis, 1979; Lewis and Casement, 1986) may selectively reflect or may impose an image that does not connect with the child's actual inner state. The result may be menacing gaps and blanks in the image of self presented to the child, and the development of an 'alien presence' within the experience of self, destroying its coherence (Fonagy, 1999a).

Summary

Kohut defined the data-gathering field of psychoanalysis as that realm which is open to introspection and empathy. He regarded psychoanalytic understanding as deriving from experience-near empathic observations, combined then with explanation within a more experience-distant formulation. Some analysts (particularly Stolorow and colleagues) have linked Kohut's empathic-introspective stance with the position of 'intersubjectivity', which rests upon the recognition that the analytic field always consists of two human subjects interacting, each bringing their own organizations of experience derived from their personal history. These theorists have objected to some elements of Kohut's framework, such as the notion of 'self' or 'bipolar self' (which they regard as reified), the concept of 'disintegration products' (which they feel denies the motivational meaning of these states), the hypothesis of 'transmuting internalization' (since they consider that healing occurs within the relationship rather than through its disruption), the vestigial drive-like idea of narcissism, and the restriction of the selfobject to the realm of narcissism (since they regard the selfobject as a much broader dimension of experience of others). However, Kohut would have defended his concept of the self on the grounds that it was derived from his empathic-introspective stance. He may also have pointed to aspects of human endeavour, such as the experience of free will and the preservation of ideals, which could not entirely be explained within the framework of intersubjectivity. Stolorow and colleagues have developed some interesting distinctions within the concepts of transference and the unconscious. For them, the transference reflects the patient's assimilation of the analytic relationship into the thematic structures of his or her subjective world (a concept similar to the Sandlers' idea of the present unconscious). They distinguish between the dynamic, prereflective, and unvalidated unconscious. The prereflective unconscious could be seen as containing the implicit memories of early interactions (again like the Sandlers' present unconscious). Recently other theorists have presented a position that could be described as radical intersubjectivity. Renik is one of the foremost advocates of this stance, and argues that analytic neutrality and a search for objective truth are illusory. Some have expressed considerable alarm that this extreme version of intersubjectivity could result in undisciplined self-disclosure, enactment of countertransference, and a general departure from a more traditional analytic stance of restraint. A wide range of positions is encompassed within the trend that has come to be called intersubjectivity.

Chapter 6
Kohut and the internal object

> . . . parental values, after first being half external, finally become fully internalized and form part of the superego. With the passage of time, however, generally over a number of generations, these internalized values may further shift from the superego to the ego: values cease to be values because they are gradually transformed into ego functions.
>
> (Kohut, 1984: 224)

Internalization of function

Kohut wrote much about the selfobject, but did he have anything to say about phenomena corresponding to an internal object – the concept arising from Freud's original writings on identification and the development of the superego, and later elaborated by Melanie Klein, Fairbairn and many others (Hernandez and Lemlij, 1999; Perlow, 1995; Sandler, 1990)? The selfobject is a relation with an other who is experienced functionally as part of the self. It is an experience that is sought and needed by the developing child, and indeed throughout life. Although the selfobject is experienced as part of the self, it does not, by definition, exist within the self; it is not carried around inside the psyche of the individual. Through the process of transmuting internalization, whereby the developing psyche gradually masters innumerable microfailures in the response of the selfobject, the *functions* of the selfobject are gradually internalized, resulting in capacities for self-soothing and the maintenance of ideals, ambitions and goals. This internalization of function does not correspond to an internal object. Kohut is describing more a process of psychological digestion, whereby the experiences with the selfobject are metabolized and made part of the subject's own structure and function:

The 'foreign protein' of the selfobject and of the selfobject's functions, whether in childhood or during analysis, becomes split up after being ingested; its constituents are then reassembled to form the self in accordance with those individual patterns that characterize the growing child's (or analysand's) specific psychic 'protein'.

(1984: 160)

By contrast, an internal object, such as the superego, implies something more like a foreign body that has been incorporated into the mind (Hinshelwood, 1997). Indeed, the superego, by definition, is not part of the ego, but is a separate structure within the mind. Although Kohut did refer to the superego, there is in Kohut's theorizing relatively little relating explicitly to an internal object or to the development of the representational world, as elaborated, for example, by Jacobson (1964) or Kernberg (1976). As Adler (1989) points out, Kohut's emphasis upon the internalization of function has meant that he left the inner world of relationship representations relatively undefined.

Transference of endopsychic structure

Kohut's theorizing was built closely upon that of Freud. The paradigm of conflict, neurosis and transference, for Freud, was the dream. As forbidden infantile wishes pushed against the repression barrier, the ego would react with anxiety. The repressed infantile wishes would be transferred to preconscious day residues. This was the original meaning of the concept of transference (Freud, 1900; Kohut, 1959; Kohut and Seitz, 1963), the passage of repressed impulses across the repression barrier and their attachment to preconscious ideas – the later more commonly used meaning, of the attachment of infantile wishes to the person of the analyst, being one instance of this more general concept. For Freud, the neurosis was essentially an intrapsychic process within one mind, a conflict between different structures of the mind (id, ego, superego). The dream itself epitomizes the one-psyche, solipsistic neurosis; the impulse, anxiety and compromise disguise all take place without any awareness of the presence of any actual other person. Kohut gives the following simple example of the analyst being experienced as a transference figure within the patient's conflict. A patient reports that he had evaded paying a bus fare on the way to the session. He also happens to mention that he 'noticed' the analyst's face seemed unusually stern when he greeted him. Kohut explains that the analyst in this instance has become the carrier of an externalized endopsychic structure, the patient's superego. A conflict that originally was interpersonal (between child and parent) before becoming internalized to form endopsychic structure, becomes re-externalized, as the unconscious superego is transferred to the image of the analyst.

The depersonified superego

Jacobson, whose work within the tradition of American ego psychology would have been well known to Kohut, wrote of the development of the superego, from early precursors to a depersonified structure:

> This is a slow process. It begins with the acceptance of 'sphincter morality'. But only at the end of the oedipal phase have the building up, the integration, and organization of superego identifications proceeded far enough to create firm moral codes. Centred about the incest taboo and the law against patricide, they begin at this stage to become independent of the parents and to displace the conflicts between parents and child onto the inner, mental stage. Then only can we observe a gradual depersonification and abstraction of the ego ideal, combined with the development of consistently demanding, directive, prohibitive, and self-critical superego functions. This is the stage at which the superego comes into existence as a new specific functional system, which replaces – at least partly – castration fear with a new danger signal: with fear of the superego.
>
> (Jacobson, 1964: 119)

From this perspective, the early fantasy precursors of the superego – frightening images of the penis, breast or other images of parts of the body, as described extensively by Melanie Klein – would be distinguished from the superego proper as a depersonified and functional psychical system.

The prestructural psyche

Following this framework which distinguished between the early precursors of the superego and the consolidated superego, as a psychical system, Kohut considered the position of the *prestructural* psyche. This is the mental organization prior to the full psychic structuring resulting from the establishment of the superego. Classical psychoanalysis, especially in the USA, tended to assume that analysis was the appropriate treatment for the neuroses of the structured psyche, but that the 'pre-oedipal' conditions required a modification of analysis. Kohut's writings on narcissistic disturbances were his contribution to showing how prestructural personalities could be helped through psychoanalysis that was not compromised in its basic stance. However, this meant that the differences between the structured and unstructured (or insufficiently structured) psyche needed to be understood and conceptualized. Kohut commented as follows:

> Persistent introspection in the narcissistic disorders and in the borderline states
> . . . leads to the recognition of an unstructured psyche struggling to maintain
> contact with an archaic object or to keep up the tenuous separation from it.
> Here, the analyst is not the screen for the projection of internal structure (trans-
> ference), but the direct continuation of an early reality that was too distant, too
> rejecting, or too unreliable to be transformed into solid psychological struc-
> tures. The analyst is therefore introspectively experienced within the
> framework of an archaic interpersonal relationship. He *is* the old object with
> which the analysand tries to maintain contact, from which he tries to separate
> his own identity, or from which he attempts to derive a modicum of internal
> structure.
>
> (Kohut, 1959: 218–19)

Arguing thus that the pathology of the unstructured psyche involves not
so much conflicts between systems of the mind, but instead expresses the
continuing search for, and fear of, nurturing relationships with others,
Kohut concludes:

> In the analysis of the psychoses and borderline states, however, archaic inter-
> personal conflicts occupy a central position of strategic importance that
> corresponds to the place of the structural conflict in the psychoneuroses.
>
> (1959: 219)

This focus on what he calls here an 'archaic interpersonal conflict' later
evolved into his concept of the selfobject – the experience of an (objectively) interpersonal relationship which (subjectively) is an extension of
self. In such situations, the patient in analysis may not be struggling with
a structural conflict but may be reacting to the analyst as the unreliable
selfobject. Kohut gives the following example:

> A schizophrenic patient . . . arrives at the analytic session in a cold and
> withdrawn state. In a dream of the preceding night he was in a snow-covered
> barren field; a woman offers him her breast, but he discovers that the breast is
> made of rubber. The patient's emotional coldness and his dream are found to
> be a reaction to an apparently minute, but in reality significant, rejection of the
> patient by the analyst.
>
> (1959: 219)

Here the patient has not externalized a systemic conflict, but is metaphor-
ically representing and reacting to the experience of the analyst as the
continuation of a rejecting and non-nurturing object from childhood.

Internalized relationships

In Kohut's emphasis upon what is missing – upon the patient's search for missing psychic structure, and for the selfobject experiences necessary for development – could there have been a danger of losing sight of what is *present* – the pathological structures or internal objects that perpetuate the neurosis and the maladaptive patterns of relationship? Whilst this may be so, the concept of internalized relationships of the past being recreated in the present relationship to the analyst must certainly be *inherent* in any notion of transference. In addition to the preservation of infantile passions, there must be preserved unconsciously an image of the object of those loves and hatreds. Kohut states that insofar as the analyst is a transference figure, then he or she is experienced as 'the carrier of the analysand's unconscious endopsychic structures (unconscious memories)' (1959: 218). Then, in a footnote, Kohut refers to the idea of the *memory trace* as a structural concept. So, is the concept of an unconscious memory the closest Kohut gets to the idea of an internal object? It would appear so.

Referring to the establishment of the transference, Kohut comments: 'once the storm breaks loose, however, the analytic situation has become the traumatic past and the analyst has become the traumatizing selfobject of early life' (1984: 178). Thus he is saying that although the patient is seeking the missing selfobject experiences, and that the analytic process is one of innumerable mournings of the loss of the sought-for selfobject perfection, he or she does retain unconscious memories of the original selfobject failures and deprivations – and that it is these unconscious memories that are transferred (through the repression barrier) to the analyst.

So Kohut wrote of unconscious memories (of a traumatizing object or selfobject) as part of what is transferred across the repression barrier, along with unconscious wishes. By implication there would, in these unconscious transferred structures, be an image of the self, associated with a wish, and an image of the object (parent) to whom the wish is directed. Indeed, Kohut's *Analysis of the Self* was set in a framework of the 'self representation', following the ego psychological framework of theorists such as Hartmann and Jacobson. But would the image of the object itself have any dynamic effect? Would it function like an internal object, a 'person' within the mind? Grotstein (1981) suggests that internal objects, as active entities within the mind, are formed by a process of projective identification whereby a part of the self is projected into an image of the object – thereby imbuing the image with a life of its own. Freud, in his concept of the superego, and Fairbairn (1952) in his concept of internalized objects, outline ways in which the prohibiting or rejecting other is taken into the self through identification with the aggressor, or through identification in response to loss (Freud, 1917).

These are not processes described by Kohut. Whilst he refers to memories of the traumatizing object or selfobject, there is no implication that such memories have a dynamic life. So in what way does Kohut portray the 'self in identification with an object' being turned against the self and giving rise to psychopathology?

Consider the situation represented by Kohut's diagram of the vertical split, on page 185 of *The Analysis of the Self*. Here he portrays the central sector of the personality, comprising a horizontal split (repression barrier), under which there is a pressure of repressed and unfulfilled narcissistic demands, related to the mother's rejection of the child's independent narcissism. On the left of this central sector is pictured a vertically split-off sector, containing openly displayed grandiosity related to the mother's narcissistic use of the child's performance for her own aggrandizement; this sector is also described as containing conscious perverse fantasies or activities. The implication is that the mother has hijacked the child's narcissism, using it for her own ends. Thus the child and later the adult continues to display and perform, as if for the mother. Presumably there is an internal image of a mother who approves of the narcissistic display. The central sector is pictured as containing the child's own narcissism which the mother has *rejected*, precisely because it repre-sents the child's own independent strivings. By implication here there is an image of a mother who disapproves.

Why are the independent narcissistic strivings maintained in a state of repression in the central sector? Kohut describes the major anxieties about revealing the repressed grandiose self as motivated: (1) by the patient's fear that his grandiosity will isolate him and lead to permanent object loss, and (2) by his desire to escape from the discomfort caused by the intrusion of the narcissistic-exhibitionistic libido into the ego where faulty discharge patterns tend initially to produce a mood of uneasy elation alternating with periods of painful self-consciousness, shame tension, and hypochondria (1971: 190-91).

Kohut argues that in the mirror transference the patient mobilizes his or her independent grandiose and exhibitionistic fantasies 'on the basis of hope that the therapist's empathic participation and emotional response will not allow the narcissistic tensions to reach excessively painful or dangerous levels' (1971: 191). Thus the patient hopes that the analytic situation will provide a buffer against psychoeconomic trauma of overstimulation. In addition, the patient 'hopes that his remobilized grandiose fantasies and exhibitionistic demands will not encounter the traumatic lack of approval, echo, or reflection to which they were exposed in childhood . . .' (1971: 191).

It appears, then, that the grandiose self is repressed because of the two anxieties, of psychoeconomic trauma, on the one hand, and of being met with lack of approval or indifference, on the other hand. The second of these is clearly an object-related anxiety, whilst the first is only mediated through a relationship but is not, in itself, a relationship anxiety. In terms of the object relational anxiety, then, there must be an image of a disapproving, rejecting or ignoring mother attached to the wish to display the grandiose-exhibitionistic self.

In neither of these two positions is there anything corresponding to a part of the self, in identification with an object, that has turned against a libidinal or narcissistic need. Instead, narcissistic needs are repressed because of the fear of overstimulation or rejection. This would contrast, for example, with Fairbairn's (1952) object relational account of a rejecting internal object and an antilibidinal ego. Just as there is little corresponding to an internalized object in Kohut's scheme, similarly there is scarcely any description of projective processes.

Kohut's concern to draw attention to the missing psychic structure in narcissistically disordered patients, and their resulting search to internalize this missing structure in micro-increments through the selfobject transference, may indeed have worked to obscure sight of the pathological structures that *are* present. Powell (1995) comments: '. . . self psychological writers seem to have said little about the acquisition of functions that are not self-regulating but self-sabotaging and indeed self-destructive' (p 90). Indeed it must surely be the case that if the need for selfobject responses is so fundamental and paramount, as Kohut argues, then it is to be expected that the early caregivers, who may or may not provide adequate selfobject functions, will be the object of powerful attachments. These attachments will often be to figures who are traumatizing and function as anti-selfobjects. In some way these recurrent pathogenetic interactions must be internalized in the form of representations, patterns or expectations of relationships. Indeed there seems every reason to assume that the phenomena Kohut described will occur alongside those that are conceptualized within the domain of theories of object relations, such as that of Fairbairn (1952). Therefore it must be important for the self psychology theory to be expanded to accommodate internal object relational processes. This point is addressed by Brandchaft, who writes 'Over the past decade I have come to recognize certain problems that call into question important concepts and common practices within self psychology' (1994: 58).

Terror of change – preservation of self

Brandchaft makes the point that Kohut clearly described resistances in analysis based upon a fear of repeating traumatic childhood experiences. He quotes Kohut as outlining the essence of these defensive manoeuvres as follows:

> . . . activities undertaken in the service of psychological survival, that is, as the patient's attempt to save at least that sector of his nuclear self, however small and precariously established . . . that he has been able to construct and maintain despite serious insufficiencies in the development-enhancing matrix of the selfobjects of his childhood.
>
> (Kohut, 1984: 115)

This dread of repeating was seen by Kohut as the most powerful resistance to exploration and resolution of the transference, and also as the source of the most resilient defensive structures designed to ensure psychological survival; for certain kinds of patients, the continuity and integrity of their very self was at stake. It concerns what Kohut called 'the principle of the primacy of self preservation' (1984: 143).

However, Brandchaft argues that 'the analysis of the defense organizations that cluster around the need to protect vulnerable self-structures is an essential but not ultimately conclusive target of the analytic procedure' (1994: 60). He draws attention to another anxiety: 'an even more pervasive fear, one more difficult to identify and engage directly and therapeutically: *a fear not to repeat*, a terror of change' (1994: 59). This is linked to a defensive structure that acts 'as a stubborn resistance to change by dismantling and preventing the consolidation of new structures of experience' (1994: 59). Rather than being evoked by an experience of the analyst as unresponsive or unempathic, it is triggered by perceiving the analyst as a reliable ally in 'sustained empathic enquiry into deepening recesses of the patient's subjective experience' (1994: 59). Brandchaft explains that the anxiety-driven dismantling of progress 'appeared whenever the process of inquiry illuminated and thus threatened some deeply entrenched unconscious principle of organization of experience of the self, a principle in which the essence of an archaic tie to a primary caretaker continued to live on' (1994: 59). This deep resistance to change keeps patients 'imprisoned in gulags of their minds' (1994: 60).

Brandchaft notes that in such cases 'treatment is complicated, for it involves an investigation into and an essential realignment of the ordering principles that shape experience and determine the nature and structure of subjective realities' (1994: 60). Mitchell makes a similar point where he writes: 'Psychopathology, in its infinite variations reflects our unconscious commitment to stasis, to embeddedness in and deep loyalty to the familiar' (1988: 273).

Brandchaft then describes examples of how a patient may experience a recurrent shift in mental state, from a briefly more free and spontaneous position to one of internal restriction and imprisonment. Why should this happen? Brandchaft explains that

> . . . the process by which one way of organizing experience is usurped by another more forceful is an internal and automatic replication of crucial developmental events of the child-caretaker experience. That point at which the shift in feeling state from enthusiasm to malaise occurs continues to mark exactly the great divide of developmental derailment. It reflects the fact that the child's attempts to use his own feelings as central organizers of experience and behaviour were stifled by attitudes and actions of caregivers. The patient cannot exit what has become a closed and noxious system. He remains trapped in the structural remains of an archaic tie.
>
> (1994: 63)

Internal sabotage

One of Brandchaft's examples is a patient called Patrick, seemingly highly successful, both in his marriage and his career, who nevertheless was plagued by feelings of emptiness and depression and a sense of life being joyless. Patrick's father had been a 'self-made man' who had risen from poverty to great wealth through relentless hard work in the business of property development. Devoted to his son, the father attempted to instil in Patrick the same values of hard work and scrupulous attention to detail that he applied to his own affairs. Every day, Patrick was given the task of sweeping up the leaves in the yard of their house; the results would be carefully inspected by the father before the family sat down to their evening meal. As Brandchaft describes: 'His father's reproaches and his own forebodings as neglected leaves were discovered and pointed to, his indolence or fraudulence thus unmasked, remained indelibly seared in Patrick's memory' (1994: 60). Although preoccupied with trying to get Patrick to emulate his own values, interests and ambitions, the father was unable to take an interest in Patrick's own initiatives, such as his achievements in baseball. Moreover, he would be upset when Patrick appeared not to be impressed by his property developments but instead viewed them as garish desecration of the environment.

Later Patrick repeated these patterns in relation to himself: 'In the tight confines of his mind there was no time and no space for the enjoyment of his superbly innovative spirit. He had to concern himself with every detail of any project he undertook, as if it were the lawn that had to be inspected by his father' (1994: 62). Brandchaft reports how Patrick would be filled with dread if he departed in any way from his ritualized existence patterned closely on his father's instructions and demands: 'He was compelled to conclude what his father had always maintained: that his insistence on' choosing his own life for himself and not accepting what his father chose for him was an unarguable demonstration of his stupidity or wilfulness' (1994: 62).

These patterns could be observed in the consulting room. Any transient feelings of hope or well-being would soon disappear in response to a self-disparaging thought: 'Then the space that had been occupied by the feeling of aliveness would be replaced by the more familiar empty malaise and joylessness that had pervaded his childhood' (1994: 62). It emerged that what was observable by the analyst replicated faithfully what took place when Patrick was alone. Brandchaft comments: 'Observing how his mental operations always came to ground zero in this repetitive self-negating process, I got a vivid sense of how like a cell Patrick's mind was. I could observe how each time the cell door opened with a fresh, innovative thought or exuberant feeling it soon clanged shut again' (1994: 62).

Brandchaft explains this process, whereby an original childhood interpersonal situation is continued as an endopsychic pattern, in terms of the existence of two separate sets of organizing principles within Patrick's mind. These two principles, operating from the prereflective unconscious (Atwood and Stolorow, 1984), express incompatible motivations. Crucially, Brandchaft comments that 'the perspective that divests the self of what is exquisitely personal is always preprogrammed to prevail' (1994: 62). The child gives priority to maintaining the tie to the caregiver, even when this conflicts with his or her 'attempts to use his own feelings as central organizers of experience' (1994: 63). This means that in order to preserve the archaic tie, the child must submit to a definition of himself determined by the caregiver; it is this that becomes and remains the dominant organizing principle, conflicting with and displacing the organizing principle based on the child's own feelings.

This, then, is the equivalent of the internal object concept that has evolved from self psychology. It may readily be linked with a definition provided by the Sandlers:

> When psychoanalysts speak of internal figures or internal 'objects', they are employing metaphors to designate hypothetical internal 'structures' – organizations or organized sets of rules – for describing what goes on in the person's inner world.
>
> (1997: 170)

Kohut emphasized the child's selfobject needs, his or her strivings for recognition and for the experience of self as a 'centre of initiative', but this focus on what is *needed* from the other may have eclipsed a view of the way in which the other is taken into the self and acts to sabotage development and autonomy from within – along the lines of Fairbairn's (1952) 'internal saboteur' in the 'closed system run on hate' (Guntrip, 1968). The emphasis on what is *missing*, on *deficit*, important though it is, may need to be balanced by an awareness of the psychopathological structures that are *present*. Nevertheless, Kohut's articulation of the child's selfobject needs has helped clinicians such as Brandchaft to discern how the faulty selfobject responses of caregivers become internalized so that the person's experience of self continues to be derailed – like an internal object that perpetuates distorted and harmful anti-selfobject responses from within. Perhaps such an idea was implicit in Kohut's formulations, such as his idea of the vertically split-off sector that perpetuates overt grandiosity – the narcissism that has been hijacked by the mother for her own aggrandizement – but it was not a concept that he made explicit.

The contemporary 'object relations' view: Fonagy, the Sandlers and the Kleinians

Commenting on current trends and biases within British psychoanalytic practice, Bollas has remarked:

> The stress on the primacy of the here and now as the core of the analysis is, in my view, the most important therapeutic advance in British technique since the discovery in the 1940's and 1950's (Heimann 1956; Racker 1957) of the precise object relational significance of the countertransference. In particular, by understanding the patient's narrative as a metaphor of the patient's ego experience of the analytic object, the clinician was suddenly alive in a field of meaningful plenty . . .
>   Now some thirty years after the diffusion of the idea that narrative material is a continuous extended metaphor of the present experience, it has become absolutely essential (at least in London) when reporting one's clinical work to demonstrate exactly how one has transformed a patient's narrative or behaviour into a here and now transference interpretation. But vital as this clinical stance is, I think it has led to the neglect of another important and previously valued clinical function; the need to collect together the details of a patient's history and to link him to his past in a way that is meaningful.
>
> (Bollas, 1989: 194)

Why has such a technical emphasis on here-and-now interpretation arisen within British psychoanalysis? In part it is because the idea of internalized representations of relations has become so central to contemporary psychoanalysis, perhaps especially in Britain. The analytic setting is seen as a theatre within which the unconscious internal roles and scripts are played out. Whilst the disciplined attention to the here-and-now interaction with the patient is certainly valuable, Bollas, amongst others, feels the approach may become unbalanced.

One influential contribution to this trend has been that of Joseph and Anne-Marie Sandler (e.g. 1984; 1997), who have developed a model of the mind which distinguishes between two forms of unconscious: the past unconscious and the present unconscious. This model, recently strongly advocated also by Fonagy (1999a), has certain theoretical and technical implications, particularly in directing analytic attention primarily to the elucidation of internal models of relationships, as played out in here-and-now interaction in the consulting room – and away from a concern with actual early experience. It is worth considering this model in some detail, as a comparison with Kohut's perspective, since it also links with other contemporary theories (especially those developed from the ideas of Melanie Klein) which give prominence to analysing present object relational conflicts and activities, whilst playing down the significance of more classic Freudian emphases upon overcoming repression, facilitating the development of a transference neurosis, and reconstructing childhood development.

The Sandlers portray the past unconscious as related to Freud's model of the system Unconscious. However, in contrast to Freud's view of this system as containing repressed instinctual wishes, they see the past unconscious as more complex and organized, involving cognitive developments as well as maturations in relationships. They view this unconscious as having evolved within a child who is developing and adapting to a specific environment:

> Above all it is an object-related child, one who has made significant identifications and interactions with significant others that have become internalized, a child with a phantasy life profoundly affected by such structured internal object relationships, including those that have been viewed as interactions with the superego.
>
> (1997: 170)

Crucially, the Sandlers consider that unavailability to conscious recall of the early experiences of life (the past unconscious) is not a consequence of repression – indeed that there is no 'repression barrier' – but is a result of the progressive cognitive development of the child. What might appear to be active repression 'is more appropriately regarded as an area of transition from one qualitatively different area of cognitive organization to another' (1997: 177).

On the other hand, the present unconscious is viewed as similar to Freud's Preconscious system, in that its contents may become conscious. However, its contents are not necessarily freely accessible to consciousness;

they may be subject to censorship before emerging into conscious awareness – rather akin to Freud's idea of the second censorship between the Preconscious and Conscious systems. The Sandlers see this second censorship as being motivated primarily by the need to maintain a sense of safety and to avoid feelings of shame, embarrassment, guilt and humiliation. They refer to 'unconscious phantasy' as a designation for thoughts, wishes, impulses and feeling states within the present unconscious. These phantasies arise in the depth of the present unconscious, but not in the depths of the past unconscious.

The Sandlers perceive the relationship between the past unconscious and the present unconscious as one in which the former provides the dynamic templates, or sets of procedures, or rules for functioning (particularly relating to interactions with others), for the present unconscious – these are perhaps the internalized object relations (and may be compared to the 'prereflective unconscious' of Stolorow and Atwood, 1992). A crucial point is that, in this model, the impulse, wish or memory that arises in the depths of the present unconscious is not one that has passed in a disguised form through a repression barrier. Instead, the censoring and defensive transformation takes place entirely within the present unconscious prior to admission to conscious awareness. Moreover, although the unconscious wish, arising within the present unconscious, may be modelled on the inner child's wishes (in accord with the past unconscious), the objects of the wish are those of the present. The Sandlers state this quite strongly as follows:

> . . . the conscious or unconscious transference wish (which may involve unconscious attempts to get the analyst – or indeed any other person – to play a particular role) is not a *transferring* from parent to analyst, but rather an attempted interaction with the analyst (in phantasy or in reality), which functions in the present according to rules set down in the patient's early years.
>
> (1997: 176)

In this model, the individual is seen as responding to the environment partly in terms of unconscious wishes and fears (in the present unconscious), given form by the past unconscious. Insofar as these responses are felt to be inappropriate or threatening to the person's equilibrium, they will be defended against, censored, and allowed to conscious experience only in a modified form created by any of the well-known mechanisms of defence.

The clear implication of the Sandlers' model is that the content of the past unconscious is inherently not available to consciousness. It exerts its influence not by emerging in disguised form through a repression barrier, but by determining the dynamic templates of the present unconscious.

Another implication is that the traditional view of transference, as a transference of past to present, is to be abandoned and replaced by the idea of the externalization, in the interaction with the analyst, of the internal patterns of relationship. What does this mean for clinical practice? Fonagy and Cooper (1999) elucidate the technical implications as follows:

> . . . interpretation of the transference should be as close as possible to the current central conflict and to the patient's immediate resistance. The present should always be interpreted before the past; if the latter is brought into the foreground, it should be done only in order to throw light on what is occurring currently.
>   Within this framework, the analyst and patient are seen as jointly creating an extended model of the patient's self and world.
>
> (1999: 19)

And how does analysis help the patient to change, according to this model? Fonagy states the process simply as follows: 'Therapeutic action lies in the conscious elaboration of preconscious relationship representations, principally through the analyst's attention to the transference' (1999b: 218). A profound shift of emphasis is hidden here in the Sandlers' model. Fonagy takes its ramifications to their logical extreme where he states:

> The removal of repression is no longer to be considered a key to therapeutic action. Psychic change is a function of a shift of emphasis between different mental models of object relationships . . . Psychoanalysis . . . is the creation of a new way of experiencing self with other.
>
> (1999b: 218)

Thus, as Fonagy's conclusions indicate, the past unconscious, consisting of the actual experiences, conflicts and development of the child, plays little part in the work of analysis in practice, according to this model.[1]

Fonagy sees the internal models of relationships as procedural or *implicit* memories (Clyman, 1996; Mollon, 1998), based on repeated interactions during childhood. He states:

> . . . what lies at the root of interpersonal problems, the transference relationship and quite possibly all aspects of the personality which we loosely denote with the term unconscious, is a set of procedures or implicit memories

---

[1.] Goldberg (2000) argues that Fonagy's position appears to privilege 'experience' in the psychoanalytic cure, contrasting this with Kohut's view that cure came about through interpretation of the selfobject transferences.

> of interactional experience . . . Individual experiences which have contributed to this model may or may not be 'stored' elsewhere, but in either case the model is now 'autonomous', no longer dependent on the experiences which have contributed to it. The models exist non-consciously as procedures which organize interpersonal behaviour but are not consciously accessible to the individual unless attention is directed to them. The models are not replicas of actual experience but are undoubtedly defensively distorted by wishes and fantasies current at the time of the experience. Thus in no sense can they be thought of as bearing testament to historical truth.
>
> (Fonagy, 1999a)

In contrast to Modell (1999), for example, who regrets the current tendency amongst some psychoanalysts to deprecate reconstruction, and who sees the persisting implicit memories of early experience in the 'dead mother syndrome' as offering support for the value and validity of such work, Fonagy sees reconstruction and concern with early experience as misguided. In his recent discussions of the therapeutic process (1999a; 1999b), it is apparent that he views declarative autobiographical memory, recovered memory, the reliving and working through of childhood trauma, and the analytic reconstruction of childhood development, as all essentially irrelevant to therapeutic change, as well as highly suspect with regard to the fidelity of their correspondence with childhood experience. Emerging memories are seen as 'of great significance, not as explanations for current patterns but as material that serves to enlighten us further about the nature of the transference relationship' (Fonagy, 2000: 169). Thus, in this view, what really matters in psychoanalytic work is simply the exploration and modification of the internal models of relationship through clarifying and reworking these in the 'transference'.

Transference as externalization of the internal world

The technical stance is similar for contemporary Kleinian analysts (e.g. Spillius and Feldman, 1989), although the theoretical basis is somewhat different. If the Kleinian theory were superimposed on the Sandler–Fonagy model, the present unconscious would be viewed as structured not so much by early interactions with caregivers, but by the predominant unconscious phantasies (driven ultimately by the innate conflict between life and death instincts). The Kleinian approach is also distinguished by the way in which the analyst will tend to interpret to the patient as if the child parts of the mind, and the infantile conflicts and phantasies, are immediately and continuously alive in the present unconscious. It is as if the Kleinian analyst would see no discontinuity between the child and adult mind.[2] The relationship to the analyst is viewed as unconsciously the continuation of the infant's relationship to the mother – although, as Spillius (1988a) points out, there has over the years been a lessening of the tendency to interpret in very concrete bodily imagery, such as breast, penis, urine and faeces. As in the Sandler–Fonagy model, the Kleinians appear to make little use of concepts of repression, regression, or the transference neurosis. For the Kleinians, the transference is not the reviving of conflicts and aspirations of the childhood past, but is the externalization of the internal world. Spillius states this clearly:

> The concept [of transference] is not restricted to the expression in the session towards the analyst of attitudes towards specific persons and/or incidents of the historical past. Rather the term is used to mean the expression in the analytic situation of the forces and relationships of the internal world.
>
> (1988a: 6)

Thus for the Kleinians, just as for those embracing the Sandler–Fonagy position, the 'transference' is the expression or enactment in the consulting room of the internal patterns of relationship. The Freudian concept of transference, as outlined in the following quote from Anna Freud, is thoroughly, albeit subtly, eclipsed:

> By transference we mean all those impulses experienced by the patient in his relation with the analyst which are not newly created by the objective situation but have their source in early – indeed the very earliest – object relations and are now merely revived under the influence of the repetition compulsion . . . The patient finds himself disturbed in his relation to the analyst by passionate emotions . . . which do not seem to be justified by the facts of the actual situation. The patient himself resists these emotions and feels ashamed . . . Often it is only by insisting on the fundamental rule of analysis that we succeed in forcing a passage for them to conscious expression . . . They have their source in old affective constellations . . . and become comprehensible and indeed are justified if we disengage them from the analytic situation and insert them into some infantile affective situation.
>
> (Anna Freud, 1937: 18–19)

Whilst for the classical analysts, the transference was *gradually* uncovered and then placed in its historical childhood context – being

---

[2.] Malcolm (1986), whilst emphasizing the way in which the past is alive in the present of the transference, does see value in linking interpretations of the here-and-now with the past. These links, she feels, help to enhance the patient's sense of the continuity of his or her life.

seen as inappropriate to the present – the Kleinians and followers of the Sandler–Fonagy position regard the transference as always existing in the here-and-now interaction of the consulting room. It follows quite logically and starkly from this that any focus on understanding childhood experience will be seen as likely to involve a collusive escape from the more affectively charged transference in the present. This is indeed the view that analysts influenced either by the Kleinians or by the Sandler–Fonagy position do advocate.

The selfobject transference from Kohut's perspective

How does this contrast with Kohut's theory? The division between past and present unconscious does not sit easily with the kind of phenomena Kohut describes. He sees a continuity between the selfobject strivings of infancy and those that are released in the adult by the process of analysis. Crucially, for Kohut, it is not the elucidation of patterns of internalized object relationships that is the vehicle of analysis. Rather, it is the renewing of the search for structure-building experiences in the selfobject transference. Although this renewed structure-building does depend absolutely on the relationship with the selfobject analyst, it is not solely a matter of modifying internal object relations. Whilst the cure does depend upon insight, the essential process is one of transmuting internalization. Bringing internalized relationships to the light of consciousness and permitting new forms of relating to evolve, as indicated by the Sandler–Fonagy model, is not the most crucial task of analysis according to Kohut. However, the exploration of the analysand's childhood history *is* seen by Kohut as an important aspect of the therapeutic work because this can enhance the patient's empathy for his or her own experience. By contrast, as we have seen, consideration of childhood within the Sandler–Fonagy framework is relevant only insofar as it illuminates current internal structures of relationships. Fonagy states:

> If we are serious about object-relations theory and consider these relations as psychic structures organizing behaviour, then it is these structures, and not the events that might have contributed to them, that need to be the focus of psychoanalytic work.
>
> (1999a: 220)

Whilst the Sandlers argue that the conflictual feelings and impulses that emerge in relation to the analyst have not passed through a repression barrier (but have arisen and been transformed within the present unconscious), Kohut believed that the narcissistic strivings expressed in the selfobject transferences have done exactly that. Kohut described the grandiose self as having undergone repression in the case of narcissistic disorders; it has undergone repression because of fears of again encountering rejection or indifference, or fears of being psychoeconomically overwhelmed. During analysis, as the selfobject transference is established, the grandiose self begins to emerge from repression.

Kohut describes very clearly in his explanation of the diagram portraying the horizontal and vertical splits (1971: 185) that the analytic work first increases the pressure of the narcissistic energies against the repression barrier, and then undoes the repression barrier itself. As the narcissistic needs and energies are released through the selfobject transference, they undergo transmuting internalization (as a result of the nontraumatic encounters with the failings and imperfections of the analyst), leading to the establishment of psychic structure (internalization of function). This involves not the exploration of 'new ways of experiencing self with other', as in the Sandler–Fonagy model, but instead requires a freeing of the archaic selfobject needs, a regression in the selfobject transference, and the building of psychic structure – i.e. the establishment of inner capacities for regulating mental states which derive from, but are essentially different from, modes of relationship with others.

The process outlined by Kohut, of benign regression and spontaneous re-engagement with aborted developmental initiatives, is similar to modes of psychoanalytic action described some decades ago by analysts in Britain, such as Balint (1968), Stewart (1989), and Winnicott (1960). Such perspectives on regression are lost in the current trend, driven both by the Kleinian tradition and the Sandler–Fonagy model, to focus on the elucidation only of here-and-now relationship conflicts. (Representing a more classical position, Arthur Couch, in a personal communication, has described this humorously as a 'here-and-now-itis' that has infected the British Psychoanalytical Society.)

Kohut, Klein and Bion: idealization, splitting and projective identification

Idealization was considered by Kohut to be part of the normal line of development of narcissism. In Britain, the notion of idealization has been associated most strongly with the theories of Melanie Klein, whose developmental framework was very different. Are there points of contact, as well as major areas of difference, between these two approaches?

Klein (1946) described idealization, not in the context of narcissism, but as part of an early defensive splitting and idealization in which, in an effort to deal with overwhelming instinctual forces of life and death, good and bad aspects and experiences of the object are in phantasy kept apart. An idealized object is sought to protect against a persecutory one. Kohut does not explicitly distinguish narcissistic idealization from idealization that is a function of splitting of good and bad perceptions of the object. Is what he describes entirely unrelated to the idealizations outlined by Klein? One clue is provided by Gedo (1981) who, drawing upon Kohut, distinguishes true idealization from pseudo-idealization – the latter seeming more obtrusive, insistent or 'noisy', perhaps being a response to the breakdown of true idealization. What Kohut seems to envisage is an initial quiet idealization, which in healthy development is optimally disrupted. Gedo remarks:

> . . . typically the omnipotent other is a symbiotic object whose availability and perfection are therefore taken for granted. This is why an idealizing trans-ference tends to be silent: insofar as it becomes explicit, it will have an impersonal quality.
>
> (1981: 127)

Thus the idealization may focus on the functional capacities of the object rather than the person per se. In the idealizing transference it may be the process or technique of analysis that is idealized. This point bears some similarity to Winnicott's (1963) notion of the 'environment mother', denoting the mother's functions as distinct from the person of the mother.

The gradual disruption of the idealizing selfobject relationship in normal development has perhaps some connection with Klein's depressive position – the stage of lessening projection, splitting and idealization in which the infant feels more separate and has a more integrated and realistic perception of its objects. According to Kohut, if the disruption is traumatic, a state of fragmentation occurs – a regression to the fragmented body imago, brooding hypochondria and emergence of archaic forms of narcissism, such as primitive grandiosity and phantasies of omnipotent objects. This may bear some relation to the splitting and fragmentation described by Klein. One difference is that Klein sees the splitting as an active defensive process, whereas Kohut sees fragmentation as a helpless falling in response to selfobject failure.

For Klein, a further aspect of the early constellation of defences is projective identification, a phantasy in which part of the self is placed in the object which is then identified with that part. This description is somewhat similar to Kohut's focus on the relation to the idealized selfobject, whereby an idealization is invested in the object with whom the subject then feels partially merged. In the negotiation of the depressive position, according to Klein, splitting is reduced. However, if development goes awry, splitting may be maintained or exacerbated and processes of projective identification are intensified. The fostering of projective identification perhaps corresponds to what Kohut has described as the increased efforts to recover the selfobject following disruption of the relation.

There are important differences of emphasis between Klein and Kohut. Grotstein (1983) points out that in the concept of the depressive position, involving the infant's concern for the attacked mother, Klein is emphasizing the infant's empathy for the mother and gives responsibility to the infant for breaks in bonding through the infant's attacks. Kohut clearly emphasizes the reverse of this. Moreover, Kohut focuses on the realities of selfobject failure rather than upon phantasies about the object. Kohut does not make use of the concept of unconscious phantasy. Nor, as we have seen, does he emphasize the formation of internal objects of a destructive and malevolent nature, of the kind outlined by Klein as developing from the infant's own 'death instinct'. Kohut's 'transmuting internalization' is the gradual microinternalization of the object's functions in response to innumerable 'microtraumas'. Goldberg (1983) distinguishes this from the massive internalization consequent on traumatic disruptions of selfobject relations. This massive internalization would give rise to an internal object. Selfobjects are not the same as internal objects – by their nature they exist in a transitional area between self and object.

Finally, Kleinian theory remained essentially a psychology of drive conflict, resting fundamentally upon the notion of innate conflict between life and death instincts – although Bion and others have developed the interactional and intersubjective potential of the Kleinian perspective. By contrast, Kohut's theory saw drive conflict as secondary to deficiency in early selfobject responses.

Kohut and Bion: empathy and projective identification

Although superficially very dissimilar, there are some surprising links between the views of Kohut and Bion. Like Kohut, Bion lays stress on the early caregiver's empathy and responsiveness. However, whilst Kohut's concept of mirroring is modelled on the parents' admiring response to the exhibitionistic child – 'After psychological separation has taken place, the child needs *the gleam in the mother's eye* in order to maintain the narcissistic libidinal suffusions . . .' (1966: 439, italics added) – Bion emphasizes the parental response to the infant's anxiety. Thus, Bion (1962) describes the situation of an infant giving expression to its distress, perhaps through crying; at this stage, the infant's behaviour is not an intentional communication – if there is mental content to it, this may simply be a phantasy of getting rid of something bad inside; however, the mother applies her thoughts – her 'alpha function' – to the baby's action and attempts to respond in a way that alleviates the distress. Through the application of the mother's thought, the baby's projective identification is returned in a modified form. In this way, Bion regards projective identification as not merely a phantasy but as an interactional activity that forms the basis of thinking and communicating (see also Grotstein, 1994b; 1995). It is clear that Bion is not talking here about the mother as a love object but is outlining some of the mother's *functions* that are required to support the infant's developing psyche – in Kohut's terms, he is describing a selfobject.

Like Kohut, Bion also describes selfobject failures of empathy and emotional responsiveness. The mother's failure to receive, think about and *detoxify* the infant's emotion – perhaps adding to it her own anxiety – results in the infant being left not with meaningful communi-cation but with 'nameless dread' (Bion, 1962). In his two papers, 'On arrogance' (1967) and 'Attacks on linking' (1959), Bion describes the internalization of an object felt to be hostile to emotional communi-cation – an internal object that attacks emotional links. Perhaps the resulting state of mind has something in common with the fragmen-tation that Kohut describes as following selfobject failures. Similarly, the state of 'nameless dread' may be the brooding hypochondria described by Kohut.

Kohut and Bion draw attention to different aspects of the required selfobject responsiveness. Although Kohut's concept of mirroring seems to rest upon the model of the exhibitionistic child and the admiring parent, it is clear from some of his writings that he is referring also to a general empathic responsiveness. Is Kohut's empathy the same as what Bion has described in terms of projective identification as communi-cation? Empathy suggests a 'feeling into' another person's experience. On the other hand, Bion's model of projective identification suggests a 'being responsive' to evocative emotional communications. 'Feeling into' and 'being responsive to' seem to be different but overlapping compon-ents of the process of early communication.

Just as Kohut and Bion are both concerned with the mother's respon-siveness to the child, so they are both interested in how the analyst listens to the patient. Bion's (1970) admonition to listen without the desire to make premature sense, to be without a 'saturated' mind, is well known. Kohut often advocates a similar attitude. For example he remarks:

> Nothing interferes more dramatically with acquiring a deep understanding of the patient than premature closure. If you think you know, then you cut yourself off from taking in more and more details with that pleasurable expectant puzzlement, until finally you see a totally unexpected configuration.
>
> (1985b: 267)

Summary

Kohut did not explicitly describe 'internal objects', apart from references to the superego. His emphasis was upon the internalization of function (which he termed 'structure') through transmuting internalization. Kohut referred to the 'prestructural' psyche, by which he meant the mind before the establishment of the superego; pathology deriving from this stage would reflect not so much intersystemic conflict, but the continuing search for nurturing selfobject relationships that would supply missing functions. However, internalized representations of relationships are *implied* in Kohut's accounts. Although Kohut's emphasis was upon structures that are missing, others working in Kohut's tradition have focused upon understanding the pathological structures that are present. Some of these structures may be compared with Fairbairn's 'internal saboteur'. A contrasting position is presented by the contemporary 'object relations' models of Fonagy/Sandlers and the London Kleinians. The Sandlers distinguish between the past unconscious (of the original child) and the present unconscious. It is the latter that is the focus of analytic attention in the consulting room. Fonagy has emphasized how this leads to an emphasis upon analysing the internal models of relationship, as these are manifest in the transference, so that the patient can develop new ways of experiencing self with other. In various ways this involves a modification of classical views of transference. Some analysts regret the implicit depre-cation of analytic reconstruction that follows from this stance, which is also apparent in the position of contemporary Kleinians. By contrast, Kohut saw the work of analysis not as lying crucially in the elucidation of internal models of relationship, but, rather, in the spontaneous re-engagement with the search for structure-building experiences leading to a strengthened capacity to regulate mental states. The vehicle of this re-engagement with thwarted developmental initiatives remains essentially interpretation of the transference, but also involves analytic recon-struction of early development.

Klein and Kohut both wrote about idealization as a normal feature of early development. Their metapsychological frameworks were very different, however. Klein's idealization arose from splitting into good and bad, driven by the conflict between life and death instincts. Kohut's idealization was part of the line of development of narcissism. The gradual surrender of idealization, through titrated disillusionment, giving rise to transmuting internalization, could be compared to Klein's notions of the giving up of illusions of omnipotence in the context of the depressive position. Kohut and Klein both envisaged early states of fragmentation, but Kohut saw these as occurring through lack of selfobject support, whereas Klein interpreted in terms of active destruction of aspects of the ego for defensive purposes. Kohut's focus on empathy and Bion's emphasis on the mother/analyst's receptive reverie are similar, albeit with subtle differences.

Chapter 7
Impasse and Oedipus: contrasting perspectives

I take the desire to be understood as rock bottom in the human mind. It is a desire so profound that I suspect, when offered counterfeit understanding, children try hard, though they know it is not the genuine article, to think that it is.

(Marcia Cavell, 2000: 51)

The psychoanalytic context against which Kohut was writing – classical American ego psychology – was one in which the oedipus complex was seen, almost by definition, as the core area of conflict determining the patient's psychopathology. Kohut questioned the primacy of the oedipus complex, suggesting that what may appear to be intense conflicts over possession and rivalry in relation to the parental couple might actually be a response to a more hidden deprivation of selfobject needs – such as to be soothed, to be related to with empathy, to feel loved and cared about and thought about. More specifically, Kohut distinguished between a normal oedipal phase of development – a step forward in development accompanied by exhilaration 'responding to a new set of experiences, however hazy it might be, characterized by a qualitatively altered and intensified affectionateness and assertiveness' (1984: 23) – and a pathological oedipus complex. The latter arises when the child's 'affection and assertiveness do not elicit the parents' proud mirroring responses (and various other empathically affirmative reactions) but eventuate instead in the parents' (preconscious) stimulation and (preconscious) hostile competitiveness' (1984: 24). Kohut notes that such parental responses may be expressed overtly, through actively rejecting and prohibiting reactions, or covertly, through withdrawal. The result is that 'the child's self becomes fragmented, weakened, and disharmonious and his normal nonsexual affection and normal nonhostile, nondestructive assertiveness becomes grossly sexual and hostile' (1984: 24). In part, Kohut saw this intensification of sexual and aggressive aims as the child's attempt to organize the fragments of the self – perhaps rather like the way that a person who has felt traumatized and shattered by a damaging event or devastating loss may temporarily derive a feeling of being held together through engaging in a fight and through generating strong feelings of one kind or another.

A deeper dread than castration

Kohut describes the primary fears of the oedipal child, not as those of castration anxiety, but of being confronted by a 'sexually seductive rather than affection-accepting' opposite-sex parent, and 'a competitive-hostile rather than pridefully pleased' same-sex parent (1984: 24). The boy's fear of castration and the little girl's conviction of having been castrated are then seen as symbolizations of deeper dreads, less easily represented than the idea of loss of a body part (similar ideas are expressed by Green, 1983). Kohut notes that 'the girl's rejection of her femininity, her feeling of being castrated and inferior, and her intense wish for a penis arise not because the male sex organs are psychobiologically more desirable that the female ones, but because the little girl's selfobjects failed to respond to her with appropriate mirroring, since either no idealizable female parental imago was available to her, or that no alter ego gave her support during the childhood years when a proud feminine self should have established itself' (1984: 21). In the case of the boy – 'the little boy's manifest horror at the sight of the female genitals is not the deepest layer of this experience but . . . behind it and covered by it lies a deeper and even more dreadful experience – the experience of the faceless mother, that is, the mother whose face does not light up at the sight of her child' (1984: 21). (This could also be compared with André Green's theme of blank experience and the 'dead mother': Kohon, 1999.)

Thus Kohut saw the pathological oedipus complex as an outcome of the failure of the background selfobject matrix of the parents to respond with empathy and pride to the child's emerging affection and assertiveness. The child's 'self' is not sustained and the result is the fragmentation into sexual and aggressive drive states. Kohut saw the results as far-reaching:

> Instead of the further development of a firmly cohesive self able to feel the glow of healthy pleasure in its affectionate and phase-appropriate sexual functioning and able to employ self-confident assertiveness in the pursuit of goals, we find throughout life a continuing propensity to experience the fragments of love (sexual fantasies) rather than love and the fragments of assertiveness (hostile fantasies) rather than assertiveness and to respond to these experiences – which always include the revival of the unhealthy selfobject experiences of childhood – with anxiety.
>
> (1984: 25)

In place of the traditional emphasis upon the oedipal child's hatred of the parental coupling, and the associated feelings of exclusion, Kohut drew attention to the effect on the child of an *absence* of an atmosphere of parental sexuality. At several points he referred to the deleterious effects of growing up in the care of grandparents who did not present the stimulation of a background of sexuality:

> The child wants to intrude into the bedroom of the parents. The doors are closed. He feels deeply rejected. That is all true. That is the tragedy of healthy pathology, and we must deal with it when it has pathological consequences. But to grow up in a family in which there are no closed doors and no sex behind doors, a family in which there are old grandparents walking around, thinking about how many more years they have to live – that is really a different atmosphere.
>
> (1996: 265)

His point was that although a family atmosphere of overstimulation, where the child is exposed to intense emotional conflicts, of rivalry and jealousy, that he or she is not able to handle, can certainly lead to disturbances of development, there is also a pathology that results from an emotionally empty family. He comments:

> . . . it is a very different pathology that a child experiences with enervated elderly parents, with parents who behave bizarrely, with parents who do not have the capacity to relate to each other or to their children, with parents who have children in order to conform to some external schema of what society demands of them, or with parents who want to solve some deep personality conflicts by having children and who then find out that they have placed more of a burden on themselves and given themselves more tasks than they can solve. It is in these families that children say, 'What kind of world is this? Here I am proudly exhibiting myself, and there is only silence.'
>
> (1996: 265–66)

Kohut was aware that his revision of emphasis in relation to the oedipus complex would evoke scepticism and criticism – and especially that he might be considered to be overlooking the conflicts stemming from a child's own desires and fantasies, and instead locating the responsibility entirely with the parents. His clearest answer to such criticisms is to be found in the following passage:

> Am I putting all the blame for a person's later psychopathology and character-ological shortcomings on his parents? Am I taking him off the hook, so to say, and in particular, am I the credulous victim of those of my patients who do not want to shoulder the responsibility for their symptoms, actions, and attitudes but waste their time accusing others, including and par excellence their parents? No I do not believe I have committed any of these errors, and I am not

simply falling in with the accusations my analysands may level against their parents even though I may listen to them respectfully for a long time without contradicting them. First and most important: the self psychologically informed psychoanalyst blames no one, neither the patient nor his parents. He identifies causal sequences, he shows the patient that his feelings and reactions are explained by his experiences in early life, and he points out that, ultimately, his parents are not to blame since they were what they were because of the backgrounds that determined their own personalities . . . It follows that at the appropriate point (usually late) in the analysis, he will demonstrate to the analysand (if, indeed, the analysand has not come to this conclusion on his own) that when the oedipal self began to crumble and lust and destructiveness began to rise in consequence of the fragmentation of the oedipal self, the analysand's perception, too began to be impaired. Thus, in response to not being experienced in toto by the parents, who saw not the child but his 'drives', the analysand, too, may have seen the parents as less human and whole than they were. As a result, he may have experienced them as seductive or hostile-competitive at times when, indeed, they had acted with warmth and tried to offer empathic parental responses to their child.

(1984: 25)

Thus it can be seen that Kohut continued to see the oedipal situation as important, but he viewed its pathology as secondary to a defective selfobject environment. He postulated that in a healthy selfobject environment, the child would be able to cope with his or her oedipal strivings and anxieties. These oedipal strivings, of increased affection and assertiveness and competitiveness, would be welcomed by the parents as indications of the child's development. They would be greeted with acceptance, but without sexual overstimulation or exaggerated hostile prohibition. The parents would not be anxious about their child's oedipal strivings and the child would feel it was safe to be affectionate, assertive and competitive. Because the selfobject environment would remain supportive and benign, the child's frustration and aggression would not be provoked to unmanageable levels, and so his or her perceptions of the parents would not be unduly distorted by projections in fantasy of the child's own impulses and emotions. In contrast to most other theorists, Kohut drew attention to the effect on a child where the home atmosphere is characterized by an absence of parental liveliness and sexuality.

Comparison with a British Kleinian approach

Could Kohut's perspective illuminate the work of other clinicians who take a different view of the oedipus complex? Obviously, any clinical material is open to a variety of interpretations according to the theoretical and personal vantage point of the particular clinician. However, differences in clinical perspective may be usefully illustrated by taking material presented as representative of a particular school and considering what questions and formulations might arise when it is looked at from a position that emphasizes the attempt to identify empathically the patient's vantage point.

For this purpose, a paper by the respected London Kleinian psychoanalyst, Michael Feldman, is considered. It is titled 'The centrality of the oedipus complex' (Feldman, 1992) and is found, appropriately enough, in a collection of several authors' work, *The Common Ground of Psychoanalysis* (Wallerstein, 1992). In addition to its interest as a representative example of the Kleinian school, the paper is of particular relevance because it appears to portray a childhood situation that corresponds to the cases of emotional emptiness and absence of parental sexuality that Kohut described.

The theoretical emphasis in the Kleinian approach tends to be upon the elucidation of complex processes of projection and introjection in the infantile parts of the patient's mind (involving the interweaving of perception and phantasy), as he or she struggles with the development from the paranoid-schizoid to the depressive position; the technical emphasis is upon the detailed analysis of these processes as they are played out in the here-and-now of the transference. Whilst it was Freud (1920) who first wrote of the death instinct and forces within the mind which oppose development, it has tended to be those analysts working in the Kleinian tradition who have emphasized such factors most.

The juxtaposition of Feldman's account alongside a self psychological perspective is intended to illustrate alternative perspectives rather than to imply that one is more 'correct' than the other. Whilst the perception from a self psychological perspective might reveal the patient's struggles to maintain a selfobject attachment, from a Kleinian perspective the Kohutian position may tend to appear lacking in a full appreciation of destructiveness and malignant anti-developmental states of mind (as described, for example, by Joseph, 1982; Rosenfeld, 1971; Steiner, 1993). Although it makes little sense to argue that one perspective is more 'true' than the other, the examination of material from different points of view can perhaps lead to a more multifaceted appreciation of mental life. (A thoughtful discussion of the contemporary Kleinian approach from the relational and intersubjective point of view is provided by Mitchell, 1997b.)

Feldman's paper on the centrality of the oedipus complex[1, 2]

Feldman begins his paper with a quote from Freud (a footnote to the Three Essays on Sexuality, added in 1920) in which he states that the

---

[1] I am grateful to Dr Feldman for helpful comments on an earlier draft of this discussion.
[2] The author's commentary is set within square brackets.

oedipus complex is the 'nuclear complex' of the neuroses. Feldman then adds:

> We have indeed come to share an understanding that the pattern of introjections and identifications based on oedipal fantasies constitutes a crucial element in the development of the personality and in the manifestations of pathology.
>
> (1992: 171)

Thus, Feldman states his belief that oedipal fantasies are a crucial element in psychopathology. He goes on to say that he and other Kleinian analysts recognize earlier and more primitive versions of oedipal fantasies, in which the parental objects are represented in a damaged and threatening state and are often not clearly differentiated from one another. The patient's negotiation of the conflicts and anxieties associated with these fantasies is considered to have a crucial bearing on his or her capacity to recognize and integrate emotions and tolerate mental pain and also in the capacity to think.

[It is apparent from this that Feldman and other Kleinians are using the term 'oedipal' to refer to any aspect of the child's relationship to the parents as a couple. This of course is different from the classical concept of the oedipus complex, in which the child wishes to have exclusive possession of one parent and to eliminate the other who is perceived as a rival, this giving rise to fears of retaliation from the rival. Thus the Kleinian usage seems to be looser.

The self psychology perspective on the oedipus complex, as argued by Kohut, is that where there is adequate selfobject responsiveness in the child's milieu, the conflicts of this stage do not lead to pathology. However, it is postulated that if the early environment is not sufficiently empathically responsive, then there may be a pathological intensification of the oedipus complex, with sexuality and aggression of a more raw and unneutralized quality. Thus for Kohut it was not the oedipus complex itself that caused a problem for the child, but the flawed responses of the child's caregivers that gave rise to a pathologically intensified oedipus complex.]

Feldman presents clinical material from a period six months before the end of a long analysis of a single woman in her mid-40s. She sought help because of recurrent difficulties in her relationships with men, becoming angry and frightened if there was a threat of intimacy, with an 'almost delusional terror of becoming pregnant'; there were also claustrophobic, agoraphobic, and psychosomatic symptoms. The analysis is described as slow and difficult, and Feldman notes that 'Any movement forward was usually followed by long periods of silence, immobility, or destructive attacks on my work and her own understanding' (1992: 173). He considers this slowness and difficulty derived partly from the patient's identification with 'primitive and damaged' images of her parents. The patient apparently conveyed the impression that she had experienced her parents as hostile to vitality and creativity – and that she defended herself against her resulting anxieties either by identifying with these damaged and threatening figures, or by 'splitting off and disowning the qualities they embodied' (1992:173). Feldman states that both these defences seriously impoverished the patient's thinking and her emotional life and led to severe inhibitions in the analysis, with 'fears of any kind of inter-action with her analyst' (1992: 173).

[Feldman indicates his view that the patient's anxieties and resulting immobility are a result of her identification with 'primitive and damaged images' of her parents. He does not indicate explicitly how these images come to be seen as primitive and damaged, but the implication seems to be, in line with general Kleinian assumptions, that this is a result of a complex interaction between perceptions of the parents' actual characteristics and the affective colouring created by the patient's hostile and envious feelings towards them – this hostility being driven partly by experi-ences of deprivation and frustration, as well as the contribution of the innate death instinct.]

The patient is described as the younger daughter of hard-working profes-sional parents. However, the family appears to have been quite abnormal. The mother is said to be 'an anxious, defensive woman who manages to cope by imposing a harsh and rigid control on herself and others' (1992: 174). Apparently the patient was regarded as a very 'good' child, who was quiet and compliant, concerned not to disturb her mother's precarious equilibrium. Of particular significance was the family's attitude towards the patient's cousin, Janet, who lived with them when she was 3 or 4, during a period when her own mother was ill. Janet was regarded with disapproval because she was lively and messy and created disorder. The family broke off contacts with Janet's family, as they had with others, when offended by some slight or critical comment; such severing of links to others were seemingly irrevocable. The patient found some relief from the bleak atmosphere in the home through turning to her grandmother, but this evoked resentment from her mother; moreover, the grandmother died when the patient was aged 8 and she was sent to boarding school soon afterwards. Although there were elements of an alliance between the patient and her father, their contacts were characterized mostly by arguments or resentful silence.

[This account implies that the patient's liveliness – her grandiose-exhibitionist self – definitely did not receive mirroring affirmation from either of her parents. Instead she may have felt that her natural grandiose self had to be repressed in order to maintain her attachment to her caregivers.]

Feldman reports that the patient's behaviour in analysis has followed a stereotyped pattern, with much silence – sometimes for several sessions in succession – and an apparent need for her to defend herself against the analyst, the analytic process, and the contents of her own mind. She would give very little overt response to interpretations. A dream was reported early in the analysis, in which a monstrous figure breaks through the garden hedge – this image appeared to be linked to the patient's mother. Six months prior to the detailed clinical material presented in the paper, Feldman had set a termination date for a year hence.

[Although the dream of the monstrous figure appears to be linked to the patient's image of her mother, it seems likely that it also expresses her fear of her own potential liveliness threatening to invade her fortress of silence and inactivity. Occurring as it does early in the analysis, it would seem to represent the threat to her fragile equilibrium posed by the analysis itself. The account of childhood suggests that she may have perceived liveliness and aggressive vigour as presenting a threat to her attachments and to survival; the lively Janet had been sent away – and it would have seemed to the child that she was sent away because of her liveliness. The patient may well have come to feel that it was absolutely essential to her survival that she maintain a very firm control over her own liveliness.]

Feldman begins his clinical material with the first session after a holiday break. The patient reported a dream in which there had been a murder. Initially it had been unclear who the murderer was, but then it had become apparent that it was the analyst. In the dream the patient had felt uncomfortable at the thought that she would have to face the analyst, knowing that he had committed a murder, and to tell him that she knew. The dream scene changed to her parents' house and both the police and the analyst were there. She said to the senior policeman that she had documentary proof upstairs and went to get it, meanwhile fearing that the analyst would have seen her talking to the policeman and would want to get rid of her by murdering or poisoning her.

> [There has been a murder. The account of the patient's childhood and of her behaviour in the analysis indicates that an original 'murder' of her grandiose-exhibitionist self had taken place because her parents could not tolerate her natural liveliness – as evidenced by the getting rid of Janet. Then the patient seemed to engage in a continual murder of her own potential liveliness, as indicated by her behaviour in analysis. Presumably the dream has some connection with the holiday break and the fact that the analyst had set a termination date – i.e. a date to get rid of her.]

The patient then described an incident that took place while her elderly parents had been staying over the holidays. Her father had been having a bath but then could not get out on his own and her mother had not been able to manage to help him out. However, her sister, Angela, was visiting and her son, Roger, had been able to help. The patient said this was fortunate because otherwise her father would have waited hours before allowing his daughters to help him out of the bath. She added that Angela had been reminded by this of a related incident from childhood. Their father had been in the bath and had called to their mother to talk to him. When the mother went in to the bathroom, Angela had wandered in as well. Their father had not immediately realized Angela was there but then shouted at her to get out in a very angry and unpleasant way. The patient said she wished Angela had not told her this.

At this point Feldman interpreted to her that her experience of being expelled during the holiday, and later from the analysis itself, led to his becoming identified in her mind as a murderer. He suggested that once she had returned to the analysis, she was attempting to relate to him more as a policeman, trying to see him as an ally in order to ward off any retaliatory attacks from him which might be provoked by her reproaches.

Feldman comments (to the reader) that in this material are represented different versions of the patient's relationship to the oedipal situation, deriving from different levels of psychic organization. He points out that the scene between the parents in the bathroom could 'be regarded as a representation of the primal scene from which the patient is excluded both by her actual parents and by her analyst during his holiday' (1992: 180). Then he argues that the experience of exclusion had provoked hatred and murderousness which were then defensively projected into the parental couple, resulting in the situation represented in the dream. Moreover, he suggests that the patient perceived the danger not only from the representation of the oedipal figures as powerful and threatening, but also from the image of them as damaged, like in the story of the helpless father unable to get out of the bath but unwilling to allow his daughters to see him vulnerable and naked. Feldman then goes on to argue 'It is as if there is something about her objects and their relationship that they cannot bear to have discovered and are willing to go to any lengths – even murder – to protect' (1992: 181). Generalizing, he then further argues that if the concept of the oedipus complex is extended to include early and primitive phantasies about the parental couple, images are found of these objects in a vulnerable and damaged state, which are even more frightening than phantasies of powerful and successful parental sexuality. Feldman sees these frightening images as posing a serious threat to the discovery of psychic truth 'about the nature of her internal (and external) objects, and her relationship to them' (1992: 182).

Feldman implies that the damaged parental figures are perceived as themselves being opposed to knowledge and truth. He states that his patient identifies with them in her fear and hatred of knowledge, exemplified in her remark that she wished her sister had not told her of the incident in the bathroom. On the other hand, he sees his patient as attempting to use the analyst as a policeman figure to help her face difficult aspects of internal and external reality.

Following his interpretation about her use of him as a policeman who could assist in her investigations, the patient told him of a further incident with her parents. Her mother had been writing the patient a cheque and had asked whether she should write the patient's single initial of 'F.' or the full initials of 'F.I.N.' On overhearing this, the father had made a joke about this signifying the end of the 'B.'s' (the surname). The patient commented that it had taken him a long time to see this play on the letters of her initials which had struck her many years ago. Turning to her mother, her father asked, 'Have you told her about Janet?' Her mother then told her that Janet, the cousin who had stayed with them when she was very young, had died. The contact with Janet and her family had remained severed but they had seen a notice in the local paper, the cause of death not being mentioned. Feldman adds at this point that the patient had recently discovered that the reason her parents had fallen out with Janet's parents was because Janet's mother had criticized their care of Janet.

Feldman interpreted to her that she was recognizing more clearly how vulnerable her parents were, and how strongly they reacted to any criticism. He also commented that although she too felt threatened by knowledge, she did communicate a desire to be helped in discovering the truth. The patient's response was to remain silent for the remaining fifteen minutes of the session.

[There could be seen to be something quite shocking in the patient's account of the interaction with her parents. Her father's joke about F.I.N. and the end of the B.'s surely alludes unconsciously to death, particularly as it is then followed immediately by a reference to Janet, who has died. Janet's actual death comes on top of her symbolic killing off when the patient's parents got rid of her in childhood because of her liveliness. The patient no doubt sees her parents unconsciously as murderers – certainly murderers of emotional links. Inherent in her account is the idea that her parents react murderously to criticism; the relationship is killed off if their position is challenged on any matter. Moreover, what is conveyed is a startling and rather chilling lack of empathy and emotion in the parents' presentation of the news of Janet's death. Almost certainly it must be this experience with her parents in relation to Janet's death that has contributed to the dream that a murder had taken place.

The self psychologist, curious to understand the patient's conscious and unconscious experience would probably have asked her what she felt about this interchange with her parents. Instead, the analyst offers an interpretation – which could carry the danger of foreclosing the patient's potential elaboration of her experience. In some ways his comments seem to slide past what may have been the most crucial aspects of the patient's experience – the shocking implications concerning the parents' ruthless reactions to criticism and their bleak lack of empathy. Is this why she remains silent until the end of the session following the analyst's interpretations?]

Then, in his comment to the reader, Feldman notes that the patient seemed to have arrived at a view of her parents as turning on Janet in a murderous fashion. However, he then uses this observation as a basis for arguing that perceptions of the actual behaviour of the parents (or analyst) may *contribute* to the internal images of the parents. That such an assumption requires justification at all appears to be a consequence of the Kleinian view that psychic reality, the internal images of others, is determined to a significant extent by the person's innately constructed and instinctually-driven fantasies, which are in turn fuelled by experiences of deprivation and frustration. Feldman states:

> What I am suggesting . . . is that although the damaged and vengeful qualities of the oedipal figures in these fantasies may primarily reflect the patient's jealous and envious attacks on the creative couple, and the projection of her own envy and hatred into them, they may be reinforced by her actual experiences and perceptions of her parents, or, at times, of her analyst.
>
> (1992: 184, italics added)

Feldman goes on to explain his view that his patient's anxiety about facing her own inner world, her psychic reality, is based on a combination of her identification with such vulnerable parental figures, and her guilt about her attacks on them. According to this perspective, the harmful impact of the actual behaviour and characteristics of the parents is that they confirm rather than disconfirm the patient's fearful fantasies about the results of her innate, instinctually driven, hostility towards them.

Feldman hypothesizes that during her childhood the patient had attempted to cope with the anxieties arising from her hostile fantasies by becoming a quiet and still child who showed no signs of hostility. This expressed her attempts to protect her parents insofar as she perceived them to be vulnerable, and also to avoid provoking their retaliation for her hostility. By contrast, Janet had not suppressed her liveliness and thus was a threat to the equilibrium of the family. Her father's comment about the end of the B.'s and the reference to Janet's death seemed to confirm the patient's view of her parents.

Feldman then states: 'These fantasies have been powerfully present in the analysis, influencing the experience of the analyst, the way she has been able to use interpretations, and her own capacity for thinking and understanding' (1992: 184–85). Thus, despite having outlined ways in which the patient's unconscious assumptions and expectations governing her characteristic patterns in relationships have been based upon her perceptions of her parents' actual behaviour and attitudes, Feldman reverts to speaking of her *fantasies*. As if to emphasize this point, he then comments on the patient's continued difficulty in facing the truth of her internal and external world: 'There remains a strong pull by something very deadly and deadening in the patient herself, which reinforces her identification with a parental object that hates and fears knowledge and understanding, and she is then driven to attack both her own thinking and mine' (1992: 185).

Feldman continues this theme of the patient's orientation towards death. He describes her as retreating into silence, making little response to interpretations, and speaking of feelings of hopelessness and thoughts of violence and death. Feldman notes that this withdrawal into silence and hopelessness had been a recurrent feature of the analysis, such that any attempt to be more constructive or hopeful seemed to arouse violence within her and an insistence that nothing could change. He comments:

> I thought the cold, deadly response to most of my interpretations during this period was the expression of the patient's own hatred of anything vital or creative, as well as her identification with the representation of the vulnerable and destructive parents.
>
> (1992: 186)

Feldman viewed his patient as projectively evoking in him the healthy aspects of herself, which were capable of interest and liveliness. The result was that the analyst was made to endure 'the painful experience of being in the presence of a cruel, almost impenetrable object, which evoked the response of wishing either to attack it desperately or to submit in a hopeless fashion' (1992: 186). Apparently the patient would become desperate and hopeless if she felt that the analyst might not be able to survive this experience.

At this point Feldman states a view that is exclusively Kleinian, in its emphasis upon innate destructive aspects of the patient's personality. He puts this as follows:

> I believe that one of the important reasons for the defensive projection of vital elements of her own personality, particularly the more healthy ones, was to avoid the disastrous possibility of the powerful destructive aspects of herself being concurrently present and interacting with more normal infantile elements.
>
> (1992: 187)

At times Feldman's account seems ambiguous in relation to the question of whether the patient's destructiveness is essentially innate or is derived from an identification with her parents. Having a few paragraphs earlier referred to 'the patient's own hatred of anything vital or creative', which he sees as distinct from 'her identification with the representation of the vulnerable and destructive parents' (1992: 186), he then comments that some more hopeful signs of progress in the analysis indicated that 'the patient had not abandoned herself to an identification with these damaged and destructive figures as completely as she had done in the past' (1992: 187). He sees this as an effect of the 'partial internalization and identification with a figure who is not too vulnerable nor too damaged, and not too threatened by the prospect of discovering something about either psychic reality or external reality' (1992: 187) – i.e. an identification with the analyst who has survived her destructive attacks.

Feldman then refers to a session in which the patient describes a situation with her boyfriend and her reaction to this. She had returned to the flat and her boyfriend, Peter, was already there watching a film. She prepared supper and lit a fire, but he remained absorbed in the film. They had sex but Peter did not seem very interested. In recounting this incident, the patient remarked that she would have liked Peter to give her more attention and support and appreciation. She then spoke of feeling that she has to manage all by herself and that sometimes she feels 'hopelessly isolated'; she then became very upset. After some minutes she spoke of expecting to feel very isolated when the analysis ended.

[This vignette based around her relationship with her boyfriend is a very clear representation of the patient's core conflicts. She wants closeness and intimacy, as well as appreciation and recognition (a combination of attachment and selfobject needs); she fears she will be ignored or abandoned; as a result she feels she must manage all by herself. In describing this she expresses feelings of desperation. Crucially, she then indicates the current context for this conflict and associated feelings: it is the imminent ending of the analysis, which had been decided upon by the analyst. From a self psychological point of view, however, Feldman's understanding appears determined by the Kleinian theoretical assumptions about the relative primacy of innate instincts of destructiveness. In his commentary he seems to oscillate between locating the source of the patient's conflicts in her experiences with her parents and viewing her pathology as deriving from her own innate destructiveness. This theoretical equivocation no doubt expresses Feldman's concern to take account of both innate factors and the patient's perceptions and experiences.[3] However, this ambiguity may also have been reflected in his interpretations to her, with the result that the reverberations in the present of the original experiences with the parents were not made entirely clear. A perspective deriving from self psychology or attachment theory might, by contrast, lead the analyst to articulate to the patient her fear that if she shows any liveliness or aggression towards him, he will abandon her – and that she has unconsciously perceived his setting a date to end the analysis as an act of murder, equivalent to the original parental disposing of Janet.]

Commenting on his patient's account of her relationship with Peter and her expression of anxiety and anguish regarding the ending of the analysis, Feldman construes her communications as an indication of progress: 'She was able to turn to me in an unusually direct and open way, recognizing how much she depended on the help and support she did get, which she could not find anywhere else, and which she would be losing' (1992: 189). However, he seems to see the problem as one of a battle between progressive and destructive forces inherent within the patient's mind, because he goes on to describe how this healthy development, of acknowledgement of dependence, is then followed by a destructive attack. He describes how the patient found herself again in the grip of a powerful silence. His interpretation was as follows:

[3.] Dr Feldman has commented that he believes it is important to keep an open mind about the relative weight of innate and environmental factors especially since the evolution of analytic work with a particular patient often leads to a revision of one's earlier view.

I commented that when she was better able to communicate with herself, and with me, this seemed to provoke a very powerful, uncompromising attack on the contact between us. She could feel safe and protected only if she remained silent and immobile, as if capitulating to the hostile force.

(1992: 189)

The patient's response was:

I was thinking about my cats, and about them dying – especially one of them. Then I thought of having them put down, if I wanted to do myself in. Then I thought of them being hit by a car, attacked by a dog – thought of burying them – the one that was dying is the more adventurous one.

Feldman notes that he found 'something quite chilling' in the way his patient spoke at this point. The determining influence of the Kleinian emphasis upon destructiveness (derived from both innate and environmental factors) is expressed vividly in his next comments:

I did not think this was simply a manifestation of a defensive withdrawal, but rather the expression of something deadly in her that became allied to the destructive aspects of her parents or her analyst. She seemed to confirm the fact that it was especially the more lively, adventurous aspect of herself that became the victim of this deadly attack. Instead of being able to tolerate the conflict and anxiety that this aroused, she seemed to ally herself with the cruel and sadistic agency that attacked her, her adventurous cat, and any progress in the analysis.

(1992: 189–90)

[The clear implication here is that there is a deadly force within the patient, which in a secondary way becomes allied to the destructiveness of her parents. What is the purpose and function of this destructiveness? Feldman gives the answer in his next comments:]

She began the next session with a another long silence. I said that I thought we had seen how she turned to a world of suicide and violent death to avoid the pain of being left out, wanting things and minding about what was happening and the fears that were aroused when her adventurousness, hopes, and wishes might be discovered. I seemed to have to bear the frustration, pain, and disappointment instead.

(1992: 190)

[What is the meaning of the long silence? Feldman seems to see it as a further manifestation of destructiveness, an equivalent of suicide. He interprets that she retreats to a preoccupation with destruction as a defensive avoidance of the pain of feeling left out. This formulation is set within the framework of the Kleinian theory of the paranoid-schizoid constellation of defences against the mental pains of the depressive position. Feldman postulates that the patient is repudiating her own potential depressive pain, of feeling left out, and is projectively evoking it, and in fantasy locating it, in the analyst instead. What the self psychological or intersubjectivist analyst is more likely to see in the patient's behaviour and communications is a clear endopsychic repetition of the original situation with the parents. She has vividly described an internalization of her parents' hostility towards her own liveliness, expressed in the thoughts of her cats dying, of her own suicide, and of being hit by a car, or of being attacked by a dog. These fantasies no doubt also become a channel for her feelings of rage, turned on herself. If she felt that the analyst was acting as a murderer, linked to her representation of her parents as murderers of Janet and the lively part of herself – and if she felt he was getting rid of her (through ending the analysis), just as the parents had sent Janet away – and if, moreover, she felt that he was not understanding her increasingly desperate communications – then she might well feel immense rage in response to a failure of empathy. In Feldman's account there is no indication of the patient's ever expressing overt anger towards the analyst. Therefore it can reasonably be assumed that she was afraid to do so, just as she would have been originally with her parents. Her rage must then be directed on herself and expressed towards the analyst only covertly. By contrast, Feldman views her aggression as an expression of her wish to avoid depressive pain. His implicit exhortation to her is that she should give up her destructiveness and tolerate her painful feelings of neediness and loss.]

Feldman reports that the patient then spoke of the fact that Peter was to go abroad for a time and she realized how much this bothered her. She added that she did not want to think about it and that her thoughts were all vague. Feldman interpreted that she was attacking her own mind, making everything vague, because she could not tolerate painful awareness of feelings about being left.

[Feldman's interpretation appears to refer essentially to an innate intolerance of depressive mental pain: because of this intolerance, the patient attacks her own mind, disabling its functioning, so that she cannot feel the pain. An alternative, object-relational formulation based on self psychology or attachment theory, might give less emphasis to intolerance of mental pain, and instead address the patterns of need/desire in relation to expectations of the response of an other – and might also describe the particular quality of what is required from the other (the selfobject needs in relation to Peter or the analyst).]

The patient then speaks of remembering that yesterday Peter had heard that his sister's baby had been born. Apparently Peter was pleased that they were naming the baby Peter. The patient had remarked that perhaps they should have given the baby its own name, and had then felt guilty that she had not kept this thought to herself.

Feldman comments that, in his view, what has taken place here is that as the analyst has been able to tolerate the patient's silence and address her destructive processes whereby she splits off or attacks her own mental functions, there has been a shift in her mental state; she has been able to speak of Peter's sister's baby – which may have been a sensitive and painful issue for her (presumably because of feelings of rivalry and envy) – and to express her sense of guilt about her lack of generosity and impulse to dampen his pleasure. He links this to the process of the previous session, in which there had been a violent attack on something alive and adventurous (the fantasies of attacks on the dog and the cat and her own self); he suggests that this destructive stance continued into this session but seemed to be milder and gave way to a position in which she appears more integrated and alive and able to look at difficult issues with less fear and hatred.

[Again Feldman gives emphasis to the patient's struggle with her own destructiveness – indeed this theme is quite central to the analysis. The analyst looking from a self psychological or object-relational perspective would be inclined to wonder first about the patient's inner experience and perceptions of Peter, his sister, her baby, and the analyst, and secondly about the recurrent pattern of hope and fear that is continually recreated and represented in the analytic material. This might lead one to wonder whether the patient's comment about the baby's not having his own name might reflect something other than destructive envy; it could express her real concern that the baby's individuality might not be recognized – a situation that she might easily be expected to assimilate to the template of the childhood experience of the parents who were opposed to her authentic liveliness. From this point of view, the patient would be seen as displaying a recurrent endopsychic repetition of the original situation of her experience of her parents. By continually emphasizing the patient's destructiveness as the essential problem, Feldman might seem to be repeatedly frustrating her attempt to explore and communicate about her early experience with her parents, now repeated in the transference.]

Feldman then reports that the patient was again silent and withdrawn. Eventually she explained that when she came into the room she experienced a muddle which she could not understand and which meant she could not speak. Feldman told her he thought that she became muddled about what kind of person he was, whether he was cold, hostile and preoccupied, in the way she had experienced her mother, or whether he was someone more benign who did care about her.

> [This interpretation has a simpler and more classical structure than many of Feldman's comments. It draws the patient's attention to the way in which she is perceiving the analyst in terms of the template derived from her experience of her mother, and implicitly invites her to consider the possibility that this perception is not accurate. In this way the patient is helped to disentangle the past and the present. The content of the interpretation is close to the self psychological and object relational view that the patient's present difficulties derive from pathological experiences with her parents, which have given rise to maladaptive constellations of hope and fear in relationships with others.]

The patient responded well to this interpretation, becoming more relaxed and speaking differently. She then quoted something the analyst had said the previous week which had made an impact on her: 'You said if I behave like this, don't talk, don't co-operate, I feel I must be hated, or some word like that. It was much stronger than you usually say or I expect; there must have been something there that I recognize' (1992: 192).

> [The patient rewards the analyst for this helpful interpretation by not only appearing more relaxed and able to talk, but also by referring to a relevant interpretation from the previous week. The clear impression of her childhood is that she felt she would be hated if she did not behave as her parents wanted. This then must be the experience repeated in the transference. When the analyst made an interpretation that helped to distinguish past and present, the patient was freed from the impasse, at least for a moment. Following this she refers to the analyst's interpretation from the previous week which had succinctly expressed this feeling from childhood, re-experienced in the present. This raises the question of why she had not been able to respond positively and with more freedom at the time the interpretation was made. The answer may be because, when given, the interpretation was framed in terms of the present relationship with the analyst, without also being explicitly rooted in a reference to her

childhood experience. A pervasive assumption in British psychoanalytic circles, particularly but not exclusively within the Kleinian group, is that interpretations should focus first on the here-and-now relationship to the analyst, and only secondarily refer to the developmental past. The argument behind this position is that references to the childhood situation can be premature and can function as a defensive retreat from the emotional heat of the here-and-now transference. However, the disadvantage may be that without the historical developmental perspective, it can be difficult for the patient to know where to go with the interpretation.]

Feldman then explained to her that what he had been addressing in the earlier session was her pain and distress associated with her belief that she was hated, and her attempts to find an explanation for this feeling. Then crucially he added that she sometimes got into a muddle because she was not sure whether this was true also in her analysis.

[Again, Feldman's interpretation is very clear, helping the patient (a) to understand the experiences of childhood and how these have shaped her self-image, (b) to see how these childhood experiences invade her perceptions of the present, and (c) to disentangle past and present.]

In response to the analyst's interpretation, the patient became visibly upset, crying for a while, and seeming to be very much in contact. Feldman comments (to the reader) that the patient's sense of being hated by her parents was clearly important. However, he makes a distinction between the patient's own attempt to explain this to herself in terms of being hated because of the way she behaved, and the more painful idea that she was unwanted and hated in a silent and cold way, without her being able to find any explanation. He considered that interpretations along these lines had enabled her to distinguish between the object whom she felt hated her and the analyst whom she did not feel hated by, and thereby made it possible for her to see the analyst as a helpful figure.

The patient began the following session by saying that she was very preoccupied with the question of what made her acceptable or not acceptable. She realized that behaviour that might be appropriate at home might not be so elsewhere. Then she referred to a dream in which she has a baby; the dream contained a sense of confusion since the identity shifted between her own self and that of an old school friend; during the dream she recalls that she has been drinking earlier, before she knew she was pregnant, and worries that this might have caused damage to the foetus. In association, she recalled that she had recently attended a working lunch where there had been a woman who was pregnant. The pregnancy was not obvious, being concealed by the woman's dress. In referring to the fact that the woman drank three glasses of wine, the patient was equivocal, at one point describing this as 'not excessive' and shortly afterwards saying that it *was* excessive. She added that she had been monitoring the amount she drinks herself.

Feldman interpreted that the patient felt that her desperate need to be acceptable had not allowed the possibility of babies and that she had disguised or eliminated her own desires in ways that she now felt were wrong; when he and she had been able to speak about difficult and painful issues the previous day, this led her to feel sufficiently accepted and supported to enable her to dream of something alive and valuable inside her, which she wished to protect from damage. Elaborating (although it is not clear from the account how much of this was said to the patient), Feldman suggests that what had emerged was a link between her oedipal preoccupations, including her feeling deprived of a baby of her own, and her questions about why it had been unacceptable for her to show any liveliness, sexuality or creativity.

[As a child, the patient had felt that her lively baby self was not acceptable – indeed was hated. Now she is able to dream of having a baby – which must in part represent a new baby self. This no doubt reflects her growing hope that her liveliness could be acceptable after all. She is worried about her own activities in the past which have endangered the potential new life inside her. There seems no reason necessarily to assume that the dream relates to oedipal wishes to receive a baby from her father, but Feldman does give it this emphasis.

At the same time, the dream may be alluding backwards in time to her sense of her parents' ambivalence towards her as a baby. This may be represented in the patient's description of the woman who conceals her pregnancy by her clothes and who drinks excessively in a way the patient fears could harm the baby. Is the woman pregnant or not? Is her drinking excessive or not? These uncertainties might express ambivalence towards a baby. The patient could indeed be considering becoming pregnant with an actual baby and be exploring her own ambivalence deriving from identification with her parents.]

Feldman then comments:

Behind the painful questions about why her father or analyst had not given her a baby, preferring sexual intimacy with another woman, there lay a much more disturbing sense of being hated and never wanted as a baby (by her parents, or her analyst) and thus never allowed to be creative. It had been important to her that I had been able to think and speak about this, as my doing so provided some reassurance against a fantasy of me as a damaged and fragile parental figure unable to face or talk about such issues, and liable to take violent revenge on her if she dared to acquire anything valuable and alive. Such reassurance was particularly important when she felt her silence, her lack of appreciation, or more open attacks had injured me and reinforced the feelings of hatred.

(1992: 194–95)

[Although Feldman posits 'painful questions about why her father or analyst had not given her a baby', the evidence for such issues preoc-cupying the patient seems unclear. The hypothesis may stem more from the analyst's own theoretical preconceptions regarding oedipal concerns. By contrast, there is abundant material to support Feldman's point that the patient felt she was hated and never wanted as a baby. Moreover, who could disagree with his comment that by thinking and speaking about these matters the analyst had helped her differentiate him from her fantasy of a damaged and fragile parental figure who would violently attack her if she appeared alive and creative? However, this central object relational constellation of hope and dread – the wish to be loved and for her liveliness to be accepted, set against the fear that she would be hated, especially for her liveliness – seems subtly to be sidelined, as if merely a footnote to a more important struggle with the vicissitudes of the patient's own destructiveness. This becomes most apparent in Feldman's next comment, which concludes his main account.]

I believe that the experience and internalization of a figure that, by addressing these feelings, made her feel accepted, enabled the patient to take greater responsibility for her own destructiveness and capacity for spoiling, and to tolerate guilt without feeling overwhelmingly persecuted by it. A more integrated and creative aspect of her could then emerge, heralded by a dream in which she was able to feel protective toward an infant inside her.

(1992: 195)

[Thus in his concluding formulating, Feldman seems to revert to a classic Kleinian understanding, in terms of the patient's becoming able to take more responsibility for her destructiveness, and devel-oping a greater capacity to tolerate guilt – i.e. achieving a firmer foothold in the depressive position. Out of this state of greater integration emerges a more creative aspect of herself, represented by the dream of a baby. Although the interplay between the parents' behaviour and attitudes, and the patient's infantile phantasies and feeling states, is considered in Feldman's account, it seems to the present writer that in the end this Kleinian perspective seems retrospectively to foreclose so much of what had emerged regarding a pathogenic early environment – one that the patient had felt to be murderous towards her own self – and the repetitions of this pattern in adult life, both endopsychically and in relation to the analyst.]

Feldman then provides a brief theoretical discussion, parts of which seem to derive relatively little from the presented clinical material. He states that he has endeavoured to 'illustrate the interaction between the patient's oedipal fantasies and the perception of her actual parents, and the way in which these fantasies, originally reflected in the symptoms which brought her into analysis, were subsequently lived out in the transference' (1992: 195). He refers to ways in which the patient could identify at times with the frightened, isolated and helpless child, and at other times with the damaged and murderous figures who were threatened by her liveliness. In addition he points to the interaction and mutual reinforcement between these fantasies (with associated impulses) and her actual experiences of her parents.

Feldman then casts the material further into an oedipal framework by suggesting that

> Any communication, thinking, and the possession of knowledge was confused in the patient's mind with a disturbed and frightening version of the parental intercourse. This made it very difficult to use her own mind properly, because of both the anxiety that resulted from thoughts and ideas coming together and the threat and betrayal this was felt to represent to the parental couple.
>
> (1992: 196)

He then refers to two particular oedipal fantasies. The first is that 'the violence of the patient's sexual jealousy has brought about irreparable damage in the oedipal couple . . . All she can do is to try to avert a murderous revenge by abandoning or concealing her own sexuality' (1992: 196). A second, more disturbing fantasy, is of 'a vulnerable and damaged oedipal couple, full of hatred and violence of an incomprehensible nature, for which she does not feel responsible' (1992: 196) Feldman notes that it was particularly when this second fantasy was addressed that an important shift could take place in the analysis. He sees the patient's progress in analysis as resting upon her gradual discovery and identification with a figure who can tolerate knowledge of what is going on, and can survive her attacks without retaliation.

[Although Feldman states that, in the patient's mind, ideas coming together were confused with frightening fantasies of the parental intercourse – an interpretation which is based on the theories of Klein and Bion – there appears little overtly in the presented clinical material to suggest this. What seems more apparent is that the patient felt that her own thinking, questioning and potential liveliness were a threat to her parents, and, in the transference, to her analyst. Her pattern of maintaining a rigid control over herself, modelled on the image of her mother, naturally became intensified in the context of the analysis. Rather than there being indications of the patient having felt disturbed by fantasies or observations of the parental intercourse, it seems likely that she would have felt reassured if there had been more evidence of the parents enjoying a vigorous and robust sexual relationship. Such an atmosphere would have left her more free to pursue her own development and give rein to her liveliness. The patient's discovery in the analysis that it was safe to think and feel and have lively desires, does not seem necessarily to require Feldman's particular Kleinian theoretical perspective.]

The self psychological view of Feldman's case

Feldman's patient gives the impression of a childhood environment that did not support and affirm her own developmental strivings. Instead, she appears to have felt that her liveliness (her *life*) and potential demandingness were threatening to her parents' well-being, especially to that of her mother. Thus she felt that she was *hated* because she disrupted their lives. She accommodated to this perception of her parents' fragility by becoming a quiet and 'good' child who caused no trouble. In Winnicottian (1960) terms this could be described as the development of a 'false self' form of adaptation. The more detailed model provided by Kohut (e.g. as represented by his diagram on page 185 of *The Analysis of the Self*) suggests a state of affairs in which an outward compliance with the desire of the mother, for a quiet compliant child, coexists, albeit separated by a vertical split, with a state in which the nuclear grandiose self is repressed, leaving a conscious experience of depletion, depression and inhibition. This repression would result in a recurrent anxiety that crude, unneutralized exhibitionism, tinged with raw aggression and sexuality, would threaten to overwhelm the fragile ego. It could well have been this anxiety that was represented in the early dream of the monster breaking through the hedge (the repression barrier).

Two anxieties within the patient would be likely in response to the parental anxieties about liveliness and disorder. First, the fear that she would be got rid of – 'murdered' – like Janet (basically an abandonment anxiety). Second, her anxiety that her own ego would be overwhelmed by the return of the repressed impulses (a psychoeconomic anxiety).

Her anxiety about the potential consequences of a more disruptive liveliness must have been greatly exacerbated by her observations and fantasies regarding the parents' attitude towards her cousin Janet. Since Janet had not been with the family since birth, she would not have learned from the beginning the importance of accommodating to the parents' needs for peace, quiet and compliance. The consequence was that the parents were critical and rejecting towards her. It seems likely that the patient perceived the departure of Janet as a doing away with her by the parents, because they found her liveliness and neediness too much to cope with. This perception or fantasy is given expression in the patient's dream of a murder having been committed.

The recurrent configurations of the patient's subjective world were played out in relation to the analyst. Potential liveliness and the communication of need were suppressed because the patient felt it would result in the analyst hating her. In turning against her own liveliness, the patient was perpetuating an endopsychic repetition of her parents' attitudes towards her. Expressions of liveliness, or of need, were followed by moods of silence and deadliness. At other times, what seemed more apparent was the enactment of the childhood pattern, with the analyst placed in the patient's original position, being made to suffer the oppression of liveliness. During the course of the long analysis, the patient gradually discovered that the conditions of her childhood, and her associated anxieties, no longer applied in her adult life. She could discover new ways of being with the other, strengthened by insights into how she had originally adapted to her childhood experiences.

What of the oedipal perspective? As we have noted, there seems little reason, on the basis of Feldman's clinical account, to assume that the patient's difficulties must necessarily be understood in an oedipal framework. However, if oedipal concerns were present, these would be construed from a self psychological point of view as manifestations of a pathologically intensified oedipus complex, deriving from the frustration of more primary selfobject needs. Because of the deprivation of basic needs for empathic involvement, the patient would have become particularly sensitive to episodes of exclusion or of being ignored. This would also have rendered her narcissistically vulnerable to evidence of indifference, lack of attention, or of being taken for granted by her boyfriend.

Perspectives on impasse

Some self psychologically inspired analysts, notably Stolorow and colleagues, have discussed ways of understanding the situations of psychoanalytic impasse which not infrequently occur at times during treatment, especially with the more deeply troubled patients. Kohut himself addressed this issue at various points, describing how the analytic work may become mired in an impasse when the analyst seems to the patient to be insisting on a particular view or theory which in some subtle way misses an important nuance of the patient's communication, and which also repeats (in the transference-countertransference) a damaging and chronic interaction from childhood. In describing his conclusions, Kohut made the following rueful observation:

> If there is one lesson that I have learned during my life as an analyst, it is the lesson that what my patients tell me is likely to be true – that many times when I believed that I was right and patients were wrong, it turned out, though often only after a prolonged search, that my rightness was superficial, whereas their rightness was profound.
>
> (1984: 93–94)

Thus the typical situations of impasse described in the self psychological literature are ones in which the analyst feels he or she is understanding the patient but the patient feels misunderstood in some important, albeit subtle way. Sometimes the failure of understanding may be hidden because it is certain features of the analytic situation itself which too closely mirror the pathogenic aspects of the original situation in childhood. This may often be the case with patients who experienced their parents as cold, aloof, rejecting of attempts at emotional or physical intimacy. With such a background experience, the typical analytic setting and stance may represent an emotional austerity that can seem like a concrete repetition of the deprivations of childhood.

There are other situations of impasse that derive from an adverse mirroring between the preconscious models of relationship (or organizing principles) of the patient and the analyst. To understand these, it may be necessary to consider the pathogenic childhood situations of both patient and analyst.

'Sarah' – Stolorow and Atwood

Stolorow and Atwood (1992) present the case of 'Sarah', a 27-year-old single physiotherapist. She sought help because of a tendency to feel like a little girl in a world of adults. Her early history involved neglect by depressed and alcoholic parents. An early memory was of crying uncontrollably in her cot, whilst her mother screamed at her to shut up and threw a feeding bottle into her bedding. In later relationships, Sarah tended to be nurturing towards men who gave little in return.

. Sarah presented a dream early in the therapy: she travelled back to the town where she had lived as a child and went into a large house, moving from room to room, finally coming to a cupboard in which an infant, covered in cuts and bruises and dirt, cowered against the wall.

The impasse

At a certain point, the therapist informed Sarah of a six week break scheduled for the following summer. Sarah showed no immediate reaction, but a few days later reported a dream in which a decrepit old animal was left lying on its back in the wilderness. When the therapist linked this to the announcement about the break, Sarah appeared clearly very frightened. The therapist gave her reassurances that he would be available by phone, and pointed out that they had several months to prepare for the break. In response Sarah became even more agitated and angry, unable to speak, eventually rushing out of the door. She then began arriving late to her sessions, had little to say, and often wanted to run away. As the therapist tried to explore and reduce her anxieties Sarah became ever more frightened. She reported recurring nightmares, in which she arrived at the building for her session, but the therapist's office had disappeared.

When the summer break arrived, Sarah refused any contact with the therapist by phone. She wrote him a letter stating her view that he had treated her with brutal insensitivity and indicating that she was terminating treatment. The therapist continued to feel bewildered, but wrote saying that he hoped she might feel able to return. After some weeks she did return. However, several similar crises occurred over the next 18 months whenever there was any interruption to the therapist's availability. A recurrent feature of the impasse was that Sarah reacted to the therapist's attempts to understand by becoming more agitated and withdrawn.

The patient's and therapist's subjective worlds

Gradually this interaction between the patient's and therapist's subjective worlds became understood. It emerged that Sarah had felt that the therapist did not show concern for her experience as a frightened and vulnerable child, and, crucially, that she perceived his attempts to be helpful and reassuring as implicit demands that she be more grown up and not feel anxious. This linked to her childhood experiences when her parents required her to tolerate difficult situations, including long separations, without displaying anxiety or need. It seemed that with her therapist she was again feeling that she had to assume a false maturity and was not allowed to be the child she felt herself truly to be. She felt that he did not understand the *depth* of her distress and despair that his vacation had triggered and perceived his attempts at reassurance as a rejection of her child-self. Moreover, she feared that displaying her longings for acceptance, love and care, would prove an intolerable burden for the therapist and would lead to rejection.

The therapist's perception of the situation was profoundly determined by his own personal history, especially the sudden death of his mother when he was eight years' old. In response to the shattering impact of this event on the whole family, the therapist, as a child, had identified with his mother's nurturing role in relation to his father and siblings, at the cost of burying his own sense of desolation. His ensuing characterological style became one of caregiving and nurturing of others, and thus avoiding his own child feelings of powerlessness and loneliness. However, his failure to rescue Sarah from her descent into despair meant that this fundamental defensive strategy was failing.

Resolving the impasse

Through the process of his own personal analysis, the therapist began to appreciate more fully the depth of his own devastation not only at the loss of his mother, but also at the ensuing emotional unavailability of his father and siblings. As he became more accepting of the extreme emotions associated with his own childhood experience, he became more able to grasp and tolerate the intensity of the patient's distress. He realized that the loneliness and despair, triggered in the transference, were simply beyond the capacity of a child to bear on her own. It was this that she needed him to understand. His premature efforts at reassurance were experienced as a rejection of her child-self, repeating the analogous traumas of her childhood.

As the therapist became more able to understand, and communicate his understanding of Sarah's suffering and anxiety, and was less compelled to rescue and reassure her, she became more relaxed and clearly felt more safe. She was able to disclose a wishful fantasy, previously too frightening to convey, of being held protectively in the therapist's arms whilst she fell into a peaceful sleep.

Comment

This example illustrates vividly the way in which reassurance, even in subtle forms, can be experienced by the patient as a rejection of the anxious and suffering child-self, as well as a communication that these intense emotions of fear and longing are not tolerable. Also exemplified is the way that an impasse involves both patient and therapist being stuck in repetitive ways of perceiving the other, each feeling driven into increasing frustration and despair. Resolution of the impasse may depend upon the therapist's arriving at an understanding of how the experiences that have formed the organizing principles of his or her subjective world may be determining and limiting the understanding of the patient's experience.

Thus, whilst Kohut rightly drew attention to the importance of empathically focusing on the patient's experience and the organizing principles of the patient's subjective world, Stolorow and other intersubjectivists have developed the point that understanding the *therapist's* subjective world can also be crucial. This does not mean that the therapist should self-disclose; rather, that the understanding, achieved in personal analysis, or in post-analytic introspection, of the contribution to the analytic process of the analyst's own subjectivity, will inform the perception of the patient's communications.

Intersubjective dimensions of diagnosis

Where is a patient's psychopathology located – within his or her psyche, or within an intersubjective realm between patient and analyst? Whilst it would be an exaggeration to assert that psychopathology varies entirely according to the intersubjective context, there may be an *extent* to which the patient's presentation will be a function of the analyst's attitude and response. Kohut remarks in a footnote:

> . . . the differentiation between neurosis and psychosis is not an immovable one. It may depend, for example, on the skill and special gifts of the therapist or on the special psychological fit between a given patient and the personality of a given therapist. A psychosis or borderline state in one situation may be a severe narcissistic personality disorder in another.
>
> (1984: 219)

The intersubjective aspects of diagnosis were explored further by Brandchaft and Stolorow (1984). Extreme positions in psychoanalysis are always best avoided. Perhaps the balanced view would be that the overt form of a person's psychopathology is a function of both intrapsychic and intersubjective dimensions.

Summary

Kohut distinguished between a normal oedipal phase of development and a pathological oedipus complex. The latter, involving an intensification of sexual and aggressive aims, arises when the child's affectionate and assertive presentation is not met with empathically affirmative responses from the parents. He describes a dread deeper than castration – the experience of the 'faceless mother' (which might be linked with André Green's 'dead mother'). A comparison is made with the perspective of a London Kleinian, Michael Feldman, who presents a detailed clinical illustration which he formulates in terms of an early form of the oedipal situation, involving primitive and damaged images of the parents. A self psychological perspective suggests that Feldman's patient had experienced her early environment as hostile to her developmental strivings, and particularly to her liveliness – with the result that she protectively 'deadened' herself as these anxieties were replayed in the transference. Self psychological perspectives on states of impasse during psychoanalysis suggest that these may occur at times when the analyst's preoccupation with a particular form of understanding seems to miss an important nuance of the patient's experience, in a way that repeats a damaging interaction from childhood. A patient's presentation may result from a combination of intrapsychic and intersubjective dimensions.

Chapter 8
Schizophrenia and depression – the fragmented self and the thwarted self

Schizophrenia: the fragmented self

Kohut regarded schizophrenia as involving a (perhaps irreversible) regression to the stage of the fragmented self, corresponding to Freud's autoerotic stage (Kohut, 1971: 29). In terms of his concept of the line of development of narcissism, through the grandiose self and the idealized parent imago, he wrote:

> In the psychoses these structures are destroyed, but their disconnected fragments are secondarily reorganized, rearranged into delusions, and then rationalized through the efforts of the remaining integrative functions of the psyche . . .
>
> (Kohut, 1971: 10)

He suggested that a psychotic regression could be provoked in a vulnerable personality by narcissistic injuries, such as traumatic disappointments in the idealized adult, or thwartings of the need for mirroring responsiveness and soothing. This fragmentation is, according to Kohut, the source of the 'deepest anxiety man can experience' (1984: 16) and therefore gives rise to the delusional reconstitution of the fragmented structures in order to restore a sense of coherence and order. In this way the paranoid person can feel relief when his or her sense of confusion gives way to delusional certainty.

Others too have described anxiety over disintegration as the core of psychosis. Jacobson (1967: 13) wrote that 'the psychotic is afraid of an impending dissolution of the psychic structure'. Sullivan (1956: 318) referred to schizophrenic terror as 'an almost unceasing fear of becoming an exceedingly unpleasant form of nothingness by collapse of the self system'. In summarizing a number of contributions, Frosch referred to 'basic anxiety', which he described as having 'an amorphous, all-pervasive quality' (1983: 205) that is difficult for patients to articulate. This appears to relate not only to the dread of fragmentation but also to the danger of being overwhelmed by affective arousal, such that 'signal anxiety' (Freud, 1926) becomes traumatic anxiety as the ego is faced with excitation it cannot master. Thus Pao referred to 'organismic panic', which he describes as 'a shock-like reaction in which the ego's integrative function is temporarily paralyzed' (1979: 221). Grotstein writes of 'a constitutionally precocious sensitivity to perceptions' which predispose the psychotic person to 'a perceptual catastrophe because of inadequate filtering' so that 'the inherent potential for terror is unfiltered and so becomes registered as nameless dread because of the failure of primal repression' (1977: 448). Eigen cites the 'sense of catastrophe that underlies psychotic experience' (1986: vii) and the feeling that 'something has gone irremediably wrong' (1986: 363) – a catastrophe that perhaps involves a breakup of the coherence of consciousness, at the level of what Damasio (1999) calls the 'core self'. Frosch points out that often the psychotic patient's experience of internal disintegration of mental structures is projected on to the external world, in the form of hallucinations or delusions of world disintegration.

All the structures and functions of mind, including the experience and structure of the self, may be altered in psychosis. Eigen comments:

> Few phenomena lead to a more precise appreciation of just what is involved in 'good enough' personality functioning than the shock of what can happen when madness appears. In psychosis, the raw materials of personality, such as the sense of self–other and materiality–immateriality, undergo startling transformations or deformations. Mental processes can speed up or slow down to such an extent that being an adequately coherent person is no longer possible. The psychotic individual may be mutely rigid, explode, then turn to putty. Clarity of ideas may oscillate with gnomic utterances. Such tendencies play a role in the mood swings of ordinary life, but in psychosis, they have a menacing finality that threatens to abandon the individual forever in shifting currents of disintegration and horror.
>
> (1986: 29)

For the person predisposed towards psychosis, either through early developmental experiences or neurobiological constitution, even the relatively normal stresses of everyday life may prove overwhelming. Managing the storms of inner affect, whilst simultaneously attending to the external world of other people, may be a task too far.

Jo and the Outside People: supportive psychoanalytic psychotherapy with a schizophrenic patient

In the following account I describe ten years of supportive psychotherapy with a schizophrenic patient, Jo. The aim of this work is not to resolve the fundamental disorder, which presumably has in part a biological and neurological basis, but instead is concerned to help the patient articulate her experience, make sense of it, and find ways of living with her difficulties.

Dread of loss of control

Jo sent me the following letter some years into the therapy, following a session exploring her potential anger. It expresses with stark clarity some aspects of her core dilemma of regulating her affective state, and also indicates the patient's sense of the safe limits of therapy.

She wrote:

> I hope I did not shock you today. I showed a glimpse of what my life would be if I had no self control. I either feel no emotion whatsoever, or I will be engulfed and suffocated. I am terrified of emotion – of passion. I live my life in a pressure cooker. Everything must be nailed down. I am stretched taut; screamingly so. I have an absolute terror of passion. I avoid it in books. I cannot bear it on television. I <u>must</u> have self control. It is all I have to survive in the 'real' world. I am terrified to consider rage. It must be driven out and squashed. I avoid feeling any emotion. Anxiety is not an emotion.
>
> If I faced my 'rage' I would be extinguished by its inferno. I would then truly be insane. Insane without an escape route back to 'real'.
>
> Do you understand me? If I felt rage I would have passed into a final maelstrom. I would be lost, unreachable. I would be truly dead. I am so scared. My life is full of violent thoughts. I have it in me to be a cold random killer. It is chilling. You never hear in the news of female serial killers but I could be one, potentially.
>
> If I thought it were a probable thing I would have to destroy myself. I must live with order.
>
> I could never visualize attacking you. You represent a state of quiet calm safe tranquillity. You are my sanity. A state of grace. I skate around the issue. This is <u>massive</u>. I am terrified of pain – I don't think I could handle all the pain I would feel. I can avoid the vicissitudes and pain of life by staying behind my walls.
>
> If you want me to realize my pain you must take me into realms I am exquisitely vulnerable to. Could you lead me through it without my destruction? The risks are massive and desperate.

Jo was referred to me a little over ten years ago, when she was aged 21. She presented as a small frightened figure, obviously intelligent, a student of a profession involving scientific work. Her family were originally from Jamaica, but she had lived in England since she was aged 2.

Jo's questionnaire

Some of what she wrote in her questionnaire before seeing me was as follows. It conveys the frightening fragmentation and fluidity of her experience, as well as her essential loneliness:

> I feel so unhappy – I think I am always full of grief – yesterday I didn't know where I was coming home – I just wandered into the road – everything was breaking up – all the outside hours, talking to people, it is someone else giving a performance – I give people the responses I believe they want to hear – or else I am reckless and do stupid things, like wanting to shout at the boss – I always have visions of violence in my head – sometimes I dream of cutting my throat in front of an invisible audience – it seems to be the only communication possible between them and me – inside my head I am screaming – and always despising my actions, ugliness, stupidity – I will sit on the bus and see myself pushing broken glass behind my eyes to get at the blackness in my head – I am pouring out blood to please the something unknown – I want to explode with rage and curl up in a bundle in a dark corner and fade away . . . I think I have always felt like this . . . I cannot continue my life the way it has been these past few years – I cannot keep it controlled or hidden anymore.

'They might hear'

In the reception area Jo would hide behind a pot plant. During her early sessions she would never look at me, but would gaze at the ground and would speak almost inaudibly and cry continually. It was extremely difficult to obtain any coherent account of her problems or their history. One day she remarked, 'It's difficult to talk because they might hear what I am saying' – her first allusion to the internal figures whom she experienced as controlling her mind – and whom she eventually told me were called the 'Outside People'. She gave the impression of an internal police state, with listening devices in every room.

Jo took to sending me letters frequently. Initially these contained accounts of her difficulties at work and other areas of her life, expressing distress which, by and large, was within the realm of normal human experience. One day there was a marked change in their content. Now they were full of florid psychotic fantasies, going on for pages. These might include grandiose ideas of being the son of God, or of having a message for the world, or ideas of extreme self-denigration, such as that she was so worthless that she deserved to die. When I talked to her about these letters and their contents it was clear that the change had not been in her mental state, but in her finding the courage to communicate her psychosis to me.

Perceptual overload

Jo's perceptual world was incoherent and overwhelming. She often appeared to lack the capacity to filter and organize the perceptual components of her experience. Her field of consciousness seemed to sprawl chaotically, as if unregulated by any function of attention. This seemed to be the case especially if she was anxious or stressed. The most confusing objects in her world were human beings, visually complex entities that moved and made noises. When faced with another person she would become distracted by details – the sound of their voice, the movements of their body, the colour of their clothes, etc. She would 'see' the sounds coming out of a person's mouth, the words making pictures in the air. However, she would be frightened to look into a person's eyes because she might disappear into them – this was the reason she avoided looking at me for a long time. Perceptual stimulation often appeared violently intrusive for her – for example, a clock in my room that made a loud tick every minute would cause her to jerk as if she had been hit.

Not surprisingly, it turned out that she preferred relationships with silent inanimate objects – such as a radiator. She eventually explained to me that a radiator would be unintrusive and accepting – it would simply be a radiator and not require anything of her, whilst she, in turn, could accept it as being a radiator. The two of them would 'radiate' loving acceptance of each other.

Dismantling the perceptual world

The calm acceptance offered by the radiator would contrast particularly with the high voltage emotional encounters with her mother, whom Jo experienced as somewhat volatile and unpredictable, and liable to bombard her with (well-intentioned) criticism. Jo described to me how she would react to these sensory and affective onslaughts by dissociating, becoming very withdrawn affectively (derealization) and *dismantling* her perception, so that her mother would then appear alien, distant and reduced to an incoherent pattern of movement, shape, colour and sound. In this state of dismantled perception, Jo would feel very calm. Having detached herself, Jo would then immerse herself in what she called her 'dreaming', which was an awake state in which she gave herself completely over to psychotic fantasy – perhaps imagining that her skin was being transformed by a process she called 'holy plastifixion' and believing that she had become the son of God.

It has seemed to me that for Jo the dismantling of her perceptions of the other, combined with dissociation, are more prominent defences than projection, although the latter is often given prominence in psycho-analytic accounts of schizophrenia.

Over the years we have come to appreciate with increasing clarity how her active psychotic states are always a response to some situation of stress – usually involving either her mother or pressure at her work. The link will have been lost to her, of course, but it is usually possible to trace back to the precipitating stress. When she is not under stress she may appear very well, with no sign of active psychosis. I have come to think of her schizophrenia as a potential which could be activated in response to stress but would remain latent when the stress was not present – a vulner-ability to react schizophrenically to stress.

Fears of encountering ambivalence

Although finding relationships with other people extremely problematic, confusing and often hurtful, Jo does maintain strong affective attachments, with her family, with certain friends and with me as her psychotherapist. However, she is inclined, as she puts it, to conduct her 'social life on the phone'. At one time she was in the habit of getting in from work and immediately phoning members of her family and a friend. Eventually, all of these, with varying degrees of tact, let her know that her continual and lengthy phone calls were intrusive and unwelcome. She described to me how she would pick up the phone, dial the number, ask a few polite questions about the other person, and then leave them to continue the conversation whilst she drifted off into a reverie. In this way she could feel in some kind of anchoring link to another person while at the same time retreating to her autistic inner world. When I pointed out that in this behaviour she was not taking any account of the experience of the other person, she was very shocked and mortified, and said she had not thought about that aspect. She then added that she never does think about the other person's mind. When asked why this might be, she replied that she thought it was because she was afraid to discover that the other person hated her – a point that can be related to the failures of mentalization and 'theory of mind' discussed by Fonagy and Target (1996a; 1996b).

This anxiety clearly related to her fear of her mother's ambivalence towards her. She longed to please her mother and evoke her love, but feared she would instead be subject to a barrage of hostility. Consequently she would anxiously monitor her mother's moods. One positive result of the years of therapy is that Jo has acquired some capacity to observe and evaluate her mother's personality more objectively.

Ambivalence towards reality

Jo's experience of her mother's ambivalence towards her is mirrored by her own ambivalence towards sanity. She referred to her 'intense fighting ambivalence' in relation to her psychosis and once remarked that in an ideal world she would be able to be sane and mad at the same time. With simple clarity she has often described the coexistence of a part of her mind that is oriented towards the reality shared with others whilst another part is engaged with an entirely alternative world of psychotic dreaming. Her emergence from psychosis has been partial, fluctuating and pervaded with pain and dread. Relationships with others frequently subject her to humiliation or bewilderment. She will venture out timidly into the world of her fellow human beings, but will shrink back into psychosis when impinged upon painfully – like a shell creature withdrawing sharply when poked. As she once ruefully put it, 'This reality is hard like steel.'

Jo shows a fundamental preference for psychotic solutions to mental and emotional problems. These are based on evasion of reality. For example, during a period when she was worried about her financial situation and the security of her mortgage, she avoided opening her mail and allowed herself to become quite uncertain about her income and outgoings. More generally it is apparent how she uses her organs of perception as sources of aesthetic pleasure rather than information. Thus she might enjoyably lose herself in perceptual sensation and private reverie, disregarding the *information* component of sensory data – rather as if a motorist were to become lost in the aesthetic qualities of the traffic light to the extent that its function as a signal is lost. Or she might settle on a solution based on concrete thinking, false analogy and mistaking part for the whole. For example, one day she told me excitedly of her plan to cut off all her hair; she explained that if her hair was sleek and sharp, then her thoughts would become clear and ordered as well. She was puzzled and disappointed that I did not share her view about this. Eventually it became clear that her excited idea of cutting her hair off was an attempt at a manic solution to having felt hurt and humiliated by a relative.

Part of what can make Jo's day-to-day experience so agonizing is precisely the coexistence of sane and psychotic points of view. She has told me how she can be in the grip of a completely mad idea, believing it to be utterly true in one part of her mind, whilst at the same time, in another part of her mind, knowing it to be false. For example, she described to me an occasion when she was driving her car and became convinced there was a time bomb in it and was terrified; she kept slowing

down to listen for the ticking. I asked what she would have said if a
policeman had stopped her because of her erratic driving – would she
have explained she thought there was a bomb in her car? She replied that
she certainly would not have communicated this because it was a *private*
idea.

Painful interactions with others

Jo has often described her experience of the world of other people as being
as if everyone else is engaged in a dance, of which she is not part, and they
are engaged in a form of communication which she does not understand. It
is clear that she has difficulty reading body language, nonverbal cues, and
emotional nuance. Instead she would like to resort to her own private sign
language. She will sometimes describe her years of terrifying dread, humiliation and loneliness particularly during her childhood and teenage years.
One horrifying incident has stuck in her memory. Her class at school had
been learning about people's need for personal space. Sadistically recognizing Jo's sensitivity, a group of them gathered around her after the lesson
and drew closer and closer, poking her and mocking. She dissociated. Such
experiences have contributed to her view of herself as an alien.

A more recent occasion when Jo was worried about participating in a
social event gave us the opportunity to examine some of her difficulties in
this area. We managed to clarify how she is inclined to use words as a barrier
between herself and others rather than as a means of communicating and
linking with others. To this end she would talk continuously, regardless of
whether what she was saying was relevant or made much sense. Her fear
was that she might otherwise be invaded by others in the spaces between
the words. However, she would have some awareness that she was misusing
words and not following the usual rules of conversation; this would lead her
into increasing panic. She would respond to her panic by talking more and
more frantically, resulting in a discharge of words that might not relate at all
to the ongoing conversation. When I put to her the possibility that she need
not put so much energy into talking continuously but instead could focus
on listening to others, she expressed genuine surprise at this novel idea. She
explained that she had focused so much on the aspect of her own performance in talking that she had given no thought to the related task of
listening to others.

Porous boundaries

Jo experiences herself as in continual danger of invasion by others or of
merger into her surrounding environment. Sensory stimulation, such as
the sound of a clock ticking in my room, can penetrate her violently. She

fears physical contact with others because her skin might blend with that of the other person. The idea of sexual activity terrifies her because she is afraid that she would become confused with the other person, both psychologically and physically. She regards her genitals as a source of intense disgust and dread. Bodily orifices are frightening holes, out of which she might fall, or into which others might invade. Sometimes she expresses a wish to seal up her vagina, perhaps with a hot iron, and make herself like a Barbie doll.

The fragile ego

Jo's dread of sexuality appears to be one example of a wider category of fears of her ego being overwhelmed. Strong affect of any kind is experienced as a danger. This applies not only to the affects usually associated with anxiety, derived from sexuality and aggression, but also those that might appear more benign and pleasurable. For example, before going on a holiday she complained of wanting to fall asleep all the time; it became clear that she was retreating to sleep because of her fear of being overwhelmed by her excitement.

Continually bombarded by sensory and affective stimulation, Jo's ego has difficulty in maintaining its coherence and integrity. She lives in dread of chaos.

Almost certainly this reflects a constitutional deficiency, a subtle neurological abnormality. Because she cannot contain her affects and emotional conflicts, and cannot therefore generate neurotic solutions, which would leave the ego intact, Jo has to resort to psychotic solutions involving compromise of the ego's integrity and function.

The reconstituted world: the Outside People

Jo's descriptions of continual experiences of emotional and sensory bombardment suggest that she has struggled throughout her life against the threat of being overwhelmed and driven into mental chaos and incoherence. One of her recurrent defences has been to dissociate and dismantle her perceptual world – i.e. she detaches herself emotionally and takes apart her perceptual experience so that it is rendered into its separate sensory components.

Whilst this is effective in dealing with psychological overload, it leaves her objectless – utterly alone and lost in psychic space. To be objectless is probably unbearable. Therefore, Jo has what she calls her 'Outside People'. These are her internal controllers, figures whom she envisages as sitting around the back of her head and whom she hears as hallucinatory voices. Although frequently hostile and denigrating towards her, Jo regards these voices as her friends. She states that she cannot imagine life without them and that they have been with her as long as she can remember.

The Outside People seem to be dedicated to drawing Jo towards psychosis and death. To this end they employ threats, lies and seduction. They attempt to undermine her relationships with actual people, especially with me, and offer her an idealized image of madness. If I challenge or disagree with the views or activities of the Outside People, Jo becomes very frightened, like a child who is encouraged to stand up to a bully, but who fears retaliation when the protective adult has left.

Jo has emphasized that the Outside People are a fundamental fact of her mental world. She has told me she regards them as analogous to vertebrae – without them she would be formless, like jelly. Moreover, she has emphasized the hopelessness of disagreeing with them – as she put it: 'Like the Pope, they are infallible.' Truly these figures are the propagandists for, and the guardians of, her alternative psychotic world based on opposition to sanity and life.

Management of shame and the regulation of grandiose excitement

On one occasion, Jo talked of her pleasure at finding she could solve a number of items in a book of intellectual puzzles. She felt reassured she was not stupid. She spoke of her hope of discovering that she had a creative or intellectual gift of some kind. All of this seemed quite ordinary and natural – an innocuous 'grandiose self' looking for mirroring and acceptance from the therapist. Next session, she reported that as soon as she had walked out of my room she had been subjected to a barrage of internal abuse from her Outside People. 'Who does it think it is?' they had begun, with typical scorn and menace. They seem consistently to aim to undermine her, destroy her confidence, and instruct her to kill herself, but they appear to be particularly provoked into their destructive activity whenever Jo becomes at all spontaneous, lively or hopeful or mildly grandiose.

I asked Jo if she had any idea why her Outside People hated her so much. She said it was that they hated her because she was still alive. I asked her to explain more. She said that they told her she deserved to die because she had done such awful things. I asked what these awful things were. In reply she spoke of her sense of innumerable experiences of shame – of repeated experiences of feeling socially inept and incompetent, of feeling *stupid*. Some of the most savage accusations by the voices were that Jo had been 'showing off' and 'making a fool' of herself. Thus it became clear that her destructive inner voices are shame-based expressions of rage against herself for her incompetence. Some degree of hatred of the self is an inherent component of shame – unlike guilt, there can be no reparation for shame – its cure depends upon empathy from others. In Jo's case the shame and ensuing self-hatred was particularly intense – and because of its intensity had to be split off in the form of her hallucinatory internal voices.

Jo's shaming voices drew some of their content from the shaming and critical voice of Jo's actual mother, who, in Jo's image of her, seemed to be continually preoccupied with Jo's shortcomings. Thus Jo's Outside People could be regarded as a psychotic form of identification with the aggressor. By using the emotional weapons of the mother against herself, and by concocting these bizarre internal objects out of bits of self and other, she could attempt to regulate her own potential grandiose excitement, as well as other affects.

The emergence of sexuality and aggression

Over the years, Jo has become more aware that she is capable of sexual sensation and desire. At one time she believed that she did not possess any sexuality and that she was indeed an alien. She would complain of 'black lightning' and pains emanating from her vagina. I explained to her that this was probably her experience of sexual feelings that she was attempting to ward off. Now, several years later, she increasingly is curious about sexual desire and even allows herself to watch erotic scenes on TV films. However, she remains extremely cautious about experiencing sexual arousal. She reports that sometimes she has dreams in which she is beginning to experience sexual arousal; she awakes in anxiety and experiences a pain in her vagina. The thought of herself engaging in any sexual activity, including masturbation, still fills her with dread, however. She imagines such experiences to be dangerously overstimulating, threatening chaos and confusion.

A later and even more anxiety-evoking awareness has been of her potential for anger and aggression. One day Jo remarked that she had been startled to notice a sudden intense feeling of rage when another motorist drove by too closely and clipped her wing mirror. This provided an appropriate opening for exploration of her anger. As she thought about this she concluded that she does not often experience violent feelings, but does observe, as if from a distance, violent thoughts and images appearing in her mind; she does not readily associate these with actual feelings. However, she has become more able to acknowledge intense and primitive violent rage – expressed in fantasies of conducting a mass killing of people at her place of work. These fantasies cause her anxiety. She commented: 'Sometimes I think I am about to get a violent thought about my mother but then I stop myself.'

Jo described how she uses thoughts of her therapist to calm herself when she experiences violent thoughts or feelings. She would think 'Dr Mollon, Dr Mollon' and this would soothe her. The letter that I quoted at the beginning indicates her terror of the consequences of a full encounter with her potential rage.

Jo's use of the therapist

Early in the psychotherapeutic work, it became apparent that Jo looked to me for help in clarifying her thoughts, sorting out her psychotic confusion, and in regulating her emotions. She would appear immensely grateful for these functions. She once remarked: 'No matter how confused I feel when I come in here, I always go away knowing what I am thinking.' She would also comment with surprise and appreciation on how calm I would appear and how soothing she would find the consulting room. I noticed that intuitively I would make my comments and interpretations short and as clear as possible – trying to compose well-formed sentences before I began to speak. Often my remarks to her would be attempts to translate her psychotic contents and processes into more ordinary and understandable human phenomena, and to present perspectives that were anxiety-reducing. She would appear immensely relieved that she could be understood by another human being – and hence that she was not an alien.

Another crucial function that I think she has sought from me is that of supporting her against the seductive pull of madness. This came starkly into focus quite early in our work. One day she turned up and excitedly asked me if I would go away with her and live in Iceland. She presented this as a serious proposition which she regarded as a solution to her problems and she explained that she had enough money in her building society to pay for our journey. I gently but firmly told her this was an idea that did not take account of reality – and explained why. In addition I said I thought she was trusting me with some of her private thoughts in the hope that I could help her distinguish what was sane from what was mad. This incident seemed to increase her trust in me considerably.

One phenomenon that used to become apparent quite commonly is that she would confuse the actual therapist with an internal version. The internal one would agree with her psychotic reasoning, or even with the views of her Outside People. She would express amazement when she discovered that the internal and external 'Dr Mollon' were different and not in agreement with each other. This confusion no longer seems to happen.

It will be obvious from what I have described that Jo has not endeavoured to use the therapy to play out a transference based on historical infantile conflicts and passions. Instead, what has been much more apparent is her use of me as a selfobject in the service of regulating her mental state – seeking functions such as soothing, the regulation of arousal, the provision of empathy, the clarification of mental processes, and the distinction between sanity and madness. I think it is the successful avoidance of historical and infantile transference and passion that has enabled Jo to find the therapy supportive rather than overwhelming.

I am in essential agreement with Kohut here. Although he did not write extensively about psychosis, he did indicate how there are natural lines of healing which do not always involve returning to the areas of deepest mental pain or chaos. He comments:

> . . . I cannot imagine that an individual would submit himself to the dissolution of defensive structures that have protected him for a lifetime and voluntarily accept the unspeakable anxieties accompanying what must seem to him to be the task of facing a prepsychological state that had remained chaotic because the selfobject milieu in early life lacked the empathic responsiveness that would have organized the child's world and maintained his innate self-confidence.
>
> (Kohut, 1984: 8–9)

Vulnerable patients will naturally avoid the threat of an irreversible regressive descent into the stage of the fragmented self – which Kohut regarded as the fixation point of schizophrenic psychosis.

Summary of the schizophrenic process

At the heart of Jo's psychosis lies a seething whirlpool of mental chaos, the fragments of affective, sensory, perceptual and intellectual debris that make no sense – the background hiss of schizophrenia, threatening continually to engulf her – with contributions from both constitutional and environmental sources. Lacking the ability to filter and repress adequately, she encounters a continual perceptual catastrophe and is able neither to be properly asleep nor fully awake, but lives in a permanent waking dream. Faced with an overwhelming world that bombards, bewilders and humiliates, Jo responds by dismantling it further.

Jo's dilemma is to be balanced precariously between the pain of coherence, attachment and relationships, on the one hand, and the dread of disintegration and chaos, on the other. Her inner psychotic world, organized around her Outside People, is a halfway house between ultimate chaos and the agony of relationships and shared reality.

Healing the soul

When I asked Jo's permission to write about her, she readily agreed and began to reflect upon the years of work. She remarked:

> I have heard it said that people with psychosis do not respond well to psycho-logical therapy – but for me it has been the best thing that ever happened to me. It seems to me that drugs help the symptoms but psychotherapy heals the soul. For me it has been like being reborn – like re-examining my life in a way that restores.

Depression: the thwarted self

> . . . classical analysis discovered the depression of the child in the adult and self psychology discovered the depression of the adult in the depths of the child . . . the depression of a lonely child is based in the dim realization that the future will not be fulfilled.
>
> (Kohut, 1981: 215–16)

Kohut indicated that the positive affective colouring of the experience of self and other – a healthy good mood and an optimistic outlook – is based on childhood support from caregivers experienced as selfobjects. Through the provision of optimum degrees of affirmation and affective response, the child grows up to feel a confidence in being understood, in being accepted and lovable, and of being able to manage the emotions evoked by whatever adverse circumstances he or she has to face. Such a person will feel committed to life, despite its potential pains, disappoint-ments and suffering. A predisposition to depression, by contrast, may reflect a sense that potential talents, ambitions and ideals have not been supported – that life has not been encouraged. An episode of acute depression may ensue when a person feels that his or her potential has been thwarted or betrayed and cannot be fulfilled in either the present or the future.

Kohut comments:

> There is something very frightening as an adult – and we know the most about late middle age – when there is a sense of not fulfilling one's basic program . . . when we go back into the past in analysis we are attempting to recognize the program that was laid down – we call that the nuclear self.
>
> (1981: 218)

Depression and death

Depression and death are closely related. The depressed person may long for death. He or she may feel dead – and may look only half alive. Life no longer holds pleasure or hope – indeed it may be only the thought of death that brings any pleasure. Sexual desire may all but disappear. The melancholic is slowed up, lacking aliveness and spontaneity. Even if she or he does not succumb to suicide, actual illness may be more likely in the wake of depression. Something has happened to the life force in the state of depression – Thanatos has overcome Eros (Freud, 1920).

Some degree of depression is a natural response to experiences of failure and loss (Bleichmar, 1996). The severely suicidally depressed person seems to experience a sense of failure that pervades the whole of their life – as if feeling that their life project itself is a failure, with ensuing rage about this. My hypothesis is that such people have indeed felt early in their development that their life project has in some profound way been thwarted or derailed – the nuclear self has come to grief. Sometimes we find this with people whose mother died early in their life – the rug being pulled out from beneath their feet, so to speak, leaving a profound sense that life cannot be trusted – and, crucially, that the life force within cannot be trusted. Or a similar response may be illustrated with those who come to feel that they can never win parental love and acceptance – decades may be spent, unconsciously endeavouring to succeed in activities that might bring the reward of the longed for love, only to result in depression when it becomes apparent that these too will fail – 'What more do I have to do?' might be the unconscious or even conscious thought. The failure of oedipal love may also give rise to a deep sense of being forever unworthy – later love objects may fail to satisfy the craving for self-esteem because they cannot erase the belief that the first love brought rejection. Of course, the female faces a double jeopardy in this respect – having to deal first with rejection of an exclusive relationship with the mother, and then with the further disappointment from the father.

Miss C – abandonment and rage

Miss C, a depressed young woman of 22, described a childhood in which she had felt rejected by both parents. She had been aware of parental discord, but had believed her mother's assurances that if they separated she would go to live with her mother. In fact, her mother left her father and Miss C for another man. In his turmoil, her father then retreated to a hippy commune in Wales. Miss C did go with him, but felt she did not belong in her father's new world. In addition to her depression, she presented with problems of promiscuity (with both sexes) and drug abuse.

In the transference she related to me ragefully, seeking evidence that I cared about her but appearing convinced that I hated her and would abandon her. She would attempt to engage my attention in various ways – by behaving seductively and offering herself to me sexually, or by shouting at me, or by threatening self-harm, or by attempting to be entertaining. She appeared to perceive me as essentially failing to keep her in mind – and clearly considered that, as with her parents, what moved me most was sexuality (a common assumption amongst people whose parents' marriage has been shattered by sexual desires for others). This general assumption also applied to her other engagements with people, as illustrated in her promiscuity. She had in fact had a sexual relationship with a doctor she had seen at another hospital.

In a manner typical of the depressed states of people with borderline personality disorder, Miss C would feel rage and hatred because she expected to be rejected – but then she would feel so full of hatred that she believed herself to be unlovable – and thus her expectation of rejection would be increased. Through this paranoid process, her rage would fuel her expectation of rejection, which in turn would fuel her hatred – and so on.

Miss C clearly felt that her desires for secure attachment were doomed to be forever thwarted. Nevertheless she did not give up hope – continually forming intense attachments to unavailable men; if she managed to seduce the man she would rapidly lose interest and her idealization of him would collapse. To assuage her original injury she had to win a lover who was unavailable, like her father and her mother, but if she succeeded she would quickly realize that he was not her father (or mother), and so the unconscious search would begin again.

At one point, following the ending of one relationship, Miss C described a kind of frenzy of promiscuity. She gave the impression of being in a state of continual sexual activity, in actuality and in phantasy. When I commented on how this contrasted with her previously expressed view that she needed a quiet period free of relationships, she recognized that she was struggling frantically to avoid having to face her feelings of depression regarding the relationship that had ended. She conveyed that she could not contain and digest her own feelings, but was compelled instead to distract herself by immersion in intense sexual scenarios with multiple partners. As we explored this pattern, it became clear that what she really longed for was to be able to talk to someone about how she was feeling – but she felt that on the whole this was not available since she believed that men are essentially interested only in sex. Thus, in lieu of a relationship of mind, she resorted to relationships of body – but she could see that these provided relief only for the duration of the activity. This mirrored the earlier stages of the trans-ference, in which she had felt she must engage me in some kind of sexual activity since she had no concept that I could hold her in mind and think about her. She went on to say that sometimes she had thoughts that she would like a sexual relationship with a woman; she felt that she wanted a more gentle and subtle kind of tactile contact than she found in sexual activity with men. I commented that this sequence in her thoughts suggested that the roots of her current motivations lay in an early childhood desire to be held, caressed and talked to by her mother, while also having her mother hold her in mind and provide thoughtful attention. Miss C responded enthusiastically to this interpretation and talked of what she had been told of her mother's post-natal depression and withdrawal during the early months of her life.

Clearly, Miss C felt that she was hated – originally by her mother who did not hold her physically or mentally, and then by every other person with whom she had any kind of emotional relationship. Her rage about this coloured her images of self and other (Jacobson, 1971; Kernberg, 1975), resulting in a variety of destructive activities towards herself, and her own body, as well as vengeful scenarios in which she would triumph over others. In such states of mind, she could envisage only hopelessly repeating patterns of pain and sado-masochism. What evoked her gratitude in therapy were thoughtful interpretations, which revealed and demonstrated to her the possibility of mentalization (Fonagy, 1997; Fonagy, Steele, Steele et al., 1991; Fonagy and Target, 1996a; 1996b)

Love versus autonomy

Sometimes the realization of failure to win parental love gives rise to pathological solutions, which contain a logic of eventual self-destruction. I am thinking of a woman, Eileen, who, having consistently failed to feel loved by her parents, aimed to create a false self (Winnicott, 1960; Mollon, 1993) based on an image of strength, always coping, never showing vulnerability. This became the basis of her sense of self-worth. She was unable to mourn any losses, because to do so would be to acknowledge emotional pain and vulnerability. She was able to sustain this false self for several decades. Later in life, her capacities began to fail. Following a fall she began to suffer fainting fits. She experienced panic because she could not control these. She arrived at a conscious decision that she must take her own life. She felt this was the only *strong* thing to do. She did not know how to be vulnerable and needy and still have self-esteem. Once she had determined upon this 'solution' of taking her own life, she felt wonderfully tranquil. She felt that this act of taking her life would be an assertion of autonomy – no one could hurt her again.

Eileen's false self was a tyrannical dictator, ruling her emotional life with a rod of iron. This is characteristic of false selves – once created they become tyrannical, suppressing the indigenous population of the mind. A false self is inherently autocratic – and opposed to psychoanalytic exploration. The false self tries to maintain a fixed view of self and the world. Thus the negative cognitions of the depressed person, challenged by cognitive therapists, are often clung to with astonishing rigidity and tenacity – as if the person is faithfully married to the belief system that has caused them so much pain.

The situation I have found common in states of sustained severe depression is a background of struggles over autonomy (Arieti and Bemporad, 1980). As a child the patient has felt that his or her own development has to be sacrificed in order to meet the needs or desires of a parent. The child learns that assertions of autonomy or anger are punished by withdrawal of love. It is often the mother who, in this way, exerts extensive control over the mind and behaviour of the child who later becomes the depressed adult. But the patient may be relatively unaware of this – and also unconscious of the extent of his or her rage at the mother. The need to assert autonomy and the rage at the thwarting of this need are both repressed; rage is continually provoked by the conditional nature of the parental love, but expressions of rage or criticism of the parent are felt to threaten love even more – so the rage can only be turned in on the self or into the body. A false self is developed based on compliance with parental (particularly the mother's) desires. The compliance is typically generalized, so that the person appears superficially obliging and pleasant in their general relationships and interactions. The problem is that the false self and the more natural self are then at war.

Parents may empathically mirror and thereby affirm and facilitate aspects of the child's development – but parents desire as well as mirror. Indeed the parents may desire that the child mirror *them*. Instead of the parents functioning as selfobjects for the child, the child becomes the selfobject for the parents.

The child who will become the depressed adult has not felt recognized and accepted as an individual. Instead, he or she is inhabited by the fantasy of the mother. This failure of external mirroring may be repeated as an *internal* repudiation of self. In general, we treat ourselves (and later our own children) as we have been treated – turning passive into active (G. Klein, 1976). The natural spontaneous self is eclipsed by the false self of compliance which assumes the dominant position. The natural self is imprisoned and suppressed – and forms a hatred of the false self.

By this point the person's mind and self has become a house divided – self against self. The defensive self has turned against the natural self, whom it regards as the enemy.

The alienating mirror

Jo's Outside People, fabricated concoctions of self and other, which intimidate from within, are a psychotic version of common phenomena. Many people, during the course of their childhood and adolescence, turn away from their more natural and unselfconscious way of being and develop a false self, based on a preoccupation with image, with how one is perceived by others, and an endeavour to present in a way that would meet with approval, liking, admiration or respect. Lacan's (1949) concept of the *mirror phase* is a wonderful metaphor for this profound alienation from the natural self that is thought by some to be inherent in human development as the infant enters the social world – the child shifts from being moved by urges from inside, to being captivated by the image 'out there'. Whilst Lacan does seem to give importance to the actual glass mirror, this can clearly also be understood as the mirror of the human community, the images, roles and expectations offered to us from outside. The false self becomes concerned with its place in relation to others, its status, achievements, possessions. With this fateful dislocation from the natural self, there is (to varying extents, depending on the individual) an alienation from the spontaneity of the life force. Indeed the values of the false self – power, control, possessions, status, image – are all essentially antilife, necrophilic (Fromm, 1965).

Whilst writers such as Winnicott (in Britain) and Kohut (in the USA) have emphasized the idea of mirroring as the affirming responsiveness of the mother's face, facilitating the development of the authentic and spontaneous self, it was Lacan's dark genius to see how the mirror of the community of others can be profoundly alienating – taking us hostage from ourselves.

The ubiquitous false self

Winnicott's original outline of the 'false self' (1960) suggests an organization that is imposed on top of a person's natural tendencies and which is opposed to those natural tendencies – and, moreover, which consists of an image based on what is felt to be of significance to others (principally the mother). It is an image of the self, derived from others – a 'looking glass self' (Cooley, 1902) – which is nevertheless believed to be true – it thereby causes a loss of awareness of natural feelings and desires.

What then is meant by a 'true self'? In fact this term is rarely heard these days. As a concept, it is usually considered too reified in its connotations – a notion that seems to miss the point that all human selves are developed in the context of relationships and are shaped by relationships. Kohut's concept of the 'nuclear self', however, recognizes both autonomy and the fact that the self is constructed through relationships. My own preference is to fall back on Groddeck's idea of the 'It', which formed the inspiration for Freud's (1923) term 'id'. This connotes the way in which we are lived by, driven by, inspired by, some force, a *source* within, which is before and beyond our sense of 'I' – '. . . man's life is not ruled by his ego, but by an Unknown Force, the It . . .' (Groddeck, 1929: 147).

The problem with the seemingly simple concept of 'false self' is that it belies the fact that *all* identities are in a sense false, insofar as we believe them to be true. This is one of the disconcerting realities of human life. We do not know what is 'natural' as opposed to culture-specific in human behaviour. Our identities are constructed out of the bits and pieces of cultural roles, images, and symbols – as well as the desires of the mother, which are themselves culturally shaped (e.g. to be a certain kind of baby, daughter, son, etc.). These ingredients of identity are given to us from outside – the distorting mirror of our families and culture. The individual is captivated by this illusory and fabricated identity, this psychic costume – and mistakenly says 'This is I.'

Once this illusion has been embraced, people will go to extraordinary lengths to protect their false perception of self. Death of the body is often preferred to surrender of the concocted identity. One need only think of Northern Ireland or other places of religious and cultural wars. Lacan (1948) pointed out that insofar as others have contributed to the very substance of a person's identity, then identity itself is paranoiac in structure – the paranoid person's 'delusions' of influence are only a more explicit expression of the way that we are constructed by others. This fundamental paranoia at the very heart of our self may result in a continual need to project the intrusive control that has formed us and which we mistake as our own self.

This is illustrated by a depressed patient I described in *The Fragile Self* – Mrs A. Her experiences of her mother, whom she described as having been 'committed to trying to get me to think the same way that she does', appeared to have contributed to the development of an internal mother who was hostile to her separation-individuation and to her making contact with her own spontaneous feelings. Thus she feared that being honest and expressing authentic feelings in her therapy would lead to internal punishment (feelings of 'guilt' and impulses to harm herself).

However, she appeared to perceive her identification with her mother's hostility towards her own self *as if it were her true self*. She would vigorously ward off the therapist's attempts to explore her feelings, protesting that she felt that what she called the 'deeply formed' parts of herself should not be altered. It appeared that she feared the therapist would want to change her into someone else – but the self she was attempting to preserve was in its very structure determined by others and was inherently opposed to her more authentic potential self.

The false nature of identity is revealed most vividly in states of Dissociative Identity Disorder (MPD: Mollon, 1996; Walker and Antony-Black, 1999), where alternative personality states take executive control at different moments. In the more florid forms of this condition, one might encounter several 'personalities' during one session, each with a separate identity and character. These quite obviously are fabrications (albeit 'believed-in' fabrications) woven out of imagination – and driven by the necessity of severe interpersonal trauma. For example, during an assessment, a patient – let us call her Alice – suddenly switched posture, announced that she was Jane and explained that she had decided to step in and help out because Alice was having such a difficult time; Jane, unlike the depressed and subdued Alice, was flirtatious, sophisticated and confident; she 'explained' that she had different parents from Alice and that her own parents lived in France. Part of the fascination and terror that multiple personality disorder tends to evoke may be because this condition reminds us of the ubiquitous confabulations in all our identities.

What is the alternative to this fabricated identity, fashioned from culturally available materials and images? Can there be a pre-cultural noble savage, whose behaviour would tell us how human beings naturally are? No human being can escape human culture, unless he/she be psychotic – and even then the content of the psychosis is woven from the unravelled threads of culture. However, in health the natural spontaneous life is expressed within the cultural forms available – and it is this balance between It and culture that defines health. Too much externally derived form and image thwarts the It, the life force within; too much unrestrained It produces something from which others recoil, whether it is regarded as autism, psychosis, gross narcissism, or psychopathy. Part of the reason we value art is that the It can be given expression within a culturally available form.

This can also be illustrated by analogy with responses to the Rorschach inkblot test. These responses are evaluated by the assessor in terms of the components such as the balance between form and colour that make up the perception. Too much response on the basis of colour, without regard for form, would be indicative of uncontrolled emotionality and impulsivity; too much attention to form, with no response on the basis of colour, would reflect a grey depressed stance devoid of emotional life.

Perhaps people may seem closest to the It when they are engaged in the most fundamental and biologically determined activities – e.g. breastfeeding a baby, smiling with a baby, making love, orgasm – but a moment's reflection will suggest that even these may contain culturally-specific shaping.

All identities are fabricated and are illusory – and yet they are necessary. To be without an identity is to be in a state of psychic agony, a mutilation of one's humanity. People's mental equilibrium becomes disturbed at points when identity is challenged – adolescence, mid-life, unemployment, retirement, etc. Earlier societies may have offered simpler and more stable identities. One might be a baker or a farmer or a miner – all roles rooted in tasks essential to life. These would be stable and clear – allowing a position of knowing who one was and one's place in the social world. Today the images, roles and tasks available in the cultural supermarket are changing rapidly. Identities are ephemeral, shifting, paper-thin – a source of inarticulate terror. And for many young people in the more desolate areas of society, there are no *viable* identities available – and thus no vehicles for the It, which then becomes powerfully destructive.

Robert

Robert is a depressed man of thirty. He is exceptionally preoccupied with the image he presents to other people. Interactions with others always feel to him like a performance. Consequently he dreads social events because he considers he has to be continually entertaining and interesting – and, understandably, he finds this exhausting. His concern with image is not confined to those whose opinion might be expected to matter to him. For example, he will sometimes quickly change the CD playing in his car if he sees people ahead on the pavement whom he suspects might be unimpressed with his choice of music. In his analysis, he endeavours to relinquish this concern with image and to be more genuinely himself since he has some awareness that this is a fundamental problem for him. Nevertheless, he finds himself preoccupied with thoughts about how I might view his clothes, his hair, his accessories (such as his mobile phone) and his political and social opinions. Moreover, on one occasion he spoke of fantasies that the pictures in my consulting room concealed secret microphones; this seemed to express a kind of Orwellian *1984* world in which all thought and behaviour is continually monitored by Big Brother, or in Robert's case, his mother.

Robert has felt himself to be dull and inhibited in most of his life. However, he contrasts this usual state of mind with a period some years ago when he was travelling and felt able to be much more spontaneous and alive. Implicitly, Robert's goal in analysis seems to be to reconnect with that natural life force within him.

During this period of liveliness and spontaneity, Robert had fallen in love with a Spanish girl. He had brought her home to see his parents. This had been a disastrous move. In the home environment with his parents he had reverted to his state of inhibition and preoccupation with image and with the approval of his peers and of his parents. His relationship with the Spanish girl rapidly deteriorated and she left him.

Robert's description of his family culture epitomized this preoccupation with image to an extreme degree. His mother, in particular, would frequently criticize him in terms of 'What would people think?' He would be discouraged from any display of spontaneity or exuberance.

At one point Robert became preoccupied with athletics and other sports. He noticed that if he played competitively against others, his performance would be significantly impaired, but if he played on his own, with no other person watching, his skill appeared very much greater. Concern with image and comparison with others clearly derailed his natural physical intelligence and skill.

He has also appeared anxious about his sexual performance and attributes, fearing girlfriends will compare him unfavourably with other lovers. On the other hand he describes a pattern of behaviour in which he would present himself to married or otherwise attached women, in an image of being a more gentle and sensitive man than their husband or partner – based no doubt on his oedipal endeavour to ingratiate himself with his mother, in rivalry with his father. The burden of this endeavour, successful though it may have been in part, is that he has felt he must try to be what his mother wanted, rather than to give expression to his more authentic inclinations. Being what his mother wanted seems to have meant inhibiting his sexual and aggressive impulses. His expressions of phallic strivings are followed by anxiety about retribution or disapproval. For example, he told me of driving his motorbike very fast – but then appeared anxious that I might be critical and antagonistic towards him. He spoke of his fear of 'cutting comments'. It seemed that he was afraid that his liveliness, his sexuality and his aggression might provoke a cutting and castrating retaliation. Therefore he has tended to settle for respectable social life, with periodic rebellions.[1]

---

[1] The role of insufficient oedipal engagement with the father in contributing to an uncertain sense of self has been explored at length in *The Fragile Self* (Mollon 1993). It is vital for the child's development that he or she be helped to accept that replacing the father and becoming the object of mother's desire is not an appropriate life goal.

In obtaining Robert's permission to publish this account, I offered to let him read the description above. He asked to do so, but then after reading the first couple of sentences handed it back in some anxiety. When we explored his reactions in the subsequent session, he articulated a fear that if he read the material he would identify with and *become* what I had written. He added that he did not like the name I had chosen for him, feeling that he was not a 'Robert'. After exploring the theme of names and their connotations for some minutes, he then told me that recently he had bought an expensive new car – a Jaguar. He had showed it to a friend, who had, to his pleasure, expressed appropriate admiration. However, he had felt dismayed when she had then commented, 'It suits you.' He feared that this meant he was seen as 'somebody who would drive a Jaguar' – and that he was therefore *defined* by his car.

Crucial themes are revealed clearly in this vignette. A name is given to the baby by the parents. The baby has no choice about this. He or she is not consulted about it by the parents (unlike the patient who is written about by the analyst). Although the given name is explicit, it is accompanied by a penumbra of *implicit* connotations, images and roles existing in the minds of the parents and wider society. These comprise the 'place' and identity to which the child is assigned. Here we find the alienating and imprisoning nature of language and culture – the person becomes defined and *confined* by the assigned identity. A baby is called 'Robert' and believes that is who he is. An inescapable feature of the human condition, the limiting effect on personality development of assigned identity seems more pronounced for some than for others. It may depend upon the capacity of the parents to recognize and accept the *unknown* potential of their child.

The dark night of the soul

A life built on image, on concern for social approval, on strivings for status and for the possessions that bring status, is like a tree torn from its roots and suspended in the air. Sooner or later it is likely to wither and die. Or it is like a military junta that ultimately must be overthrown from its illegitimate rule. The term 'mid-life crisis' is a relatively innocuous-sounding cliché that fails to convey the 'dark night of the soul' (Backhouse, 1988) when nothing seems to work anymore. All the previous means of seeking pleasure, security, reassurance and love now fail. The person feels utterly resourceless and helpless. This is a dangerous time. A person in a mid-life crisis may turn to drugs, alcohol, promiscuity, gambling, risk-taking and other forms of stimulation and distraction from the mounting despair and dread. Physical pain may be sought because it gives some evidence of being alive. Night-time may be terrifying, when the rest of the world is asleep, and when the distracting stimulations of the day and the evening are no longer available. Suicide may appear as a serious and welcome possibility at this time.

The urge to destroy the self in suicide is an expression of the rage against the false self which has usurped the person's life and potential. Image had replaced life – and now the image, the distorting mirror, must be smashed. There is a recognition of having been dislodged from life, from the source, set adrift and shipwrecked on a desert island of false goals and false gods. In fury there then may be an angry turning against life, the life-giving breast, the nipple, the mother, the heart. Death may be idealized as representing peace, the womb, a reunion with the loving mother of life who existed before the separation and eventual alienation. Moreover, to take one's life may appear as the ultimate assertion of autonomy and final despairing triumph of the self whose life energies have been thwarted.

In the severely depressed person, the Lacanian ego, the lie at the heart of the personality, has usurped the It. Instead of constructing an identity as a vehicle for the It – the life force – the demands of parents and the surrounding culture have been incorporated, like a Trojan horse, to conquer the It.

Therapy for depression

The task of psychoanalytic therapy for a person who has been imprisoned by a constructed self is not to enable him or her to live without a culturally determined identity – that would be impossible whilst living within a human society. However, one aim might be to facilitate an understanding of the origins and content of his or her constructed self in the images, desires, expectations and humiliations presented by the early environment. This is then to open up a realization that *all* such identities are fabricated rather than inherently real, and therefore can be changed – to enable the person to discover that there can be choice about values and goals, and modes of relating to others. In this way can a person find some degree of freedom from history and illusion. Through clearing the stranglehold of false self, the new life of the thwarted It – the unknown self – can begin to emerge, making possible more adaptive and creative ways of relating to others – of being a subject in relation to others who are also perceived as subjects.

An adolescent patient, who was beginning to emerge from her severe depression as a result of a lengthy period of psychotherapy, put this very simply. She said, 'For the last few years I have tried to be like other people or to be what I thought other people would like – but now I'm beginning to realize that I can be what I choose to be.' Succinctly she stated the reason for her depression and its solution.

Summary

Disintegration anxiety and the threat of mental chaos may be a core feature of schizophrenia. In Kohut's framework, schizophrenia may involve a regression to the stage of the fragmented self. A person suffering with schizophrenia may experience the perceptual world as overwhelming and incoherent. He or she may also live in dread of being overwhelmed by strong affect. As a defensive strategy, there may be a dismantling of this perceptual world, and a dissociation from emotion. An alternative psychotic world may then be created, fabricated from elements of self and other. This alternative world may contain strong controlling figures that are opposed to relationships of dependence with external others.

Depression and death are intimately connected. The depressed person may have felt that the selfobject supports necessary for the unfolding of their potential have been denied to them – with ensuing rage. This rage floods the representations of self and other. Failures to obtain selfobject support in childhood may give rise to the development of a tyrannical false self which provides internal structure, albeit of a pathological nature. The psyche becomes a house divided, false self opposed to the natural self. Psychological mirroring can be nurturing and affirming, but can also be alienating. A depressed person may have excessively identified with images and roles presented by others. The urge toward suicide may express a wish to destroy the false self. Psychoanalytic therapy can help a person to become more free of imposed identities and to evolve new and more satisfying ways of being a subject in relation to others as subjects – to discover intersubjectivity.

Chapter 9
The developmental neurobiology of the selfobject relationship[1]

> . . . attachment is, in essence, the right brain regulation of biological synchronicity between organisms.
>
> (Schore, 2000a: 11)

One of the remarkable findings of recent neurobiological explorations of infant–mother interactions is that the patterns of early attachment provide not only learning experiences but also affect the developing brain itself. Adverse selfobject experiences are in effect 'hard wired' into the brain, leading to chronic difficulties with affect regulation – and leaving a legacy of permanent vulnerabilities when the later adult is faced with emotional stress or pain. The mother's empathic attunement to her infant, now seen to be crucial to the regulation of the child's affect, is also recognized as playing a vital role in brain development (Schore, 1994). Indeed, Schore (2000a) has argued that 'the self-organization of the developing brain occurs in the context of a relationship with another self, another brain'. A period of brain growth spurt exactly overlaps the period of the formation of early attachment and intense emotional interaction with the mother during the first one and a half years of life (Schore, 2000a). Such observations give rise to the notion of *the social construction of the human brain*. In this way the developmental neurosciences are confirming Kohut's insights into the selfobject origins of the capacity to regulate affect. Moreover, one recent definition of attachment is 'the dyadic regulation of affect' (Sroufe, 1996) – a concept very close to that of the selfobject – reflecting the way in which the infant looks to the caregiver to assist in the modulation of affect, enhancing positive arousal and minimizing negative.

---

[1] This chapter is based predominantly upon Allan Schore's very substantial work of synthesizing psychoanalytic and neuroscience data (Schore, 1994). For a critical review of Schore's conclusions, see Nahum (1999).

By analogy, one could say that if early childhood is the emotional factory producing the later adult brain, then the selfobject experiences provide the 'factory settings' for crucial aspects of brain function. These settings may be very difficult to modify later.

Selfobject catastrophes

Schore gives a vivid illustration of how a noxious or anti-selfobject experience can result in catastrophic escalation of dysphoric affect (1994: 383–84). He quotes a study by Gaensbauer and Mrazek (1981) which describes a highly aroused angry infant in interaction with a mother who amplified her distress rather than offering soothing. The infant displayed tantrums and other expressions of anger during separation from the mother. Then, at reunion, the infant's anger actually increased. She moved initially towards the mother but then aggressively resisted being held. In response the mother teased and humiliated the infant. This frightened the child, resulting in an intensification of screaming, accompanied by running away and hitting and spitting. In turn the mother's response was further anger. Thus the mother, humiliated by her infant's rejection, reacted with rage, rejecting and teasing the infant in retaliation, thereby driving the child into an increasing state of hyper-arousal and explosions of rage. Schore notes that in later life a child subject to repeated experiences of that kind will become an adult whose relationships are extremely conflictual, needing constant reassurance, yet displaying clingy hostility which drives the other away, provoking the very abandonment that is feared, which then precipitates overwhelming rage. Obviously this is a description of an adult borderline personality disorder.

Instead of the soothing responses that the child requires, the interaction with the mother, in this example, generates further arousal. This is an anti-selfobject process. Such episodes, especially if repeated, will be registered in the brain, forming expectations that generate real neurochemical and physiological effects in both the brain itself and in the autonomic nervous system of the rest of the body.

Mother–infant attunement

From approximately 2 months of age, infant–mother interactions are rapid affect-laden interpersonal experiences which provide the infant with extensive emotional-cognitive information. The mother tends to follow the infant in mirroring and amplifying the latter's facial and vocal gestures. Synchrony develops between the interacting partners such that each develops an inner *psychophysiological* state similar to that of the other. In developing this synchrony, the mother must become attuned not so much to the outward display of the child, but to his or her internal state as reflected in the more overt behaviours. This attunement to the infant's internal state is indicated by the process of cross-modality processing of emotion (Stern, 1985). For example, the mother may reflect with her facial expression the emotion her infant communicates vocally, or vice versa. This cross-modal interpersonal processing of emotion between human beings can be extremely rapid and can take place below awareness. Thus emotion expressed vocally will elicit electromyographically measurable changes in another person's facial expression of emotion, at speeds as fast as 300–400 milliseconds (Hietanen, Surakka and Linnankoski, 1998; Stenberg, Wiking and Dahl, 1998). It has been suggested (Bruner, 1994; Schore, 2000b) that this rapid mimicry of emotional expression not only facilitates bonding between partners but also functions to send signals back into the emotion-processing brain, which then helps to bring about appropriate arousal which mirrors that of the other person (or infant); thus the surface automatic mimicry helps to produce the internal physiological mirroring. The tendency towards empathic attunement appears to be built into the human brain.

Misattunement and recovery

Studies show that empathic misattunements and disconnections are common in early proto-conversations, but what characterizes healthy relationships is a pattern of *re-establishing* attunement after it has been lost. Schore (2000a: 8) describes this as follows:

> In this reattunement pattern of 'disruption and repair' the 'good-enough' caregiver who induces a stress response in her infant through a misattunement reinvokes in a timely fashion her psychobiologically attuned regulation of the infant's negative affect state *that she has triggered*. The key to this is the caregiver's capacity to monitor and regulate her own affect, especially negative affect.
>
> (2000a: 8–9)

This corresponds to the process that Kohut considered to be crucial to the mutative action of analysis – the recurrent loss and regaining of the empathic link between patient and analyst. Kohut's term for the positive developmental impact of this is 'transmuting internalization'. Another way of expressing this might be to say that the child or the patient gradually gains increasing confidence that empathic understanding can be restored, that communication of affect is possible, and that the empathic connection can provide regulatory soothing.

A further observation (Schore, 2000a) is that mothers and infants will, during intense facial interactions and proto-conversations, mutually reinforce positive affect states, reaching a crescendo and then subsiding. The mother's allowing the subsiding of affective arousal, so that the infant can enter quiet states, seems to be very important. If the infant is not allowed periods of quiet recovery from affectively intense experiences, then he or she may become chronically over-aroused and agitated. This ebb and flow of affective intensity may also have its parallel in the adult consulting room, where there may be islands of acute engagement between analyst and patient, emerging within a broader ocean of introspection and quiet reflection.

Early selfobject experiences and the orbitofrontal cortex

The earliest selfobject experiences involve the modalities of touch, sound and, above all, vision. Although the sound – the prosody – of the mother's voice is important in conveying emotional information, the linguistic meaning of her utterances is obviously not of relevance to the infant. Vision appears to play a major role in the affective engagement between mother and infant. The infant's visual focus is perfectly adapted for locking on to the mother's face during breast feeding. Moreover, the right hemisphere of the brain is more highly developed than the left during the first two years of life (Chiron, Nabbout, Lounes et al., 1997) and it is this right hemisphere which is specialized for processing the visual emotional information provided by the mother's face. Infant and mother both engage and bond with each other primarily through their right brains (Manning, Trivers, Thornhill et al., 1997).

Of particular significance in the processing of information through the right cortex is the orbitofrontal regulatory system, which is more extensively developed in the right than in the left hemisphere. Schore (2000b) argues that this corresponds to the executive regulatory control system postulated by Bowlby (1980). The orbitofrontal cortex is particularly involved in the processing of social signals (from the mother's face) and other attachment functions. It is crucially located at the hierarchical apex of the limbic system and thus is positioned to manage the interface between the externally arising emotional information (from mother's face) and the emotional responses arising internally from the sympathetic and parasympathetic nervous aspects of the autonomic nervous system. Thus the orbitofrontal system of the right hemisphere acts in executive control of physiological and endocrinological functions that are involved in survival and coping with stress. It is through this system of the right brain that the selfobject interactions with the mother shape the infant's developing neurophysiology.

Later, the orbitofrontal cortex is involved with the assignment of emotional meanings to thoughts and impressions (Joseph, 1996; Teasdale, Howard, Cox et al., 1999) and also plays a crucial role in self-awareness and self-reflection. Its activity is essential to the empathic perception of the mental states of others and thus is concerned with 'theory of mind tasks with an affective component' (Stone, Baron-Cohen and Knight, 1998: 651). Schore (2000b) concludes that the functioning of the orbitofrontal control system 'is central to self regulation, the ability to flexibly regulate emotional states through interaction with other humans – interactive regulation in interconnected contexts – and without other humans – autoregulation in autonomous contexts'. Thus it seems that the evidence suggests that the selfobject functions are mediated through the orbitofrontal cortex.

One-brain intrapsychic vs. interpersonal relational psychoanalysis

Much of the diversity of psychoanalytic theorizing organizes into two broad paradigms: first, the intrapsychic model of Freud, based essentially on the position of one person's brain in isolation; and, second, the relational models (object relational, attachment, self-psychological) based on the assumption of a brain in communication with other brains. This division parallels the point made by Blatt and Ford (1994) that personality development involves two fundamental tasks – (1) the estab-lishment of a differentiated and stable sense of self, and (2) the development of stable and satisfying relationships. Different theories may emphasize one or other of these different but complementary dimen-sions of development.

Freud's model was influenced by the theories of the neurologist Hughlings Jackson (Sulloway, 1979), who saw the brain as functioning according to a vertical hierarchy of interrelated systems and structures – in contrast to other neurologists who were more inclined to think in terms of localized functions. Jackson proposed that ontogenetically earlier maturing structures are progressively subsumed and regulated by later-developing higher cortical structures (see also Luria, 1980). According to this model, the lowest functions are those of the autonomic nervous system – 'the physiological bottom of the mind'. This progression in development, from lower to higher brain functions, was seen as having occurred in the evolution of the human species, but also as forming part of the development of each individual brain. Jackson also considered that the lower functions of mind – preverbal and visceral – are temporarily set free from higher cortical control during sleep and dreams (rather like Freud's idea of the primary process mode of thought found in dreams). According to Jackson, psychopathology involved a loss of the higher inhibitory functions (negative symptoms) and the release of lower functions (positive symptoms) – i.e. essentially a regression to develop-mentally earlier processes. It can be seen that Jackson's model – of a hierarchical brain with the potential for regression – became the basis of Freud's theory of dreams and of psychopathology: dreams involve a regression to primary process modes of thought during sleep, and psychopathology involves a regression to lower or earlier modes of bodily and mental impulse, resulting in anxiety and attempts to reassert higher control (the ego's mechanisms of defence). Moreover, Jackson's emphasis upon developmental stages of brain function became metamor-phosed in Freud's scheme into the idea of the stages of sexual development (oral, anal, phallic and genital) in which, again, the later stages subsume and organize the earlier ones. Jackson's idea of the autonomic nervous system being the physiological bottom of the mind finds expression in Freud's emphasis upon the somatic basis of the instincts (the 'id') which provide the energy for the mind – and his idea of the unconscious as the link between psyche and soma. Schore comments:

> Jackson's ideas, far ahead of his time, are directly relevant to contemporary neuroscience and psychoanalysis, especially as both are now intensely focusing upon the problems of affect and motivation.
>
> (Schore, in press)

Whilst the one mind model is inadequate as a complete framework for understanding mental life, it does have a place. At times people do process emotion when alone, without interaction with others. In many respects the brain *can* be seen as a system of structures for regulating and expressing emotional arousal. Emotion arises from the activation of the limbic system and the sympathetic and parasympathetic aspects of the autonomic nervous system. It is then modulated and organized by the higher cortical structures. For adults, no longer contained within the emotion-regulating care of the mother, autoregulation of affect is crucial. The achievement of the capacity to experience, contain and express affect appropriately is one of the marks of mental health. If the brain is injured, affect regulation suffers – the person may display emotional lability, catastrophic emotional storms, increased or decreased anxiety, and tendencies towards depression or inappropriate high spirits. Moreover, psychopharmacological treatments that are aimed at negative affective states are also based essentially on the task of improving autoregulation of affect – and thus assume an isolated brain.

Schore comments:

> . . . current neurobiological studies which highlight the essential role of the adaptive functions of right hemispheric control centers in regulating drive centers in the hypothalamus . . . and of the right brain in the metacontrol of fundamental physiological and endocrinological functions . . . support the notion of an unconscious mind operating in a 'one person' autoregulatory strategy. This mode does represent one organizational configuration of an unconscious mind, a mode that is accessed when one is processing emotion but not transacting with external social objects.
>
> (Schore, in press)

On the other hand, the emerging view of the 'social construction of the human brain' indicates that a relational perspective is also essential for psychoanalytic theory if it is to take account of the reality of the intersubjective world of the infant. Perhaps the point is that both an intrapsychic and a relational perspective are necessary. This would be congruent with Grotstein's (1983) idea of the 'dual track' and his emphasis that the infant (and perhaps human beings throughout life) are experientially both separate and merged with others. Indeed, Kohut considered that, although human beings achieve a cognitive separation of self and other, we continue to require selfobject connectedness with others throughout life.

The right brain unconscious

Schore (1994; 2000b) has drawn together much evidence that the right hemisphere can be equated with Freud's unconscious mind and is particularly concerned with processing emotional information. Damage to the right hemisphere can be associated with difficulties in both the perception and communication of affect (Bear, 1983; Fricchione and Howanitz, 1985; Voeller, 1986; Weintraub and Mesulam, 1983), and with the establishment of love relationships involving recognition of the other as a whole person (Solms, 1999). The emotion-processing right brain hemisphere is actually dominant in human infants (Chiron et al., 1997) and there is much evidence that it is particularly affected by early social experiences (Denenberg, Garbanti, Sherman et al., 1978; Schore, 1994). Some evidence suggests right brain to right brain communications are predominant in early infancy. For example, females (but not males) show a tendency to cradle infants on the left side of the body (relating to the right brain hemisphere), irrespective of handedness. This may be to do with facilitating the flow of affective information from the infant through the mother's left eye and ear to the emotion-processing right hemisphere (Manning et al., 1997) – and may also reflect the fact that the substrate for the mother's response of soothing and comforting her infant is later-alized in the right hemisphere (Horton, 1995). The infant's own right hemisphere is more adapted than the left to processing information concerning the mother's face and in recognizing emotional facial expression (Deruelle and de Schonen, 1988; Nelson, 1987), as well as in early language development (Locke, 1997; Schumann, 1997). Semrud-Clikeman and Hynd (1990) comment:

> The emotional experiences of the infant develop through the sounds, images, and pictures that constitute much of an infant's early learning experience, and are disproportionately stored or processed in the right hemisphere during the formative stages of brain ontogeny.
>
> (p. 198)

This dominance and rapid development of the right hemisphere coincide with a period of intense socio-affective learning in the first couple of years of life. It is then superseded by the maturation of the linguistic left hemisphere – which then becomes the dominant medium for consciousness. This biphasic maturation of the right and left hemispheres can be taken as part of the neurological basis of infantile amnesia. Whilst our conscious thought becomes predominantly linguistic, the right brain continues to process emotional information holistically and rapidly but less consciously.

The left hemisphere plays its part in processing emotion later when linguistic communication becomes more important. Under optimum developmental conditions the mother helps the child to express feelings in words, which can then become the vehicle for empathy. Probably what is crucial neurologically in this process is interhemispheric communication (Kitterle, 1995; Parker and Taylor, 1997) so that the *emotional* meanings of words are processed and combined with other sources of affective information such as facial expression and tone of voice.

However, the right brain appears fundamental in *perceiving* emotion from both internal (one's own emotion) and external sources (the other's emotion). Jackson (1931) grasped the perceptual functions of the right brain many decades ago. Luria, the Russian neuropsychologist, who was greatly interested by Freudian psychoanalysis (Kaplan-Solms and Solms, 2000; Solms, 2000) comments as follows:

> Nearly a century ago, Hughlings Jackson postulated that the right hemisphere
> . . . participates directly in perceptual processes and is responsible for more
> direct, visual forms of relationships with the outside world. This hypothesis
> failed to attract due attention for many decades, and it is only recently that it has
> been begun to be appreciated. First of all it was noticed that the right
> hemisphere is directly concerned with the analysis of direct information
> received by the subject from his own body and which, it can easily be under-
> stood, is much more closely connected with direct sensation than with verbally
> logical codes.
>
> (Luria, 1973: 165)

Thus Luria is emphasizing the right brain unconscious's functions of both
perceiving the outside world and also of communicating with the body.
The right hemisphere is particularly adapted to perceiving external
emotional information – originally from the mother's face. This
emotional information is processed holistically and much more rapidly
than the linguistic left hemisphere is capable of – and much more rapidly
than can be registered consciously. At the same time the orbitofrontal
cortex, particularly expanded in the right hemisphere, extends down to
the emotion generating limbic system. Moreover, connections to the
autonomic nervous system are highly lateralized to the right brain
(Schore, 1994). Because of this, the right orbitofrontal cortex – the
neurological unconscious – can act as a go-between, accessing information from both the body (the autonomic nervous system and the
limbic system of the brain) and the external emotional world. As Damasio
comments:

> The overall function of the brain is to be well informed about what goes on in
> the rest of the body, the body proper; about what goes on in itself; and about
> the environment surrounding the organism, so that suitable survivable accom-
> modations can be achieved between the organism and the environment.
>
> (Damasio, 1994: 90)

As described earlier, the selfobject processes are mediated originally
through the orbitofrontal system of the right brain. The fact that the right
brain appears to be the basis of the unconscious mind suggests that, to a
large extent, selfobject processes are indeed largely unconscious – silent
unless disrupted – as Kohut indicated.

The right brain contribution to 'true' and 'false' self

This neurological unconscious is essentially perceptual, scanning the
internal and external environment for emotional information. The
original and paradigmatic external source of emotional information is
the mother's face. Indeed, the idea that facial expression is a crucial

form of emotional communication has roots in Darwin (1872), whose work was well known to Freud. The intricate and rapid interplay of visual and auditory affective signals between mother and infant – the intersubjectivity of the mother–infant dyad – can be regarded as a means whereby each informs the other of their respective brain states, and each becomes attuned to the other's brain state. By becoming attuned – mirroring or resonating to – the infant's brain state, the mother can then lead the infant away from noxious brain states (over- or under-stimulated states) and facilitate positive arousal (Feldman et al., 1999). In this way she becomes what Bollas (1987) called a transformational object.

Schore emphasizes the importance of the mother's respect for the child's autonomy, her willingness and ability to follow the infant's lead:

> . . . the more the mother tunes her activity level to the infant during periods of social engagement, the more she allows him to recover quietly in periods of disengagement, and the more she attends to the child's reinitiating cues for re-engagement, the more synchronized their interaction.
>
> (Schore, 2000a, pp. 7–8)

This supports Winnicott's (1960) position regarding the significance of the mother's response to the child's initiative (in facilitating the true self) and the deleterious consequences of consistently imposing her own (in fostering a false self). Again this responsiveness appears to involve particularly the right brain. Using EEG and neuroimaging data, Ryan, Kuhl and Deci conclude:

> The positive emotional exchange resulting from autonomy-supportive parenting involves participation of right hemisphere cortical and subcortical systems that participate in global, tonic emotional modulation.
>
> (1997: 719)

A succinct way of stating the gist of these findings and speculations is to say that the mother's right brain regulates the infant's states of affective arousal through the medium of the infant's right brain. The infant is immersed in an intersubjective system of finely tuned and exquisitely timed visual and auditory exchanges of affective communication. This is Kohut's selfobject. Its function, as Kohut described, is a *psychoeconomic* one, of regulating affective arousal.

From this neuropsychological and developmental research perspective, it is possible to reframe the meaning of the selfobject as outlined by Kohut. The three main forms of selfobject – the mirroring, the twinship, and the idealizing – can all be seen as offering different aspects of the affect regulating functions of the infant–mother dyad. Thus the mirroring function may relate to (or at least be analogous to) the synchrony of visual and gestural matching between infant and mother. The twinship function – giving rise to the sense of there being an other who is like the self – may relate to the infant's perception of the mother's matching brain state, a mirroring or resonance of *internal* state between the two partners. Idealization can be seen as offering the opportunity to merge with a representation of strength, calm and perfection – and thus may relate to the infant's experience of being soothed, calmed and protected by the mother, who manages to be attuned yet leads the infant back to a more positively toned brain state.

Selfobject failures and traumatic impingements

What happens if the intersubjective infant–mother system (selfobject) fails to regulate the infant's affective arousal within tolerable limits? The infant will be subjected to aversive brain states, of negative affective tone, of over- or under-arousal, or of disorganization. If instead of soothing a distressed child, the mother adds her own agitation, fuelling the child's rage or anxiety and disorganization, then arousal may rise to catastrophic levels, resulting in wild, extreme and impulsive forms of behaviour. Repeated episodes of this kind will be stored in the right hemisphere as implicit memories of aversive and dangerous interactions; the message will be that turning to another person for help may lead to further distress. Profound distrust will be deeply etched into the neurological circuits. (This may correspond to both the insecure-avoidant and the disorganized-disoriented patterns of attachment described by Main, 1991.)

Or, less damagingly, what if the mother's attunement to her child is well-intentioned but simply incompetent or based upon a distorted or inaccurate assessment of the infant's mental state, so that she persistently misjudges or mistimes her emotional response? The infant may again learn that attempts to engage with another person are likely to result in subtle forms of frustration, and discouragement, leading the child to turn away; the message of such repeated experiences may be that people always misunderstand one another and that attempts to communicate are hopeless (which may correspond to the insecure-ambivalent pattern of attachment described by Main, 1991). One result of repeated failures or active hostilities of the early selfobject environment may be the excessive reliance on transitional objects (Taylor, 1987), such as a soft toy or blanket which is used for comfort and self-soothing, or the resort to hard sensation-based forms of containment (Tustin, 1981, 1986; Ogden,

1989); these are all attempts at affect regulation in the absence of a selfobject partner.

In addition to such episodes of aversive interactions with a caregiver, another form of noxious selfobject failure is the situation of the child who is left alone too long without an interactional partner. Here the brain is left to its own devices, under-stimulated and under-organized. Dysphoric states of boredom and emptiness may result, with cravings for stimulation and excitement. There may then be a resort to self-stimulation, either masturbatory or through infliction of pain or orally (through repeated turning to confectionery, for example). Another attempted solution may be through excessive reliance upon television or electronic games. All these may have the strong potential to become addictive. Later, in adolescence and adulthood, addiction may move to computer games, sex, or alcohol or substance abuse. All forms of addiction can be regarded as pathological substitutes for the selfobject relationship of infancy and as attempted solutions to problems of affect regulation (Taylor, 1997).

The selfobject responsiveness of the mother must involve more than just a capacity to notice facial, vocal and gestural cues from her infant. The sensory data of perception – phenomena – must be given emotional meaning in order to form the basis of empathy and symbolization – a process that Bion (1962) designated 'alpha function'. Without this hypothetical process of alpha function, the interpersonal perceptual data remain merely phenomena, devoid of affective significance. An example of this was given by an alexithymic patient, Mr T, who had difficulty in identifying and thinking about his own emotions as well as those of others. He described an interaction with his new girlfriend during which 'her face creased up and her eyes started watering'. Having mentioned this, Mr T moved on to recount further events, presenting a purely descriptive narrative without indication of any its emotional significance. The analyst asked what Mr T's understanding was of why his girlfriend had reacted in this way. He replied that he had no idea. Puzzled, the analyst enquired whether Mr T had asked his girlfriend why she was upset. Mr T replied that he had not. It became clear that not only had Mr T been unable to register his girlfriend's facial expression and tears as signifying her distress, he had not even realized that facial and bodily expressions do in general indicate an inner emotional state, As a result, Mr T experienced human emotional displays as profoundly puzzling. These were experienced not as signifiers of emotion but as 'things in themselves', which Bion (1962) termed beta elements. According to Bion, alpha function depends upon the mother's capacity for reverie, which is an expression of her love for her infant:

> . . . reverie is that state of mind which is open to the reception of any 'objects'
> from the loved object and is therefore capable of reception of the infant's
> projective identifications whether they are felt by the infant to be good or bad.
>
> (Bion, 1962: 36)

Using Bion's insights, it is possible to understand that failures by the primary caregiver to receive and process (through the right brain) the primitive affective proto-communications of the infant – to give them meaning through her thoughtful attention and thus transform the raw sensory data (Bion's beta elements) into the currency of symbols and significance (Bion's alpha elements) – may result in the infant's experiencing not an introduction to the world of human discourse and empathy, but instead an immersion in sensation, experienced at best as indifferent and at worst as hostile. If the mother's alpha function fails to catalyse that of the infant (sometimes because of constitutional or neurological deficits in either partner), the result can be that anxiety is denuded of meaning, becoming instead a nameless dread or terror (Bion, 1962: 96), a subtle and incommunicable agony in which the person feels imprisoned in a fragmenting vortex of sensation-based experience falling outside the realm of symbolization – a state of mind that Grotstein (1990; 1991) has evocatively termed the 'black hole' of non-meaning.

Perhaps this is something like Kohut had in mind when he wrote of the 'unspeakable anxieties' (1984: 8) of the schizophrenic state of the fragmented self, which he saw as the ultimate dread – 'the deepest anxiety man can experience' (1984: 16) – a 'prepsychological state' (1984: 8) which he believed lay outside the therapeutic reach of psychoanalysis. Such a state can also be produced by extreme trauma and terror (van der Kolk, Pelcovitz, Roth et al., 1996). It may also play a role in conditions of chronic derealization or depersonalization. Although inherently beyond the realm of normal communication and empathy, this 'black hole' state of mind is profoundly aversive, giving rise to insistent efforts to avoid or escape its hell. Such efforts may include overwork, compulsive over-activity, avoidance of sleep, and the seeking of intense sensation.

Sexual and addictive enactments of selfobject dysfunction

Many forms of sexual enactments that are experienced as addictive, or at least as imperatively driven, may be considered as pathological attempts at selfobject regulation – as well as representations of earlier traumatic (anti)selfobject experiences.

A good source of detailed descriptions and insights into these is the work of Stoller (1976; 1986; 1991; 1992). In his earlier work, Stoller (1976) outlined ways in which a transvestite man may be endeavouring to master childhood experiences in which he felt his masculine identity was under threat from a hostile female (the mother or sisters); the mechanism being one essentially of identification with the aggressor, turning passive into active, so that the original danger is now brought about deliberately and is manically perceived as the source of the greatest sexual pleasure.

Following Stoller's lead, let us consider the likely psychodynamic and developmental basis of the activity in which a person (mainly but not exclusively men) voluntarily submits to various forms of torture or physical abuse by a woman (dominatrix), usually involving some kind of restraint or interference with bodily movement or natural functions – or those instances whereby a grown person asks to be dressed and treated as a baby (Stoller, 1991). One striking feature of such activities is that they involve handing over to an other the regulation of affective arousal and the experience of pain and pleasure. The 'client' deliberately surrenders his (or her) own autoregulation to a dominant other whom he knows will bring about aversive affective states. Of course, he knows that ultimately he retains some control since he is the customer and in the end it is a kind of theatre, a form of desperate 'play' and therefore not 'real'. Why is this done? It seems likely that what is enacted somewhat compulsively is the early experience of affect and arousal having been misregulated by the caregiver – the experience of being helplessly at the mercy of a caregiver who does not come, who leaves the infant in pain or terror, or who imposes her own agenda which is not congruent with the infant's needs, or who fails to soothe but instead exacerbates the distress and adds further suffering, either through misperception or deliberate cruelty and sadism (and perhaps we should not underestimate the potential for sadism evoked in the caregiver by the helplessness of the baby, especially if there is no other adult to act as an inhibiting presence). There may be another component as well. States of emptiness (alexithymia) may give rise to efforts to seek selfobject stimulation based on the original dysfunctional experiences of affect (dys)regulation. Then the imperative need to surrender regulation to a dominant other, in a commercial transaction, may combine the search for selfobject stimulation with the attempt (unconsciously) to master the original trauma.[2]

[2.] Sado-masochistic activity may also be driven by feeling-states of isolation and disconnection. Benjamin comments:

> . . . erotic domination, for both sides, draws its appeal in part from its offer to break the encasement of the isolated self, to explode the numbness that comes of 'false' differentiation. It is a reaction to the predicament of solitary confinement – being unable to get through to the other, or be gotten through to . . .

(1988: 83)

Such compulsive re-enactments of early trauma of (anti)selfobject (mis)regulation of affective arousal may also be a factor in substance addiction. The use of a poisonous substance may be more than just an attempt to regulate affective arousal in the present. Its toxic qualities may precisely represent and recreate noxious aspects of early experiences with caregivers whose regulation of the infant's affect was dysfunctional.

The internalized models of interaction which organize the brain

The emerging data of neuroscience indicate that early experiences of interaction with the caregivers form representations within the brain which have far-reaching functions in organizing the activity of the brain. In this respect, neuroscience and developmental psychology are forming conceptual bridges with psychoanalysis, which, for decades, has made use of concepts of internalization of relationships. Now this idea is used by non-psychoanalytic theorists and researchers as well as those within the psychoanalytic tradition. For example, Wilson, Passik and Faude (1990) describe the internal representation of affect-regulating experiences with the caregiver; Beebe and Lachman (1988) write of representations of 'self-with-other' appearing at the end of the first year of life; Trevarthen (1993) refers to 'relational scripts'; and Forgas (1982) refers to 'internal representations of social interactions that guide interpersonal behaviour' and 'episode cognitions' which act as integrative schemata for organizing social information. Schore (1994) points out that the establishment of an internal model of the external world is an important aspect of functioning systems of whatever kind that interact with the surrounding environment, and is congruent with 'the general cybernetic principle that the inclusion of a dynamic internal model of the outside world in a control component of a feedback regulator is responsible for internal stability and output regulation' (Schore, 1994: 194).

The classic psychoanalytic concept of the inner representation of an external figure is that of the superego, a structure based upon the image of the prohibiting father, which Freud regarded as the legacy of the oedipus complex. This was the first version of the concept of the internal object and contained the idea that an internal representation could be based upon both phantasy (driven by the child's own impulses) and actual experience with the external figure. Later this was developed further, but in different ways, by Klein and Fairbairn.

Klein postulated a complex inner world of unconscious phantasy, populated by an extensive range of figures, including 'part object' images of parts of the body such as breast and penis. However, she saw this inner theatre as deriving predominantly from the infant's own instinctual drives. Fairbairn (1952) by contrast, regarded internal objects as derived essentially from 'bad' experiences with the primary caregiver.

In the USA, ego psychologists Hartmann (1950) and Jacobson (1964) developed the idea of internal representations of self and other – images that could be cathected with various qualities and quantities of aggressive or libidinal drive energy – whilst in Britain, Sandler and colleagues (Sandler and Rosenblatt, 1962) developed the concept of the 'representational world'. Developing attachment theory, Bowlby (1980) presented the concept of internal working models of relationships – elaborated further by other attachment theorists (see Seganti, Carnevale, Mucelli et al., 2000). Stern, a psychoanalytic developmental researcher, wrote of 'repetitive interactions that have become generalized' – RIGs (Stern, 1985), as well as 'schemas of being-with' (Stern, 1995).

A clear trend in theorizing has been a shift from the original idea of the internal object to a concept of the internal representation of a *relationship* of self and other. A related feature of these emerging models is to regard the internal representations as *abstractions* which generalize from a range of subjective experiences associated with interactions with significant others (Zeanah and Barton, 1989). Thus, for example, Bollas comments:

> . . . infants do internalize the mother's actual idiom of care, which is a complex network of 'rules for being and relating'. These rules are procedures for processing internal and external reality, and their regularity eventually leads to their structuring in the ego . . . Isn't ego structure a form of memory, and its structure a testimony to the logic of its formation rather like a building recollects an architect's intent?
>
> (1989: 195)

Stern and his colleagues in the Boston Process of Change Study Group (Stern, Sander, Nahum et al., 1998) point out that these internal abstractions or generalizations are forms of *implicit relational knowing*; they are forms of knowledge that are implicit rather than conscious and declarative, although psychoanalytic therapy can obviously enable a person to become aware of their internal models of relationships.

In general, those theorists who study children directly have given more emphasis to actual experiences with caregivers than to the influence of the child's own impulses and affects in generating the internal representations (Tronick, 1998) – although an interaction between the two is usually acknowledged. However, Kernberg (1976; 1984), who has developed an elaborate theory of personality development based around internalized structures of self and object, each with an affective link, follows Klein in seeing these as derived primarily from the vicissitudes of the individual's own libidinal and aggressive drives.

As we have seen, Kohut did not develop a theory of internalized relationships. Instead he emphasized the internalization of the affect-regulating *function* of the selfobject. However, as Schore and others have argued, the data of neuroscience increasingly demonstrate that it is the internal representations of experiences with others (selfobject representations) that perform the functions of regulating affect – or, in other cases, of generating aversive states of affective arousal.

Schore (1994) has proposed that the most basic elements of the internal representation of self-with-other are abstractions of the infant's physiological-affective response to the emotionally expressive face of the mother. Thus this representation would consist of a facial image and a physiological state. As Wright (1991) has commented, 'At the very beginning – before separation, before there is an object at all – the mother's face is already there.' The infant's perception of facially expressed emotion can become abstracted and generalized to act as 'face icons' (Bowers, Blonder, Feinberg and Heilman, 1991) or 'mother icons' (Kraemer et al. 1991) which function as social and neurobiological 'guidance systems'. Schwalbe (1991) has suggested that the mother's face, which consistently provides stimulation to the infant, creates a neural network based on pulses of electrochemical energy at developmentally critical moments:

> As these pulses flow through the brain, synaptic connections are established and strengthened and the firing rates of groups of neurons are set. The result is that certain kinetic pathways are established, making it more likely that these patterns will guide energy flows in the future . . . The initial configuration of the matrix may influence the possibility of capturing certain kinds of information later; its initial form may affect the vividness and completeness with which different kinds of imagery (visual, tactile, olfactory, auditory) can be captured.
> (Schwalbe, 1991: 280; quoted in Schore, 1994: 185–86)

Schwalbe suggests that this neurologically captured imagery 'works in the same way as cognitive schemas' (1991: 283) and thus regulates the flow of social and affective information through the brain. The neural networks would also act to select which emotional imagery is attended to and which is less easily registered.

Here in the emphasis upon the infant's experience of facial imagery forming the basis of internal representations of self-with-other is the neuropsychological underpinning of Kohut's proposition that the 'gleam in the mother's eye' provides the foundation of the child's self-esteem and narcissistic economy – the establishment of positive affect regulation.

Summary

The mother's empathic attunement to her infant, which is crucial to the regulation of his or her affect, also plays a part in the development of the brain. By means of repeated selfobject experiences, the infant internalizes representations of self with other, which continue to exert a persisting and considerable effect on brain state – as if a virtual 'hard wiring'. Healthy mother–infant relationships involve not an absence of misattunement, but a rapid re-establishment of attunement after disruptions have occurred. The orbitofrontal cortex appears to play a particular role in the processing of emotional information, both externally derived – from the mother's face – and also from the limbic system and the autonomic nervous system of the body. This orbitofrontal system may also be involved in assigning emotional meanings to thoughts and perceptions, and in theory of mind tasks to do with perceiving the mental and emotional states of others. An intrapsychic model of the mind, linked to a hierarchical model of brain function, may still be necessary alongside a model of the 'social' regulation of the brain. The functions of the right hemisphere of the brain can, in many ways, be equated with the unconscious mind. It processes emotion and perceives holistically, contrasting with the linguistic functions of the left hemisphere. The mother's right brain regulates the infant's affective state through the medium of the infant's right brain. Selfobject failures, where the mother does not regulate the infant's states of affective arousal, but creates further disorganization and under- or over-arousal, may be linked to Bion's concept of alpha function and its failure. Addictive or compulsive sexual enactments may be considered as pathological attempts at selfobject regulation and the mastery of early traumatic interactional failures of affect-regulation. Many variants of contemporary psychoanalytic and developmental psychological theorizing make use of the idea of internal representations of relational experiences. These can be linked with neuropsychological evidence to provide a broader underpinning to Kohut's concept of the selfobject and the 'gleam in the mother's eye'.

Chapter 10
Self psychology perspectives on childhood trauma

> You know everybody is fragile somewhere. The question is where is the
> breaking point . . .
>
> (Chicago Lecture, 25 October 1974: Kohut, 1996: 148)

Kohut himself did not write extensively about patients who suffered
severe and repeated gross trauma or abuse. Most of his clinical illustrations are of patients whose childhood traumas were relatively subtle,
albeit far-reaching in effect. Nevertheless, Kohut's observations regarding
the structure and development of the self, the lines of development of
narcissism, and the crucial role of the selfobject environment, are readily
applicable to the circumstances of those whose trauma was extreme and
repeated (Brothers, 1995).

The experience of self in childhood trauma

Abuse by a caregiver acts as a profound reversal of the selfobject conditions required for optimum development. It functions to prevent
maturation of narcissism and the establishment of a coherent sense of
self. The child may be thrust back to the brink of the position of the
fragmented self. All manner of dissociations, and distortions of
perception of self and other, may be resorted to in order to preserve a
semblance of coherence of experience.

A parent or other caregiver is one to whom the child turns for soothing
and empathy when hurt emotionally or physically. When the caregiver is
the *source* of the trauma then this selfobject function is fundamentally
compromised. It can work only if the child's perceptions are dissociated,
such that one area of experience is kept apart from another area of
experience which contradicts the first. An example of this is a patient with
a Dissociative Identity Disorder who had some personalities who
reported that a stepfather had abused her sexually over many years of

childhood, whilst other personalities maintained an unequivocally positive view of him and would speak of all the ways in which he made her feel special and loved. Rather than a self making use of repression – or horizontal splitting – to avoid awareness of a disturbing experience, there has here been a resort to an *alteration in the self* as a central and coherent organ-ization of experience – a vertical split. Thus there is not just an alteration in the *content* of consciousness, but, crucially, a change in the very structure of consciousness and the self. Compartmental-ization, and forcible unintegration of contradictory experiences, may result in multiple representations of self and other.

Under circumstances of the reasonable provision of selfobject functions, the child develops a self having coherence and cohesion – a sense of 'I' that persists through varying and conflicting experiences and which has continuity across time. By contrast, in states of extreme organized dissociation, the experience may be of having no central self, but instead a group of disparate personalities, each of which at any particular moment may regard him/herself as *the* self. The more extreme the dissociation, the more each fragmented part of the self is likely to assume an egocentric position. Each part may feel haunted or inhabited by the intimidating voices of the 'others'.

The experiences of numbing and detachment, which are part of the dissociation found consistently in response to trauma in adulthood, are also a feature of a child's reactions to abuse – even if the more extreme and elaborate condition of dissociative identity disorder does not arise. As a result, the child's experience of self and of the surrounding world becomes unfamiliar. If such a situation is repeated or chronic, the sense of connection to self and other, which is a normal feature of background experience when there is a good enough selfobject environment, will be dislocated, giving rise to unrooted particles of consciousness that do not cohere in the normal way. This disruption of self-experience is, of course, objectively invisible to others, but an empathic immersion in the commu-nications of patients extensively abused in childhood will reveal, I suggest, a pervasive backdrop of anxiety against which there is a limited sense of the continuity of self. I have previously (Mollon, 1998) described these as 'mutilated states of consciousness'.

As well as coherence, cohesion and continuity in time, the self experience of those who have grown up with adequate selfobject avail-ability and reliability is also of having *depth*. Thus some aspects of self are clearly visible to others – and could be described as being above ground, so to speak; other aspects are more hidden, both from consciousness and from others – although these hidden depths may gradually be discovered, for example through psychoanalysis. Part of the sense of depth, of having roots, or foundations, may lie in the early experience of safety (Sandler, 1990) – the feeling of being supported, held securely, or 'backed up', as connoted by Grotstein's (1981) concept of the 'background selfobject of primary identification'. However, the person whose early life has been pervaded by terror, pain and betrayal (Freyd, 1996) may lack this background of safety and experience of soothing. Instead of being able to surrender securely, for example during sleep, the person may experience a dread of falling into a nightmare. What should be a bedrock of safety becomes infiltrated with the uncanny, a distorting mirror that offers not soothing but mockery.

Without this reliable background selfobject, the experience of self is analogous to that of Alice in Wonderland, who is left without stability, predictability or consistency, as she encounters continual change in her own dimensions whilst all around the inhabitants behave in bizarre and cruel ways that are completely devoid of empathy. She comes across a cat whose body dissolves, leaving behind only its grin. It is as if the very fabric on which the tapestry of self-experience is to be woven is absent, or so flimsy that it is full of tears and holes. Lacking a stable backdrop formed by reliable selfobject support, the experience of self will be incoherent.

Like Alice, the child repeatedly traumatized by caregivers experiences a continual dread of falling. The ground is not secure and there are no firm foundations to the personality. As Balint (1968) conveyed, the metaphor of a structural fault can be very apt.

Dissociation in response to trauma

A core feature of responses to trauma – i.e. to experiences that overwhelm the individual's normal coping capacities – is that of dissociation. This can include a variety of forms of detachment from the immediate trauma, ranging from states of depersonalization to the development of elaborate alternative personality states, as found in Dissociative Identity Disorder (DID: Mollon, 1996; Sinason, in press). In the DID state, the child makes use of pretence and imagination – 'This is not happening to me; it's happening to someone else' – to establish distinct personality states, amnesically bounded to varying extents, each with their own identity, style of cognition, mood tendencies, memories and general attitudes. Although dissociative disorders used to be considered extremely rare and were not well conceptualized, it is now recognized that most victims of childhood sexual abuse show some degree of dissociative reaction, although mostly this falls short of the fully developed DID.

The development of a full state of DID may require the combination of a number of factors. Kluft (1994) theorizes that four key components interact to produce the multiple personalities of DID. These are:

- A capacity for dissociation. People vary in their natural propensity to dissociate, to become detached and absorbed in fantasy (Vermetten, Douglas-Bremner and Spiegel, 1998).
- Life experiences that traumatically overwhelm the child's non-dissociative defensive/adaptive capacities.
- The dissociative defences make use of the *substrates* for divided-ness that are already present in the environment or in the child's psychobiological constitution. Such substrates may include: state-dependent and mood-dependent memory (the tendency for memory of experiences to be more readily available when in the same mood or mental state as when the experiences originally occurred); contradictory parental demands and parental behaviour (such as when a parent is abusive at certain times, but behaves in seemingly benign ways at other times); double binds (the parent requiring incompatible emotional and behavioural responses from the child); the child's identification with a parent's multiple personality; the child's use of autohypnosis, as a means of escaping from pain and unbearable perceptions.
- The child is not provided (a) with adequate protection against further overwhelming experiences, and (b) with appropriate soothing and opportunities to express and process their pain – i.e. the necessary selfobjects are not available.

Kluft's theory highlights the role of the absence of selfobjects. It is the non-availability of caregivers who can provide empathy and soothing which means the child abused within the family must resort to patho-logical forms of internal escape through dissociation. Probably children can survive all manner of trauma, or abuse by strangers, provided there is reliable and empathic support within the family. But without this soothing by reliable and consistent caregivers, the trauma-tized child is unable to regulate his or her mental state and restore emotional equilibrium. Pathological solutions, in terms of the disso-ciative sequestering of traumatic experience are developed instead. DID could be said to be one form of pathology of psychoeconomic regulation, deriving from childhood trauma in the context of selfobject unavailability.

Disturbances in the regulation of affect

For the incestuously abused child, the caregiver had acted not as a source of soothing but of trauma – an anti-selfobject. As a result the child cannot gradually internalize an image of a soothing selfobject. The affects of rage, anxiety and depression are overwhelming for the person who has been incestuously abused. Pathological forms of affect regulation must be used. These include not only dissociation, but also the turning of rage on the self, giving rise to depression, self-hatred and impulses to harm the body through cutting or overdosing. Such impulses, which can be very difficult to resist, may be aroused particularly by any reminders of the abuse. Overdosing may be perceived as a means of evoking feelings of peace and relief of tension, whilst cutting may paradoxically be experienced as immensely soothing and reassuring. Actions of this kind against the body may be understood as substitutes for the availability of selfobjects. The more healthy alternative, of seeking soothing from others, may be quite unfamiliar to the person who has been abused in childhood.

The distortion of narcissistic maturation

As Ulman and Brothers (1988) have emphasized, childhood trauma and abuse is likely to play havoc with the normal maturation of the line of narcissism. Instead of the normal development of grandiosity and idealization into ambitions and ideals, through the mediation of the selfobjects, as described by Kohut, there may be a hijacking of these by the perverse narcissism of the abuser. This is particularly the case where there has been sexual abuse involving extensive manipulation and control of the child's mind by the perpetrator. The child's own illusions of perfection, omnipotence and invulnerability are utterly shattered. In the wake of betrayal by a caregiver, the splintered fragments of narcissism may be regathered by a fantasy of merger with an idealized abuser – a manoeuvre dependent on denial. A second solution to the catastrophic demolition of narcissism is through identification with the aggressor, a perverse grandiose self modelled on that of the abuser. The latter may be a route whereby the abused becomes an abuser. Failing these desperate attempts to resurrect some semblance of lost perfection, the person abused by a caregiver in childhood may succumb to a boundless depression.

Distortion of sexuality

Kohut described, in many places, the way in which unmet selfobject needs may become sexualized and concretized. Sexual preoccupations and sensory stimulation are sought in lieu of the experience of being related to with empathy. A child who is lonely, and who feels unrelated to by interested and admiring selfobjects, may turn to autoerotic sexual stimulation and fantasies that in some way capture in a concretized way the selfobject longings; for example, Kohut's 'Mr E' developed his homosexual voyeurism during an episode at a country fair when his mother, ill with hypertension, was unable to respond to his grandiose excitement whilst on a high swing. Deflated, the young Mr E had wandered off to a lavatory where he had sought sight of a large adult penis, trying in that sexualized way to establish a concretized version of a merger with an idealized selfobject. Lacking the needed experience of empathy from his mother or father, he had resorted to idealization of the adult man's penis, and attempted to form a merger with this body part. The body of the other was used in place of the mind of the other.

Stoller (1976) described a related process whereby perverse forms of sexuality develop as an attempt at sexualized mastery of childhood traumas that threaten the sense of self and gender identity in a profound way (building on ideas first presented by Freud, 1924). For example, he showed how, in some cases, transvestism develops as a result of a male child's efforts to overcome the injuries to his masculine self perpetrated by repeated feminizations by a dominant mother or sisters. Through the process of sexualization, the source of the deepest anxiety (of castrations and of being turned into a female) becomes the context for the greatest sexual excitement and pleasure – and thus the anxiety is repudiated, again and again compulsively. In this way, Stoller portrays how sexuality scavenges the most psychologically noxious experiences – of the anti-selfobjects which *threaten* the self rather than facilitate its development – and uses these to form the content of its desires and fantasies.

Where the child is subject to sexual abuse by those who should function as selfobjects, his or her sexual development is subject to distortion by pressures from two sources. First there are the tendencies within the child towards sexualization of selfobject needs, as described by Kohut, along with the sexualization of anti-selfobject experiences, as described by Stoller. Then, in addition, there is the fact that sensory experiences are offered by the abuser in place of the needed responses of interest and empathy. Although toxic, these sensory experiences provide a link and moments of quasi-interest from the perpetrator. In some cases – prior to being overwhelmed with the sense of betrayal – the sensory pleasure can also be used as a bulwark against the threatening engulfment with depression and feelings of emptiness. Sexuality – the usurper – is offered in place of the needed selfobject availability. Bodily contact is substituted for a relationship of mind.

In these ways, the sexuality of the child sexually abused by caregivers is hijacked, overstimulated, and misused by the concretized selfobject desires of both child and abuser.

Further damage to the experience of self resulting from sexual abuse

In an earlier book (*The Fragile Self*), a taxonomy was described of seven dimensions of disturbance in the experience of self: the differentiation of self; the subjective self (the sense of agency); the objective self (self-esteem and self-image); structure-organization (the sense of cohesion, coherence, and integrity of the self); balance between the subjective and objective self (the extent of excessive accommodation to the other); illusions of self-sufficiency; the sense of lineage (connection to a sense of origins). All seven of these may be damaged by experiences of sexual abuse by a caregiver.

An abuser who has regular access to a child may set out systematic-ally to distort the child's sense of reality, undermining his or her confidence in their own perceptions. This 'grooming' strategy, whereby abusers seek to control and manipulate the victim's mind, has been extensively described in recent years (e.g. Salter, 1995; also material presented in workshops by sex crime specialist Ray Wyre). The child's perception of abuse and betrayal may be in conflict with the abuser's message that the abuse is love, or that the abuse does not actually take place. Under such circumstances, the child may surrender his or her own perception of reality in favour of the false version offered by the abuser (Freyd, 1996).

A woman talked to her psychiatrist of having been sexually abused for many years by her father. When she disclosed to her parents that she had done so, they told her she was telling lies and that they loved her and that the psychiatrist was making her worse, and, moreover, that she would get better once she accepted that her accounts and memories were false. She retracted her allegations. Later her father made a deathbed confession that he had in fact abused her.

Another woman would talk to her therapist of her abuse, but would often feel she must whisper because of her sense that her domineering and abusing father could somehow overhear her and would punish her for telling.

The person who has been extensively abused by a caregiver will tend to inhabit the version of reality presented by the abuser. Such a vision may include the illusion that the abuser will always have control over the victim. The 'walled garden' sequestering of reality which invisibly imprisons the abused one, will contribute to disturbances particularly in the two areas of *differentiation* of self, and the sense of *agency* (or subjective self). This is because the victim will experience his or her self as insufficiently differentiated from that of the abuser, and will feel relatively powerless, particularly in relation to the abuser.

In the realm of the *objective* self, the abused child's self-esteem will be negative in the extreme. He or she will assume responsibility for the abuse, believing that they must have been very bad for the abuse to have occurred. Moreover, because of the incomplete separation of self and other (resulting from the control exerted by the abuser), the child cannot hate the abuser without also hating the self. This could be described as state of merger, not with an idealized selfobject, but with a denigrated anti-selfobject. If the adult victim experiences dissociative internal voices (as many do), these may scream that he or she deserves to die, thus generating violent internal propaganda directed at undermining self-esteem even further. Moreover, there may be self-hatred in response to the self-perception of having failed to prevent the abuse taking place.

The abused child will identify with the image forced upon him or her by the abuser. As a shorthand, one might describe this as a process of projective identification – or, as I should prefer to call it, *imposed identity*. The abuser perceives the child in a particular image (helpless, bad, etc.) and behaves in such a way as to force the child to experience him or herself in terms of that image – to identify with, and be defined by, the projected representation. A significant part of the motivation of the abuser may be to evoke projectively in the child the unwanted negative images of the self – to make the abused one feel utterly helpless, humiliated, shamed, violated and abject – and to bring about a near annihilation of the true self of the abused. Such an intrapsychic and interpersonal manoeuvre is carried out in order that the abuser does not have to feel that way himself. Because this defensive activity, of projectively forcing noxious self-experience into the victim, provides only temporary relief, it has to be repeated again and again addictively.

The child's development of a *coherent* sense of self depends upon experiences of security and empathy, wherein his or her feelings, needs and inherent autonomy are recognized and supported. These conditions are not present for the child who is abused within the family. Such a child may grow up with what is effectively a shattered self – a chaotic plethora of self-images, lacking coherence and integration. For example, the person may be at one moment an abused and frightened child, at another moment a triumphant aggressor, then an adult in denial of abuse, then a sexual predator, then an asexual 'latency' character, and so on, in an endless movement between states. During therapy, such a person may oscillate wildly between states of mind, even within one session. In extreme instances, there may be dissociation into multiple selves, distinct personality states, each with a different attitude, identity, mode of cognition and memories (Mollon, 1996).

The abused person is often flooded with feelings of *shame*. This experience is in itself a trauma, an overwhelming of the ego's coping capacities. Extreme shame is analogous to a tidal wave, violently sweeping away all vestiges of self-esteem. In the state of shame, the person loses all empathy for the self, giving rise to wishes to punish the self severely. He or she becomes then an abuser to the self – highlighted in those instances where the person takes sadistic pleasure in hurting him/herself. Shame impacts negatively on every area of self-experience to some extent (Mollon, 1993).

The *balance between subjective and objective self* is inevitably skewed towards accommodation to the other in the child who is extensively and repeatedly abused by a caregiver. Surrendering to the abuser's will is an inherent part of the experience, giving rise to a pervasive expectation that meeting the other's desire or agenda is always required. Performing as a debased selfobject for the other becomes the life-role of the abused child.

The abused child's *sense of lineage* will be permeated with shame and self-loathing, especially if the perpetrator(s) were a parent. This is because the sense of origin is linked to (a) having been abused and therefore a victim, and (b) being the child of an abuser.

Damage to relationships to others

The person whose early environment has provided not protection, soothing and security of attachment but instead malevolence and betrayal will not easily be able to form relationships of trust and healthy depend-ence. There are likely to be deep messages or procedural memories established, which warn that the traumas of the past must never be experienced again. Intimacy, dependence, or the seeking of selfobject responses from others will be perceived as profoundly dangerous. Instead the person may seek *illusions of self-sufficiency*, taking flight, or sabotaging relationships whenever attachment or trust is threatened. In therapy, the paradox may arise that the more the patient feels trust towards the therapist, the more he or she feels in danger – because to trust is felt to be utter folly, inviting betrayal.

As a result of the massive failures of the protective functions of the early caregiving environment, many abused people will have established in their minds secret organizations of 'controllers', which operate like a sort of internal police state or mafia (Rosenfeld, 1971). These may be considered as radical internal controls and boundary-keepers, developed in lieu of the more gentle regulation normally offered by selfobjects in more benign environments. They may become violently active under certain conditions, such as when the person reveals secrets about the abuse, or if he or she moves towards a position of trusting the therapist. Bringing about change in these harsh internal organizations may be as difficult as the challenge of overthrowing a repressive political dictatorship.

Forms of defence in reaction to sexual abuse trauma

Dissociation and related forms of detachment, including depersonalization and derealization, are among the most fundamental reactions to trauma. If childhood trauma or abuse is repeated, and if the abuser is a caregiver, so that the child has nowhere to run and no one to turn to, then internal escape is resorted to – the child learns to dissociate more easily and in a more organized way. In this way, the personality system preserves at least parts of itself from the impinging trauma or violation, by sequestering, or sealing off, the area of damage.

One patient, who had managed to develop a very extensive Dissociative Identity Disorder, described how this was done, from the perspective of her internal experience: 'I would withdraw more and more, until I could not see or feel the experience; then a space would be left, and this would be filled with a new personality.' This description was given by one 'personality', which claimed to have had a fundamental role in generating the other personalities within the system of personalities.

The dissociation within the personality, or system of personalities, is often modelled on dissociations inherent in the abusive environment. Abuse may take place, whilst at other times, or even at the *same* time, the abuser and other family members may behave as if everything were normal. The abused child may be punished for speaking of the abuse. He or she may be encouraged to present a 'normal' image to the outside world. In these ways the experience of abuse may be invalidated by the environment (Palef, 1995). As a result, the episodes of abuse may come to be felt as unreal. The child will have difficulty thinking about the abuse. Since the awareness of abuse and betrayal is inherently painful, the child will be motivated to forget, to avoid thinking about it, and to dissociate and sequester the aversive experience. There will be internal invalidation. The person may behave much of the time as if nothing untoward had happened in childhood. For example, in one state of mind a patient spoke of her parents as having subjected her to all manner of abuse and cruelty, whilst in another state of mind she spoke of them as the most kind, caring and respectable parents one could hope to have.

Although parts of the child's mind *will* perceive the abuse and betrayal (Freyd, 1996), it appears to be more or less impossible for a child fully to accept the perception of the caregiver as abusive. Thus, almost all abuse victims will be inclined to take the blame, engaging in elaborate cognitive distortions so as to attribute responsibility to the self. In this way, the victim preserves some semblance of a sense of control – better to feel guilty than helpless.

Fairbairn (1952) may have been the first to describe this 'moral defence' clearly:

> . . . the child would rather be bad than have bad objects . . . he is really taking upon himself the burden of badness which appears to reside in his objects . . . The essential feature, and indeed the essential aim, of this defence is the conversion of an original situation in which the child is surrounded by bad objects into a new situation in which his objects are good and he himself is bad.
>
> (Fairbairn, 1952: 65, 68)

Fairbairn notes that abused children often appear to have difficulty in reporting the sexual assaults:

> At one time I used frequently to have the experience of examining problem children; and I remember being particularly impressed by the reluctance of children who had been *victims* of sexual assaults to give any account of the traumatic experiences to which they had been subjected. The point that puzzled me was that, the more innocent the victim was, the greater was the resistance to anamnesis. By contrast I never experienced any comparable difficulty in the examination of individuals who had *committed* sexual offences.
>
> (Fairbairn, 1952: 63)

He concludes that thinking about the experience of sexual assault within the home would be resisted by the child 'because this memory represents a record of a relationship with a bad object' and 'a bad object is always intolerable, and a relationship with a bad object can never be contemplated with equanimity' (1952: 63). Fairbairn uses the term 'bad object' to refer to a caregiver who functions as an anti-selfobject. He is making the point that it is not so much the traumatic experience itself that creates profound malformations of personality, but the fact that it occurs in the context of a crucial relationship – a relationship that generates panic rather than security. The child resorts to substituting his or her 'badness' for the badness of the relationship.

Related to the processes described by Fairbairn, identification with the aggressor and turning passive into active are also commonly used defensive strategies. The therapist's countertransference may offer a clue as to the quality of the patient's early experiences. Sometimes the therapist is subject to states of considerable anxiety, dread and confusion, as if his or her sanity and sense of reality were under attack. For example, during one phase of therapy a patient would often appear to hint at potential threats to the therapist from those who had abused her, giving the impression that intimidation might take place, designed to discourage the therapist from continuing. No tangible threat did ever materialize, but the resulting state of mind induced in the therapist gave some suggestion of what may have been a chronic or recurrent experience of the patient – of living in dread, of not knowing what was truth and what was fantasy, of doubting one's own perception and experience, and of uncertainty whether the person one was in the room with was benign and could be trusted or was intent on betrayal. Sometimes the betrayal and the patient's identification with the aggressor becomes very tangible. Amongst patients who report extensive childhood abuse by caregivers, there is not uncommonly a tendency ultimately to turn on the therapist, pursuing complaints or litigation – the patient has become the abuser and the therapist is her victim (even though the situation is presented as if it were the reverse of this).

The defences of turning active into passive and identification with the aggressor are also exemplified in the various forms of recreating the trauma, deliberately but unconsciously. Prostitution and promiscuity may sometimes have this motivational basis. Attacks on the body, such as cutting, burning, overdosing, or the painful inserting of objects into the vagina, are also common amongst those abused in childhood. Such attacks on the self are in addition emergency ways of discharging overwhelming rage. Being overwhelmed with rage is probably ubiquitous amongst victims of abuse by caregivers. This is because those whom the child needed to function as soothing selfobjects instead did the opposite – a reversal of selfobject function, such that rage and other dysphoric affects were fuelled rather than calmed. This would be analogous to firefighters throwing petrol instead of water on the flames.

Summary

The coherence, cohesion, continuity and depth of the experience of self are all affected by repeated childhood trauma perpetrated by caregivers.

Numbing and detachment give rise to mutilated states of consciousness. In extreme cases, dissociation can be elaborated into dissociative identity disorder, resulting in multiple selves. Disturbances in the regulation of affect, arising from defective soothing by selfobjects in childhood result in self-hatred and impulses to harm the body. The normal process of narcissistic maturation may be 'hijacked' by the narcissism of the abuser, leading to idealization of the abuser or the development of a perverse grandiose self based on identification with the aggressor. Sexualization of both selfobject needs and also of anti-selfobject experiences may develop from sexual abuse, as well as the substitution of sensory experience for a relationship of mind. Damage occurs in all seven areas of the taxonomy of disturbance in the experience of self: the differentiation of self; the sense of agency; the objective image of the self; the sense of structure-organization; balance between the subjective and objective self; illusions of self-sufficiency; the sense of lineage. Profound distrust of dependency will be deeply rooted in the person abused in childhood. Along with dissociation and identification with the aggressor, the *moral defence*, described by Fairbairn, is common in those who were sexually abused – this is based on the preference for feeling guilty rather than helpless. Turning passive into active may be manifest in prostitution, promiscuity and attacks on the body, as well as in victimizing the therapist.

Chapter 11
Further reflections on psychoanalytic cure

> Self psychology is at one with the technical principle that interpretation in general, and the interpretation of transferences in particular, is the major instrumentality of therapeutic psychoanalysis.
>
> (Kohut, 1984: 210)

As I reflect upon the experience of psychoanalytic work when it appears to be going well, certain qualities stand out: new understandings and perspectives emerge regarding the patient's conflicts, phantasies and anxieties; these are genuinely 'new' in the sense that neither party has thought of them before; the understandings are not clichéd formulations derived from existing theory (although they may on reflection be understood as congruent with particular theories); they are satisfying to both patient and analyst; both feel that 'work' has been done; the patient experiences some sense of an internal change as a result of the understanding; gradually changes are apparent in the patient's outer behaviour, inner experience, and reactions to events and circumstances. These developments appear to be dependent upon an attitude in the analyst of not presuming to know, of being capable of surprise. The rigid application of a theory marks the death of the 'spirit' of psychoanalysis. I believe this spirit is rooted in a stance of relentless enquiry, in which clinical observation and tentative formulation continually enrich each other. Freud's own work displayed this stance throughout. Psychoanalysis seems to work best for patients who, at least in part and despite resistances, are able to share this valuing of enquiry.

There have been many perspectives on the therapeutic process of analysis (Sandler and Dreher 1996), beginning with Freud's (1940a) own emphasis on expanding the domain of the ego, through Strachey's (1934) formulation of the modification of the superego (by a process of projection and reintrojection as this internal object is made more benign by its sojourn within the analyst), and the Kleinian perspective on the movement towards the depressive position and greater integration of the ego (Joseph, 1989), to the more contemporary emphasis upon the transformation of internal models of relationships (derived from attachment theory, object relations theories, and the intersubjectivists: Stern et al., 1998). Within this broad spectrum, Kohut stands out for his attention to the particular significance of empathy – both in child development and within the therapeutic process.

The channel of empathy

Here is how Kohut summarized the therapeutic process from the point of view of self psychology:

> How does self psychology perceive the process of cure? The answer is: as a three-step movement, the first two steps of which may be described as defence analysis and the unfolding of the transferences, while the third step – the essential one because it defines the aim and the results of the cure – is the opening of a path of empathy between self and selfobject, specifically, the establishment of empathic in-tuneness between self and selfobject on mature adult levels. This new channel of empathy permanently takes the place of the formerly repressed or split-off archaic narcissistic relationship; it supplants the bondage that had formerly tied the archaic self to the archaic selfobject.
>
> (Kohut, 1984: 66)

A little later he states the results of successful analysis as follows:

> . . . analysands who had originally been restricted to archaic modes of self–selfobject relationships because the development toward maturity in this sector of their personality had been thwarted in childhood became, in the course of successful analyses, increasingly able to evoke the empathic resonance of mature selfobjects and to be sustained by them.
>
> (Kohut, 1984: 66)

Thus Kohut describes a maturation in the line of development of selfobject relations. In place of reliance on fantasies of merger with idealized and omnipotent selfobjects, or of an imperative need for perfect mirroring, the person becomes more able to seek mature and appropriate empathic responses from others – and also able to *give* such responses to others.

The selfobject and the therapeutic frame

Why does empathy facilitate development? Empathy appears to be soothing, enhancing a person's sense of connectedness to others, and rendering distressing emotional experience more manageable. By contrast, the absence of the availability of an empathic other can greatly exacerbate the unmanageable nature of a person's distress, giving rise to radical and pathological attempts at affect regulation. A vulnerable person (for example, with a borderline personality disorder) who suffers a serious assault to their self-esteem, and who is not able to find relief with an empathic friend or partner, may resort to alcohol or substance abuse, compulsive sexual activity, cutting or other self-harm, or detachment and dissociation. A child who repeatedly does not experience empathy from caregivers will not develop the capacity to be empathic with self. Without the availability of empathy from others and the capacity to be empathic with oneself, a person will not be able to process emotional experience and create a verbal narrative. Bion's alpha function and the integrative linking between cognition (including dreams and fantasy), affect and behaviour will not develop.

Although interpretation may be regarded as the privileged function of the analyst, a good deal of other important activity takes place in the consulting room. The patient talks and thinks about experience – and as he or she does so, new thoughts, observations and feelings come into awareness. To draw upon a concept from cognitive psychology, we might say that the 'global workspace' (Baars, 1988) of consciousness is expanded – with increased internal 'publication' of emotional information – enabling enhanced processing of affective experience and the discovery of new solutions to emotional conflicts and dilemmas. From this point of view, the analytic setting is a *space for thinking*. Moreover, the thinking space may be said to exist *between* analyst and patient, since both contribute to the thoughts that emerge.

The thinking space depends upon maintenance of the boundaries of the analytic frame – such that thought rather than action is facilitated (Gabbard and Lester, 1995). Some analysts (e.g. Casement, 1985; Langs, 1976) place particular importance upon the analyst's monitoring of the patient's unconscious commentaries and prompts regarding the maintenance of the frame. This responsiveness to the patient's unconscious corrective messages often seems to be experienced as being of considerable significance for the patient – in a way that is perhaps similar to the importance Kohut gives to the analyst's recovery of empathic understanding following a breach. Part of its significance may be that the patient is thereby affirmed as an active agent – a subject – in the communicative process. What commonly happens in the analytic process is that there is, through role responsiveness (Sandler, 1976), first a repetition, in a modified and symbolic form, of an original early dysfunctional parental response to the child. This is then followed by the analyst's eventual correction of this (conveyed by interpretation), so that the patient is able to re-experience the original trauma in a more manageable form, such that it can be processed and integrated within the global workspace of consciousness.

Analysts who follow this model are sensitive to the patient's attempts to correct the frame through unconscious communication. Others, perhaps particularly certain Kleinians, give more emphasis to ways in which the patient may attempt to *subvert* the frame.

Setting the patient free

There is another important element implicit in Kohut's descriptions of the therapeutic process – the freeing of the patient from the tie to the noxious anti-selfobject. For example, in the diagram (on page 185 of *The Analysis of the Self*) showing the 'flow of narcissistic energies' in a particular form of narcissistic disturbance, Kohut portrays a tie to the mother and her narcissistic use of the child. This tie, associated with conscious grandiosity and perverse activities or fantasies, is vertically split off from the reality ego. It reflects the mother's narcissism rather than the child's own authentic initiatives of exhibitionism. The child's own natural grandiosity and exhibitionism has been hijacked – thus overt grandiosity (false) coexists with depression (at the thwarting of authentic initiatives). Through analytic work, the vertical split is gradually undone. This results in the patient's expressions of 'astonished estrangement' as he asks 'Is this really me?' or 'How did this get into me?' (Kohut, 1971: 184). Kohut notes that this feeling of astonishment and estrangement 'is due to the fact that for the first time the central sector, with its own goals and its own aesthetic and moral values, is now truly in contact with the other self and is able to behold it in its totality' (Kohut, 1971: 184)

However, Kohut envisages more than merely undoing a split and thereby facilitating integration. He also sees the analytic process as puncturing the repression barrier which has held back the authentic infantile narcissism. Once released into the transmuting vessel of the transference, these energies become available in the person's general life – giving rise to creativity, ambitions, ideals, humour and empathy. Thus this is a two stage process: the liberation from the tie to a development-impeding anti-selfobject; and the releasing of the authentic initiatives of the self. This takes place through the relationship with the selfobject analyst – a relationship that sets the self free.

The alienating mirror

Another perspective on this process is inspired by Lacan's idea of the alienating function of the mirror. Lacan (1949) wrote of the infant's mimetic identification with the image seen in a mirror or through sight of another child. Inherently this is a false identification – the child misperceives him/herself as the image 'out there'. More crucially, it paves the way for identification with the social mirror, the images offered by family, society and culture. Thus Lacan saw a split, an alienation, as inherent and inescapable in the human condition.

It seems to me that it is possible to envisage *degrees* of alienation, dependent upon the extent to which a 'true' or 'false' self (in the Winnicottian sense: 1960) is fostered by the early caregiver. In many of the examples given by Kohut, the analysand has been imprisoned by an identification with an image imposed by the mother, according to her desire for a particular kind of child, or her projection of a disowned aspect of herself. The child's own potential and autonomy has not been fostered. By contrast, in more healthy development, the child's autonomy and talents have been responded to and encouraged.

Of course this is not an absolute distinction. There is no such thing as a 'true self' existing outside of a relationship with the caregiver. Development, including the nurturing of talents and interests, always takes place within the context of (indeed is dependent upon) the relationship with caregivers (including teachers and other influential adults). This relationship will include the caregiver's desire – even if it is a desire to encourage autonomy in the child. Therefore the particular shape of the child's personality, emerging from the array of innate potential, will depend on the selective responsiveness of the caregiver. A great musician will probably have benefited from not only an innate talent, but also encouraging and appreciative parents. However, there is a difference between the selective responsiveness that favours one of the child's initiatives over another (e.g. music rather than visual art), and a parent's imposition of an image which does not derive from the child's initiative. Kohut's 'desire' would be to free the analysand from the captivation by a false image (or phantasy in the mind of the mother) and set in motion a developmental pathway of individuation in the context of the facilitating other (the selfobject analyst).

Imposed identity and cognitive imperialism

The invalidation of those who are stigmatized (as mentally ill, or as a member of a racial, religious or sexual minority) has long been recognized (Goffman, 1968). However, the imposition of an alien image or identity is a form of psychological violence that is extremely common in all kinds of human families, organizations and societies – so common indeed that it is easy to be blind to the pervasiveness of this ubiquitous aggression. The essence of imposed identity is that one person implicitly says to another: 'I shall view you and define you in this particular way and completely ignore your own experience of who and what you are; moreover, I shall force you to define yourself, and experience yourself, in the way that I choose to define you.'

Such activity may be readily observed in the realm of politics. Opposing sides will attempt to define the other and impose a particular (negative) image upon them, whilst claiming a particular identity for themselves – and at the same time endeavour to resist the identity the other side is attempting to impose on them. However, the same struggle to impose or appropriate a particular identity can be found in every area of human society and organization (including psychoanalytic societies!). Racism, tribal and group loyalties are all based on this aggressive assumption of one identity for the 'in-group' and imposition of another identity on the 'out-group'. The earliest cauldron for the manufacture and imposition of an identity is the family – and indeed a child's image and identity may be established whilst he or she is still in the womb. This is not an inevitable process, however, and families may, to varying extents, be able to accommodate the child's autonomous development and individuation.

A protest against being seen as a 'sex object' is a commonplace form of resistance to imposed identity. The 'victim' attempts to assert that she is a person with her own experience and is not to be defined merely in terms of being an object for the other's sexual desire. A particularly violent form of identity imposition is found in cases of childhood sexual abuse – the child is made to feel that he or she is, in essence, defined as the defiled object whose function is to provide sexual and sadistic gratification, and to be a virtual toilet bowl for evacuated feelings of humiliation and self-hatred of the powerful adult.

A phenomenon related to imposed identity is that of the aggressive expansion of one's own perspective, theory or belief system. Religious wars or 'cold wars' between competing political ideologies are obvious examples of these. Everyday arguments where one person attempts to impose their view on the other are trivial and ubiquitous examples. More subtly, this also pervades scientific disputes. This was strikingly apparent in the debates (in both the popular and academic media), in the mid-1990s, regarding recovered memory and false memory (Mollon, 1998; 2000). Many scientists and clinicians found that 'discussion' was often not constructive because so much time would be taken up with the necessity of correcting distortions of their position as presented by others who held different views. Usually there appeared to be pressure force-fully to identify people as belonging to particular 'camps'. The virulence of identity imposition in this debate becomes less puzzling when it is recognized that the subject matter itself was essentially to do with struggles over imposed definitions and identities. Thus, there were people claiming to have been 'objectified' through sexual abuse in childhood; there were others who complained that they had been falsely saddled with the identity of perpetrator of abuse; as a result there were familial and legal battles over whether a person's 'memories' were to be defined as 'true' or 'false'; and finally, there were those whose imposed identity was that of 'recovered memory therapists' and who were accused of having imposed on their patients a false identity as victim of sexual abuse.

These are just some examples of the pervasive phenomenon of aggressive imposition of identity and definition – aggressive because it involves an attempt to supplant or displace alternative or competing identifies and definitions. Thus Greenwald (1980) wrote of the 'totalitarian ego' and presented experimental evidence for the general tendency for people actively to distort information in order to impose and maintain their own assumptions about self and the world. It seems that we are all (potentially) cognitive imperialists – driven perhaps by an unconscious awareness of the inherently flimsy nature of our symbolic impositions on an essentially unknowable reality (Bion's 'O', Kant's 'thing-in-itself' and Lacan's 'Real' – see Grotstein, 1997c)

On not presuming to know

Much of Kohut's work can be seen as a corrective to the damaging developmental impact of cognitive imperialism. For example, in his last book, Kohut gives a lengthy clinical vignette from the analysis of a man who had made several previous attempts at analysis before breaking off each (1984: 178–84). During this treatment with Kohut – which, unlike the others, he did not break off – the patient developed extreme somatic reactions of prolonged severe headaches, but, more alarmingly, eventually appeared increasingly paranoid and angry following a break. In this state of mind, the patient rejected Kohut's interpretations of reactions to the break. Kohut describes his efforts to maintain an analytic stance – although he had not at that time explicitly formulated the principles of self psychology:

> I had grasped, intuitively, that even serious states of self fragmentation, if they occur as an intrinsic aspect of that layer of the therapeutic action which I later designated the selfobject transferences, are less dangerous than they appear to be if – a crucial 'if' indeed! – the analyst retains his analytic stance and, open-mindedly and nondefensively, attempts to resonate empathically with what the patient is experiencing . . . That my own reactions were imperfect, that I often

became defensive under the barrage of attacks, is understandable since the patient always reproached me for real flaws in my emotional responses and intellectual performance. And I learned – again of course imperfectly – not even to respond by telling the patient that however germane his criticisms might be, they were exaggerated and disproportionate. The patient as I finally grasped, insisted – and had a right to insist – that I learn to see things exclusively in *his* way and not at all in *my* way . . . To hammer away at the analysand's transference distortions brings no results; it only confirms the analysand's conviction that the analyst is as dogmatic, as utterly sure of himself, as walled off in the self-right-eousness of a distorted view as the pathogenic parents had been.

(Kohut, 1984: 182)

Thus Kohut emphasizes here his flaws and failures of understanding and allows the patient his own sphere of cognitive imperialism. Paradoxically, this then allows the patient eventually to relinquish his need to control the analyst's perception. In this particular case, material emerged that indicated a transference based on experiences with a cognitively tyran-nical father. Kohut comments:

The father and I – through my originally erroneous transference interpretations – insisted on being looked up to and imitated. The son had wanted the father to respond to his own (i.e. the son's) potentials, suggestions and ideas; he wanted to have the father's experience and knowledge as an aid in his own growth and in the realization of his own potential.

(Kohut, 1984: 183)

The son had needed the father not to impose his views but to facilitate the development of his own. A paranoid reaction in the transference (as repetition of a historical experience) is understandable because a parent's cognitive imperialism is, in effect, a psychological murder of the child's development and autonomy. Kohut seeks to free the patient's potential and development of autonomy through the provision of a facili-tating (selfobject) relationship – as well as by analysing and unravelling the shackles to the anti-selfobject.

A more extensive example is given in Kohut's (1979) renowned account of *The Two Analyses of Mr. Z.* – both analyses being conducted by Kohut, but the first along classical lines, whilst the second was informed by his emerging concepts of self psychology. Mr Z presented initially with feelings of isolation, some somatic symptoms, and masochistic sexual fantasies of being in the service of a domineering woman. Significant features of his background were that his father had left for a couple of years to live with another woman, but returned when Mr Z was five years' old. Kohut noted that the most conspicuous theme in the first year of analysis was a 'regressive mother transference', associated with what appeared to be the patient's 'unrealistic, deluded grandiosity and his demands that the psychoanalytic situation should reinstate the position of exclusive control, of being admired and catered to by a doting mother who . . . in the absence of a father who would have been the oedipal rival, devoted her total attention to the patient' (Kohut, 1979: 399). Interpretations along these lines, which Kohut saw as in keeping with a classical psychoanalytic understanding, were met with intense opposition and rages. Nevertheless, the patient appeared to make some progress over the years and the analysis was concluded seemingly satisfactorily. Indeed, Kohut felt quite certain of the correctness of the theory and of the analytic work based upon it: 'To my analytic eye, trained to perceive the configurations described by Freud, everything seemed to have fallen into place' (Kohut, 1979: 408).

Four and a half years later, Mr Z contacted Kohut again, indicating that he was experiencing further difficulties. During the ensuing second analysis, a deterioration in the mental state of Mr Z's mother threw new light on her personality and her influence on his development. Kohut notes that the picture of her that Mr Z had presented in the first analysis was essentially that of the image she presented to the world outside the family. However, what emerged was a much darker picture of her, which both Mr Z and his father knew but not at a level of awareness that would have enabled them to talk to each other about it:

> They knew that the mother held intense, unshakeable convictions that were translated into attitudes and actions which emotionally enslaved those around her and stifled their independent existence . . . The mother's emotional gifts were bestowed on him under the unalterable and uncompromising condition that he must submit to total domination by her, that he must not allow himself any independence, particularly as concerned significant relationships with others.
>
> (Kohut, 1979: 417)

Mr Z had initially presented an idealized picture of his mother – along the lines that she herself presented. With the support of the analyst, he became able to 'question the formerly unquestionable':

> And as he gradually became able to rid himself of the sense of the sacrosanctity of the outlook on their relationship with which the mother had indoctrinated him, he began to recognize a certain bizarreness . . .
>
> (Kohut, 1979: 419)

For example, Mr Z recalled his mother's obsessive interest in his faeces and in his skin – and particularly in the possible presence of blackheads which she would search for in minute detail every Saturday afternoon.

Kohut asks the question as to why this material had not emerged more clearly in the first analysis. His answer is that a crucial aspect of the transference had remained unrecognized. He explains:

> Put most concisely: my theoretical convictions, the convictions of a classical analyst . . . had become for the patient a replica of the mother's hidden psychosis, of a distorted outlook on the world to which he had adjusted in childhood, which he had accepted as reality – an attitude of compliance and acceptance that he had now reinstated with regard to me and to the seemingly unshakeable convictions that I held.
>
> (Kohut, 1979: 423)

Kohut mentions one dream in which Mr Z's mother appeared: 'a starkly outlined image of the mother, standing with her back turned toward him – it was filled with the deepest anxiety he had ever experienced' (1979: 431). Various levels of the meaning of this dream were explored. However, Kohut states that the deepest meaning was contained in its invisible part, 'the unseen, the unseeable frontal view of the mother' (1979: 432). Mr Z experienced intense anxiety when he tried to think about this. Initial interpretations in terms of the horror of castration, fantasies of blood and mutilation and so on, seemed relevant but did not appear to capture the essence of the anxiety. Eventually Kohut suggested that what the mother had lost was not her penis but her face. Mr Z responded with prolonged silence, but then appeared noticeably more relaxed. Kohut concluded that 'Although . . . the archaic fear to which he was exposed defies verbalization, I think that my attempt to define it came sufficiently close to the psychic reality of his experience to allow him a degree of mastery' (1979: 432).[1]

Kohut approaches here the presymbolic dread, the absence of form and meaning, which lay behind the apparent certainty of the mother's position. He comments:

> All in all . . . the conclusion we ultimately reached was that the unseen side of the mother in this dream stood for her distorted personality and her pathological outlook on the world and on him – of features, in other words, that he was not only forbidden to see but whose recognition would in fact endanger the structure of his self as he knew it. The dream expressed his anxiety at the

---

[1] The dream image of Mr Z's mother, with her face obscured, might be compared to Green's account of the 'blank anxiety' associated with the experience of 'the dead mother'. Like Kohut, Green distinguishes between anxiety on the paradigm of 'castration' – 'a bodily wound associated with a bloody act' (Green, 1983: 145) – and forms of anxiety based on absence.

realization that his conviction of his mother's strength and power – a conviction on which he had based a sector of his own personality in intermeshment with her – was itself a delusion.

(Kohut, 1979: 432)

In these and other accounts, Kohut demonstrates how the patient has been the prisoner of imposed identity and a parent's cognitive imperialism. Under these developmental circumstances, the child has built a sector of personality around the identity or cognitive framework imposed by the parent. This 'false self', to use Winnicott's term (1960), is in opposition to the child's authentic potential and autonomy. One danger in analysis, as Kohut describes with the first analysis of Mr Z, is that this pattern will be repeated invisibly in the transference, such that an adoption of the analyst's framework will form another version of false self. In recognizing this danger, and guarding against it, Kohut adopts a stance that places central importance on the analyst's not presuming to know – and which in fact sees the analyst's errors, and acknowledgement of these, as the very vehicle of therapeutic progress.

Freedom through the analyst's errors – transmuting internalization

This may well be part of the reason for Kohut's emphasis on transmuting internalization (resulting from the analyst's failures of understanding) as the essential curative process. He describes this as follows:

> In response to the analyst's errors in understanding or in response to the analyst's erroneous or inaccurate or otherwise improper interpretations, the analysand turns back temporarily from his reliance on empathy to the archaic selfobject relationships . . . the analyst takes note of the analysand's retreat, searches for any mistakes he might have made, nondefensively acknowledges them after he has recognized them (often with the help of the analysand), and then gives the analysand a noncensorious interpretation of the dynamics of his retreat.
>
> (Kohut, 1984: 67)

Thus he outlines how he looks for the analyst's contribution, in terms of errors of understanding or interpretation, to the patient's withdrawal or regression. He then offers the patient an explanation of what has gone on between them. Such sequences lead, he argues, to therapeutic progress:

> . . . each small scale, temporary empathic failure leads to the acquisition of self-esteem-regulating structure in the analysand – assuming, once more, that the analyst's failures have been nontraumatic ones.
>
> (Kohut, 1984: 67)

Kohut, in essence, is saying that the patient makes progress through the analyst's errors and his or her acknowledgement of these. Although many of those sympathetic to self psychology have disagreed with the concept of transmuting internalization (e.g. Orange et al., 1997; Shane, Shane and Gales, 1997), Kohut himself clearly regarded it as crucial. Perhaps this was because it captured the need for the analyst to eschew certainty and cognitive imperialism – and placed this at the centre of his theory. He emphasized the importance of listening open-mindedly and commented:

> By listening open-mindedly, I mean that he must resist the temptation to squeeze his understanding of the patient into the rigid mold of whatever theoretical preconceptions he may hold, be they Kleinian, Rankian, Jungian, Adlerian, classical-analytic, or, yes, self psychological, until he has more accurately grasped the essence of the patient's need and can convey his understanding to the patient via a more correct interpretation.
>
> (Kohut, 1984: 67)

Without memory and desire

Some comparison may be made here with the analytic stance advocated by Bion (1970). Although his recommendation that 'memory' and 'desire' be eschewed in the consulting room is sometimes dismissed as unrealistic, my own feeling is that, in this formulation, Bion managed to capture something fundamental about a truly psychoanalytic attitude. Moreover, I believe that Bion and Kohut, however different their heritage and writing styles, had much in common in their basic observational stance. It is worth looking more closely at what Bion meant. His position is stated as follows:

> . . . the capacity to forget, the ability to eschew desire and understanding, must be regarded as essential discipline for the psycho-analyst. Failure to practice this discipline will lead to a steady deterioration in the powers of observation whose maintenance is essential.
>
> (Bion, 1970: 51)

He explains the reason for this in terms of the need to allow the emergence of the unknown:

> . . . to spend time on what has been discovered is to concentrate on an irrelevance. What matters is the unknown and on this the psycho-analyst must focus his attention. Therefore 'memory' is a dwelling on the unimportant to the exclusion of the important. Similarly 'desire' is an intrusion into the analyst's state of mind which covers up, disguises, and blinds him to the point at issue: that aspect of O that is currently presenting the unknown and unknowable . . . This is the 'dark' spot that must be illuminated by 'blindness'. Memory and

desire are 'illuminations' that destroy the value of the analyst's capacity for observation as leakage of light into a camera might destroy the value of the film being exposed.

(Bion, 1970: 69)

Bion suggests that memory (thoughts about what is already known, or formulations in terms of clichés based on existing theory) and desire (to move the patient in a particular direction) act to block the emergence of what is new in the patient. The emergence of what is new, and the freeing of the patient from imprisonment within false identifications and beliefs, is the psychoanalytic concern of both Kohut and Bion, even though each formulates this differently.

Bion addresses the question of whether the suspension of memory would be an abnormal mutilation of the analyst's mind:

. . . it may seem impossible to have a link with a patient without remembering who he or she is; but such recognition does not depend on memory, nor does psycho-analysis . . . We are familiar with the experience of *remembering* a dream; this must be contrasted with dreams that float into the mind unbidden and unsought and float away again as mysteriously. The emotional tone of this experience is not peculiar to the dream; thoughts also come unbidden, sharply, distinctly, with what appears to be unforgettable clarity, and then disappear leaving no trace by which they can be recaptured. I wish to retain the term 'memory' for experience related to conscious attempts at recall. These are expressions of a fear that some element, 'uncertainties, mysteries, doubts' will obtrude. Dream-like memory is the memory of psychic reality and is the stuff of analysis.

(Bion, 1970: 69–70)

Thus Bion advocates a state of mind in the analyst that is akin to reverie, a deep immersion in the experience of being with the patient, which allows an openness to what is new and hitherto unknown. By not imposing a theory, a memory, a belief or a desire, the analyst can be receptive and responsive to the patient's spontaneous movement. Such eschewing of illusions of knowing by the analyst can also help the patient gradually to relinquish their own false knowledge of self.

Kohut describes a similar state of mind in one of his Chicago lectures in 1975, drawing upon Freud's original recommendations:

Evenly hovering attention by the analyst is the counterpart . . . to the patient's free associations. It should not be defined primarily in the negative as is generally done, as a suspension of preconscious or conscious activities. Rather, evenly hovering attention should be defined positively by pointing up the expansion of the analyst's psyche, its partial encompassing of the patient's psyche, and its reverberation with the analysand's preconscious and unconscious material. Ideally . . . the listening that an analyst does is a listening in

depth and the insights one arrives at are closures that establish themselves
spontaneously without the active will of the analyst.

(Kohut, 1996: 369)

Kohut emphasizes that theories are necessary for the psychoanalyst, but
they must be put out of intentional conscious awareness when with the
patient. Just as Bion described the way that dreams and dream-like
thoughts may float into consciousness, so similarly theories may be
triggered by the patient's communication – but these must be a *response*
to rather than *imposed* on the patient's material. Kohut comments:

> . . . an observer needs theories in order to observe . . . these theories must be
> the helpmates of the observer, not his masters. If an analyst is convinced that a
> particular set of theories has ubiquitous applicability and relevance at all times,
> he will often misinterpret his patient's reactions and, in compliance with his
> unshakeable convictions, will look upon their protestations as resistances.
>
> (Kohut, 1984: 67)

The subtly coercive imposition of theories and meanings can clearly be
harmful to the psychoanalytic process and the patient's development
(Casement, 2000) and is a misuse of the analyst's authority (Mitchell,
1997a). It can even drive the patient mad, as Searles (1959) describes.

In order for spontaneous, autonomous and authentic potential –
Winnicott's 'true self' or Kohut's 'independent centre of initiative' – to
unfold within the analysis, the patient must be protected from the
analyst's capacity for cognitive imperialism, but also freed from the
cognitive imperialist within himself. The analyst too must be freed from
his psychoanalytic false self – his identification with particular theories
and his desire for left brain categorization – and instead be open to the
spontaneous promptings of image, feeling, thought and dream, the gifts
from the right side of the brain – the neurological unconscious (Galin,
1974; Schore, 2000).

It is worth noting that this stance involves the surrendering of illusions
of omnipotence and omniscience, which Klein saw as crucial elements of
the move from the paranoid-schizoid (dis-integration) to the depressive
(integration) position. Something must be allowed to happen, the unconscious must be allowed to speak, and the internal parents must be
allowed to have their intercourse. Money-Kyrle comments:

> Remember that in the inner world, parthenogenic creativity is a megalomanic
> delusion. All you can do, and surely this is enough, is to allow your internal
> parents to come together and they will beget and conceive the child.
>
> (Money-Kyrle, 1971: 442)

The internal primal scene – intercourse between left and right hemispheres

The phantasy of an internal primal scene need not be thought of exclusively in terms of internalized parents in intercourse. It can be taken as a paradigm for the creative coitus and communication of different elements within the mind – relating particularly to the communion between right and left hemispheres of the brain. Just as we may commonly speak of the young child's envious and fearful desire to control or prevent the intercourse of the parents, so it is possible to envisage an envious relationship between left and right hemispheres of the brain. One might think of instances where it is as if the left side of the brain, operating with a 'rational', linguistic, logical, categorizing mode of cognition, attempts to subjugate or deny the more holistic, imagistic, emotion-processing right brain.

There are, in fact, empirical demonstrations of the potential independence and opposition of the two hemispheres – perhaps corresponding to the dual track consciousness emphasized by Grotstein (1981). Some years ago there were instances of patients whose corpus callosum – the connection between the two hemispheres – had been surgically severed because this was found to alleviate some cases of epilepsy. No immediately obvious impairment of brain function was found, but investigations showed that such patients acted essentially as if they had two brains, with two different modes of processing information. Whilst most studies with split-brain patients concerned cognitive and perceptual tasks, there are also some anecdotal observations reported regarding emotional information processing. Two of the investigators, LeDoux and Gazzaniga, made the following comments about one patient:

> The day that case P.S.'s left and right hemispheres equally valued himself, his friends, and other matters, he was a calm, tractable, and appealing adolescent. On the days that the right and left sides disagreed on these evaluations, case P.S. became difficult to manage behaviourally. Clearly, it is as if each mental system can read the emotional differences harboured by the other at any given time. When they are discordant, a feeling of anxiety, which is ultimately read out by hyperactivity and general overall aggression, is engendered. The crisp surgical instance of this dynamism raises the question of whether or not such processes are active in the normal brain, where different mental systems, using different neural codes, coexist within and between the cerebral hemispheres.
>
> (Quoted in Springer and Deutsch, 1989: 329)

Springer and Deutsch (1989) draw attention to the idea that the right brain is able to express itself more freely during dreaming because the left hemisphere does not dominate or interfere. Psychoanalysis has always attempted, in effect, to facilitate the expression of the right brain; not only through consideration of dreams, but also by creating the setting for free-association whereby the normal concern for linguistic logic and the rational channelling of thought is set aside. Arthur Koestler, in *The Act of Creation* (1964), argues that creativity occurs through the suspension of conscious intention and control. He sees creativity as arising from the mode of cognition of the unconscious, Freud's 'primary process' (Matte-Blanco, 1975; 1988) – in effect the suspension of left brain dominance: 'a temporary liberation from the tyranny of overprecise verbal concepts, of the axioms and prejudices ingrained in the very texture of specialized ways of thought'. These insights suggest a human tendency to have lost contact with the creative spontaneity of the right brain through the overdominance of the left brain.

Indeed, Jaynes (1976), in his theory of the bicameral mind, suggests an evolutionary misalliance between the hemispheres such that early mankind misinterpreted internalized speech arising from the right brain's attempts to communicate to the linguistically developing left brain – giving rise to auditory hallucinations and commands from the 'gods'. Using Bion's (1970) metaphor of container–contained, we might consider that the linguistic left brain acts as a container for the communications of the right brain, attempting to give these an appropriate form. The spontaneity of the unconscious can be given expression and form through free-association, through art, and perhaps through certain kinds of meditation. All these are known to have psychotherapeutic applications. Each is a different way of drawing back the controlling dominance of the left brain so as to give freer rein to the play of the right brain unconscious – and thus can be seen as vehicles of the 'true self'.

Winnicott (1988) discusses two kinds of artists, who give expression to the true (or 'secret') self by two different routes. The first, who starts with the false self, is able to make an exact representation of external reality and uses this gradually as an ability that can express the true and secret self: 'If there is success, the artist has not only produced something recognizable to others, but also something which is individual to the artist's true self' (1988: 109). By contrast, the other kind of artist 'starts off with crude representations of the secret self phenomena or personal aliveness which are pregnant with meaning for the artist but at first have no meaning for others' (1988: 109). The task for this second kind of artist is to express his or her personal meanings in a form that is intelligible to others. However, this may give rise to a sense of having betrayed the true self, and the artistic creations may be felt by the artist to be failures no matter how much they are appreciated by others: 'in fact if they are appreciated too widely the artist may withdraw altogether because of the sense of having been false to his true self. Here again, the main achievement of the artist is his work of integration of the two selves' (1988: 109–10). Perhaps it would not be entirely conceptually cavalier to suggest that the right hemisphere is the source of the 'true self' whilst the linguistic left hemisphere – which must work with the pre-existing language of the family and culture – expresses the social or 'false self'.[2]

Winnicott and Kohut both drew attention to the way in which psycho-analysis – which is meant to facilitate *free*-association and spontaneity – can itself become infected by the left brain impulse to control and dominate, so that interpretations are given dogmatically, imposed on the patient's material, resulting merely in compliance and a subtle reweaving of the false self. That such dangers are ubiquitous in psychoanalysis is illustrated by Kernberg's (1996) outline of 'Thirty methods to destroy the creativity of psychoanalytic candidates'!

Edward de Bono, the originator of the concept of lateral thinking in relation to creativity, has some relevant observations regarding a funda-mental antagonism that can sometimes exist between two contrasting cognitive styles:

> If the necessity to be right at every stage is one limitation of vertical thinking, another one is the necessity to have everything rigidly defined. The compul-sively logical mind likes everything to be cut and dried. Such a mind is uneasy with variation: a word must always mean the same thing and cannot change its meaning temporarily in order to accommodate a flow of ideas. A lateral thinker may step fleetingly on a word, using it only as a brief foothold in his passage: the vertical thinker must balance squarely on it, acknowledging its firm rigidity. The vertical thinker is for ever classifying things because this way vagueness can be controlled. The vertical thinker is more interested in seeing on what basis he can pull things apart, the lateral thinker is more interested in seeing on what basis he can put things together.
>
> (de Bono, 1967: 97–98)

Thus de Bono describes the contrast between the 'fixed cathexis' (Freud, 1900) of the secondary process mode of thought – whereby a word's meaning is relatively fixed – and the 'mobile cathexes' of the primary process, which finds expression most vividly in dreams, but also in all forms of creativity. De Bono also notes that vertical, or linear, thinking is associated with rigidity and a need to control, to be certain, and to be right. He also implies an inherent aggression in linear thinking – the desire to pull things apart.

[2.] The neuroscientist Jaak Panksepp (2000) argues that the left hemisphere is the inter-preter of the 'true' affective experience processed in the right hemisphere and, moreover, is the source of confabulation, rationalization and 'lies' – perhaps like the Lacanian ego.

In contrast, the concept of transmuting internalization privileges uncertainty, not knowing, and the analyst's failure of understanding. The analyst must understand enough, empathically, to establish an affective connection with the patient, but must fail to understand enough to allow the patient the space, and the impetus, for his or her own mental growth. Many years ago, Bob Hobson, who originated the 'conversational model' of psychotherapy, remarked to me that he thought what really facilitated development was not the analyst's understanding, but optimal *misunderstanding* – this is very similar to Kohut's insight. What is remarkable in Kohut's perspective is the idea that this optimal misunderstanding – and the subsequent tracking of the vicissitudes of this in the transference – has a real effect on the patient's brain, in that affect regulation is enhanced. Kohut states this clearly:

> . . . psychoanalysis cures by the laying down of psychological structure. And how does this accretion of psychological structure take place? . . . psychological structure is laid down (a) via optimal frustration and (b) in consequence of optimal frustration, via transmuting internalization.
>
> (Kohut, 1984: 98)

Kohut goes on to clarify what he means by this psychic structure which transmuting internalization lays down. He explains that he is not referring to the structures of the Freudian mental apparatus, nor any of its constituents, but to the structure of the self. Whilst a metaphor of psychic structure can be tautological, it serves as an aid to thought and communication. Thus Kohut comments:

> It allows us to speak of the attributes of the self in general terms, without specifying whether we have in mind its cohesion, its strength, or its harmony – that is without specifying whether we refer to a person's experience of being whole and continuous, of being fully alive and vigorous, or of being balanced and organized . . . And it allows us to evoke, again without being specific, such diverse yet defining attributes of the self as those given by our abiding sense of being a center of initiative, of being a recipient of impressions, of having cohesion in space and continuity in time, and the like.
>
> (Kohut, 1984: 99)

Kohut states here that transmuting internalization – through the analyst's failure (and subsequent recovery) of understanding – leads to improvements in such aspects of self-experience as feeling whole, continuous, balanced, organized, alive, vigorous, having cohesion in space, and continuity in time. These attributes suggest a psychobiological organism that is well-regulated in terms of the management and transaction of internal and external emotional currency. Thus, according to Kohut, the analyst's surrender of illusions of omniscience and refraining from the dogmatic imposition of meaning give rise, in time, to the most far-reaching changes in the analysand's experience of self.

Towards discovery of the subjectivity of self *and* other

If an analyst always provided accurate and perfectly attuned empathic understanding, an illusion could be sustained that he or she is not a separately experiencing and desiring person, but exists only as a selfobject. It would be possible to misunderstand Kohut's position as implying that under ideal therapeutic conditions, the analyst is indeed reduced to a function – that of selfobject – and is perceived by the patient as having no separate subjectivity. Benjamin (1988; 1990) has cogently drawn attention to the tendency in psychoanalytic theorizing to conceptualize the other as an 'object' of the individual's instinctual drives or attachment needs – a habit of thought that has tended to deflect attention from exploration of the implications of recognizing the other as also being a centre of experience and initiative. As Benjamin comments: 'An inquiry into the intersubjective dimension of the analytic encounter would aim to change our theory and practice so that "where objects were, subjects must be"' (1990: 184).

Benjamin espouses a developmental intersubjectivity perspective, arguing that 'the other must be recognized as another subject in order for the self to fully experience his or her subjectivity in the other's presence' (1990: 186) and that this depends upon a capacity for mutual recognition, which is acquired only in the course of development. To some extent, this developmental achievement is addressed in the work of Stern (1985), who describes how the child comes to recognize that the mother can have a similar emotional and perceptual experience. However, Benjamin points to something beyond this – the child's becoming able to appreciate that the mother has her own subjectivity which may not coincide with that of the child. She points out that in Kohut's theorizing it can appear to be that the self is the receiver and never the giver of empathy. She asks: 'The responsiveness of the selfobject, by definition, serves the function of "shoring up our self" throughout life; but at what point does it become the responsiveness of the outside other whom we love?' (1990: 186). Thus she is looking at the inherent tension between the experience of the other as selfobject and the other as one who is loved as a separate person.

However, despite very different conceptual language, this concern with the child's recognition of the mother's subjectivity is absolutely central to the British Kleinian tradition. It is found in the conceptualization of the 'depressive position'. Although some derivatives of Kleinian theory, such as Kernberg's (1976) object relations theory, place emphasis predominantly upon the developmental attainment of integration of loving and hating feelings, and of the hitherto split images of the loved and hated mother, Klein and her followers also focused upon the child's struggle with the painful recognition that the mother is a separate person. Thus Segal (1973) comments on the infant's recognition of the mother as a 'whole object':

> He begins to see that his good and bad experiences do not proceed from a good and a bad breast or mother, but from the same mother who is the source of good and bad alike. *This recognition of his mother as whole person* has very wide implications, and opens up a world of new experience. *Recognizing his mother as a whole person means also recognizing her as an individual who leads a life of her own* and has relationships with other people. The infant discovers his helplessness, his utter dependence on her, and his jealousy of other people.
>
> (Segal, 1973: 68; italics added)

Segal is indicating here that the child's discovery of intersubjectivity can be the source of considerable distress and conflict – particularly as it becomes focused in oedipal and sibling rivalries. By contrast, Kohut's implication is that if the child's own subjectivity is given sufficient recognition then he or she does not experience intolerable distress in sibling or oedipal jealousies.

This apparent incompatibility of view, between Benjamin and Segal, on the one hand, and Kohut, on the other, might not be as stark as it at first seems. The concept of transmuting internalization, so central to Kohut's theory, provides the bridge. It is through the analyst's well-intentioned failures (of empathy and understanding) that the patient is confronted with the analyst's separate subjectivity – *'Here is an other being, who looks human, like me, but does not understand me, and therefore I am all alone with my own experience.'* However, providing there is no impasse and entrenched empathic misattunement, the patient also recognizes that the analyst is *endeavouring* to understand his or her subjectivity – the implicit thought might be *'Here is another being, human like me, separate from me, yet trying to understand me from my point of view, and sometimes succeeding; therefore it is possible for us to be quite distinct individuals, with our own thoughts, feelings and desires, and yet be able to understand each other, to imagine ourselves in the other's position, at least to some extent.'* The other is encountered as a subject who is trying to relate to the patient as a subject. Thus, in the interplay of empathic attunement and disruption, through the process of transmuting internalization, the patient continually experiences the separation of subjectivities, as well as the background presence of selfobject continuity. Here we find the 'dual track' consciousness emphasized by Grotstein (1981; 1983), the coexistence of separation and fusion, of other-as-subject and other-as-selfobject.

Intersubjective suffering

Prolonged and deep analytic work seems to involve mutual suffering. Analysis of conflicts, of unconscious phantasies, and so on, which does not involve the analyst, as well as the patient, in suffering, appears to characterize only early and relatively superficial stages of the work. My own experience is that even with patients who are comparatively healthy, there comes a point when a particular quality of mental pain is encountered, which in some way is unbearable – *and the analyst feels responsible*. Although this is most clearly the case when the patient has experienced severe abuse or neglect in childhood, it may well be to some degree ubiquitous. It cannot be entirely reduced to issues of sadism and masochism, or of a patient's stance of malignant entitlement (Freud, 1916; Rothstein, 1980). At a deep level of the unconscious (Matte-Blanco, 1975; 1988), the analyst *is* responsible for the patient's suffering. Grotstein drawing on Meltzer's (1978) formulation that 'transference' involves the transfer of mental pain from the patient to the analyst, proposes the idea of 'potential parental and analytic guilt for birthing children when one cannot guarantee them "safe passage" through the straits of the "Real"' (1997a: 197). And who has not at some point rebuked his or her parents for giving birth to a life that contains pain? Grotstein refers to a paper by Kubie and Israel (1955), which describes how a mute child suddenly began to speak after Dr Kubie, during a presentation, was inspired to say to her 'I'm very sorry!'; immediately the girl exclaimed to each member of the audience, 'Say you're sorry!' The demand for an 'apology' may be a universal unconscious archetype. Grotstein comments that the analyst 'like the infant's mother, applies reverie, patience and "dream-work alpha" to process and to translate the pain into its ultimate meaning for the infant/patient' (1997a: 211). He adds:

> In doing so, the analyst suffers the patient's pain in the depressive position and thereby allows the patient to resuffer the pain once again but on a more tolerable level – as the patient's own pain – in the patient's own depressive position.
>
> (Grotstein, 1997a: 211)

The suffering 'belongs' to the patient, but in order for it to be transformed through analytic work, it must be shared. The analyst's sharing of the pain and feeling responsible for the patient's suffering cannot simply be dismissed as transference and countertransference. Although it is part of transference-countertransference, it must *also* be experienced as real. Grotstein comments:

> The subjective medium is the transference effigy, that is, an invisible image of the object that is transposed between the analytic subject and the analyst, one that the subject cannot distinguish from the analyst without the analyst's interpretive intervention. The analyst, on the other hand, though able to distinguish between the image and him/herself, is nevertheless caught up in the dilemma of feeling both connected to (identified with) and disconnected from (nonidentified with) the effigy object.
>
> (Grotstein, 1997a: 211–12)

The suffering of the analyst – and the patient's perception of the analyst's struggle with the transferred pain (Carpy, 1989) – is an implicit but not explicit feature of Kohut's formulations of the empathic stance.

Releasing the unknown self

During the analytic process, the transference effigy is eventually unravelled, revealing the reality behind it. The patient gradually is able to differentiate the analyst, as a person, from the imposed identity of the historical transference (based on the templates of childhood experience), or the projective transference (based on projection of an internal image or self or 'object'). In this way there develops a groping and uncertain move from an initial position of perceiving both self and other in terms of imposed images (effigies), to a recognition of self and other as persons, each with their own subjectivity, and each continually evolving – and therefore each with an unknown centre of spontaneous initiative.

The 'true' self is indeed an unknown self. It is a *source* which cannot itself be viewed or defined – a subject which can never be an object (Grotstein, 1997). Bollas comments:

> Unlike the latent thoughts which constitute a manifest text, or the chain of signifiers that link the freely associated, or the familiar, if various, constellations of defences, the true self cannot easily be isolated as an object of study . . . As the true self is . . . only a potential, it comes into being only through experience. It does not have an established meaning (unconscious or otherwise), as its significance is contingent on the quality of object experience.
>
> (Bollas, 1989: 15)

and, he adds:

> In our true self we are essentially alone. Though we negotiate our ego with the other and though we people our internal world with selves and others, and though we are spoken to and for by the Other that is speech . . . the absolute

core of one's being is a wordless, imageless solitude. We cannot reach this true self through insight or introspection. Only by living from this authorizing idiom do we know something of that person sample that we are.

(Bollas, 1989: 21)

Although psychoanalysis can be an effective treatment for a variety of mental health problems (Fonagy, 1999c), it can do something more, of infinitely greater value. As practised by those who endeavour diligently to eschew certainty and illusions of knowing – who can say with Goldberg, 'The beckoning feeling of certainty and comfort is the worst affliction of the mind of the analyst' (1994: 29) – it becomes a unique vehicle for freeing the individual from the tangled web of inherited and received discourse. These words, opinions, attitudes, values and images of parental and societal voices are indeed *chains* of signifiers, which invisibly colonize, shackle and imprison, and, worst of all, are mistaken for the subject's own self. It is not that an individual can sanely live outside a (mostly pre-existing) social structure, but psychoanalysis can enable a person to choose his or her place in that structure with more awareness – and with a recognition that all ways of saying 'I am thus' are temporary and ultimately false – a freezing of a moment, like identifying with a photograph. The temptation to re-intern the self is ever present, however, for the emergence of the unknown is a source of profound disquiet as well as joy. Even a small increase in the capacity to tolerate contact with 'O' (Bion, 1970) can result in unexpected riches of new development – but so quickly the evolving unknown self is recaptured, imprisoned in a representation, a word, an image, or a theory. For these reasons, all psychoanalytic theory is suspect – useful for but a moment, and then to be discarded, as we await what next comes to mind.

Summary

Many aspects of the therapeutic process have been described since Freud's original emphasis upon expanding the domain of the ego. Empathy, as highlighted by Kohut, has various functions: such as soothing, enhancing the feeling of connectedness to others, and enabling the processing of emotional experience. Analyst and patient together create a space for thinking, an enhanced 'global workspace', within which emotional information can be 'published'. In addition to Kohut's emphasis upon the role of empathy in the curative process, he also described the liberation of the patient from the internal tie to the noxious anti-selfobject. This restricting tie can be linked to Lacan's insights into the alienating mirror (of the images, identities and roles provided by others) and Winnicott's account of the origins of the false self (in excessive adaptation to the desires and expectations of the mother). Imposed identity and cognitive imperialism may be ubiquitous aspects of the human endeavour to flee from presymbolic dread. During analysis, the patient may emerge from imposed identity by mean of the analyst's *errors* of understanding and the acknowledgement of these. Through the disruption in the representation of the analysand something new is enabled to unfold. In this way, the unknown potential of the analysand is released from the shackles of identity imposed by self or other. This process of 'transmuting internalization' involves the surrender of illusions of omnipotence and omniscience (by both analyst and analysand) – and can therefore be linked to Klein's depressive position. In the depressive position, the internal parents are allowed to have their creative intercourse. Similarly, the right and left hemispheres of the brain must engage in a co-operative intercourse in order for unknown potential to emerge. Commonly, the linguistic modality of the left hemisphere may exert dominance over the emotional and primary process modality of the right hemisphere – the latter being in many ways equivalent to the unconscious. Psychoanalysis provides a unique method for supporting the communications from the right brain unconscious – including the communicative transference of suffering. By the gradual release from the constraining constructions imposed by the left brain linguistic modality and the obscuring function of the 'transference effigy', the state of intersubjectivity is eventually achieved, whereby the analysand is able to experience self and other as subjects – centres of initiative – evolving from an unknown source. Psychoanalytic theorizing can help this process, provided that it is repeatedly discarded after use – to be replaced continually by new thoughts and insights.

Appendix
A note on Kohut the man[1]

Heinz Kohut was born on 3 May 1913, in Vienna, and died 8 October 1981, in Chicago.

In Vienna – as 'the quintessential young Viennese intellectual, frequenting the coffeehouses that were centres for discussion and debate' (Cocks, 1994: 7) – he knew and was interested in Freud's work. At the University of Vienna he studied medicine. His family were middle class and music was an important part of their life. His father, Felix, worked in the paper business – he was also a talented pianist. His mother, Else, was an accomplished singer. Kohut's first published psychoanalytic paper, in 1950, was entitled 'On the enjoyment of listening to music'.

Some impressions of Kohut's early life are given in his famous paper *The Two Analyses of Mr. Z.* (1979) – now, according to Cocks (1994), believed by his wife and son, as well as other friends and colleagues, to be essentially autobiographical. Mr Z's mother is described as highly dominant, controlling and paranoid, taking an intrusive and hypochondriacal interest in her son's body. She also subjected him to continual criticism. At the same time the father is portrayed as relatively absent – and Mr Z felt that he had abandoned him to his crazy mother. Like Mr Z, Kohut himself was an only child, and his mother did later develop an overt paranoid illness.

With the Nazi annexation of Austria in 1938, Kohut and Freud both fled, within a few months of each other. Freud left for London in June 1938. Kohut departed in March 1939 to London en route to Chicago. He actually witnessed Freud's departure on the train and later recalled, 'I had the feeling of a crumbling universe' (quoted in Cocks, 1994: 8). Almost all his relatives died in Nazi concentration camps (letter, 2 June 1946).

---

[1] The best source of material regarding Kohut's life is the collection of his letters edited by Cocks (1994).

Like Freud, Kohut began as a neurologist, before moving to psychiatry and then to psychoanalysis. After an internship at Roseland Hospital in Chicago, he received his Illinois medical licence in August 1941, becoming then a resident in neurology at the University of Chicago Hospital the same year. Then, from 1947 to 1950, he was an assistant professor of psychiatry at the University. In 1946 he commenced training in psychoanalysis at the Chicago Institute, graduating in 1950 and becoming a member in 1953. He married a social worker (Betty Meyer) at the Institute in 1948.

Kohut's own analysis was with August Aichhorn (in Vienna) and then Ruth Eissler (in Chicago). This was a cause of some financial hardship. In 1946, he wrote in a letter to Aichhorn:

> Although I have been employed for more than five years at the University of Chicago (my official title is Instructor in Neurology and Psychiatry) and have a salary of $3000 per annum, I have to pay for my analysis and that amounts to about $1200 a year so there's hardly anything left over.
>
> (quoted in Cocks, 1994: 48)

In a further letter to Aichhorn, he describes some uncertainty regarding the direction of psychoanalysis as taught at the Chicago Institute:

> Dr. Eissler is of the opinion that the Institute here which is under the direction of Franz Alexander has little to do with analysis in the Freudian sense – the people with whom I work at the hospital . . . think that the European analysts who have come to America are unnecessarily traditional and conservative and reject progressive experimentation. It is simply impossible for me to come to any halfway reasonable conclusion.
>
> (Cocks, 1994: 50)

During the 1950s, Kohut became a major figure at the Chicago Institute, where he was generally regarded as a brilliant teacher. He became president of the Chicago society from 1963 to 1964 and president of the American Psychoanalytic Association from 1964 to 1965 – when the APA had about 1100 members, in total seeing about 11,000 patients a year. He was very much an establishment figure, becoming affectionately known as 'Mr Psychoanalysis', famous for being a staunch public advocate of the scientific validity of psychoanalysis.

Kohut's seminal contributions to the new understanding of narcissism began in 1960s, with papers such as: *Forms and transformations of narcissism* (1966); *The psychoanalytic treatment of narcissistic personality disorders* (1968); *Thoughts on narcissism and narcissistic rage* (1972). These ideas regarding the separate line of development of narcissism, the narcissistic transferences, and the concept of the selfobject, evolved into his three books: *The Analysis of the Self* (1971); *The Restoration of the Self* (1977); and *How does Analysis Cure?* (1984).

His creative energy and sense of urgency were fuelled by the fact of being diagnosed with lymphatic cancer in 1971. Then in 1979 he underwent a coronary bypass and suffered various complications. This probably meant that in his efforts to articulate and clarify his own ideas within the available time left to him, he did not read a great deal of the work of British analysts, such as Winnicott and others within the British Independents Group (Rayner, 1991), with whom he has been compared.

Kohut's novel formulations received a mixed response. In a letter to his son and daughter-in-law in 1978, he wrote:

> My professional position is peculiar. I get buffeted around by nasty rejections and warmest praise – I could do with less of both but must admit that I am sometimes quite upset about it all.
>
> (Quoted in Cocks, 1994: 23)

One of the recurrent criticisms of Kohut was that he ignored the centrality of the oedipus complex. Actually, he did not, but he did give emphasis to a different aspect of it. He commented:

> Is it not the most significant dynamic-genetic feature of the Oedipus story that Oedipus was a rejected child? . . . The fact is that Oedipus was not wanted by his parents and that he was put out into the cold by them.
>
> (Quoted in Cocks, 1994: 31)

The final letter in Cocks's collection is to his son, Tom, and is dated August 17th 1981. He writes:

> My mind is ok, my courage unbroken, my work proceeds.
>
> (Cocks, 1994: 433)

He died less than two months later, at the age of 68.

References

Adler G (1989) Uses and limitations of Kohut's self psychology in the treatment of borderline patients. Journal of the American Psychoanalytic Association 37: 761–85.

Aichhorn A (1936) The narcissistic transference of the 'juvenile' imposter. In Delinquency and Child Guidance: Selected Papers by August Aichhorn (1964) New York: International Universities Press.

Alexander F, French TM (1946) Psychoanalytic Therapy: Principles and Applications. New York: Ronald Press.

Arieti S, Bemporad J (1980) Severe and Mild Depression. London: Tavistock.

Atwood G, Stolorow R (1984) Structures of Subjectivity. Explorations in Psychoanalytic Phenomenology. Hillsdale, NJ: Analytic Press.

Baars BJ (1988) A Cognitive Theory of Consciousness. New York: Cambridge University Press.

Bacal HA, Newman KM (1990) Theories of Object Relations: Bridges to Self Psychology. New York: Columbia Universities Press.

Backhouse H (1988) The Dark Night of the Soul: St. John of the Cross. London: Hodder and Stoughton.

Baker R (2000) Finding the neutral position: patient and analyst perspectives. Journal of the American Psychoanalytic Association 48(1): 129–53.

Balint M (1968) The Basic Fault. London: Tavistock.

Bateman AW (1998) Thick- and thin-skinned organisations and enactment in borderline and narcissistic disorders. International Journal of Psychoanalysis 79: 13–26.

Bear DM (1983) Hemispheric specialisation and the neurology of emotion. Archives of Neurology 40: 195–202.

Beebe B, Lachman FM (1988) Mother–infant mutual influence and precursors of psychic structure. In Goldberg A (Ed) Progress in Self Psychology, Vol 3. Hillsdale, NJ: The Analytic Press. pp 3–25.

Beebe B, Lachman FM (1994) Representation and internalisation in infancy: three principles of salience. Psychoanalytic Psychology 11: 127–65.

Benjamin J (1988) The Bonds of Love. New York: Pantheon.

Benjamin J (1990) Recognition and destruction: an outline of intersubjectivity. Psychoanalytic Psychology 7 (suppl): 33–47. Reprinted in (1999) Mitchell SA, Aron

L, (Eds) Relational Psychoanalysis: The Emergence of a Tradition. Hillsdale, NJ: Analytic Press.

Bion WR (1959) Attacks on linking. Reprinted in (1984) Second Thoughts. London: Karnac.

Bion WR (1962) Learning from Experience. London: Heinemann. Reprinted in Bion WR (1977) Seven Servants. New York: Aronson.

Bion WR (1963) Elements of Psycho-Analysis. London: Heinemann. Reprinted in Seven Servants. New York: Aronson.

Bion WR (1965) Transformations. London: Heinemann. Reprinted in (1977) Seven Servants. New York: Aronson.

Bion WR (1967) On Arrogance. In (1984) Second Thoughts. London: Karnac.

Bion WR (1970) Attention and Interpretation. London: Tavistock. Reprinted in (1977) Seven Servants. New York: Aronson.

Blatt SJ, Ford RQ (1994) Therapeutic Change. New York: Plenum.

Bleichmar H (1996) Some subtypes of depression and their implications for psycho-analytic therapy. International Journal of Psychoanalysis 77: 935–61.

Bleichmar H (2000) Attachment and intimacy in adult relationships. Paper presented to conference of the International Attachment Network. London, 15 July.

Bollas C (1987) The Shadow of the Object: Psychoanalysis of the Unthought Known. London: Free Association Books.

Bollas C (1989) Forces of Destiny: Psychoanalysis and Human Idiom. London: Free Association Books.

Bowers D, Blonder LX, Feinberg T, Heilman KM (1991) Differential impact of right and left hemisphere lesions on facial emotion and object memory. Brain 114: 2593–2609.

Bowlby J (1980) Attachment and Loss, Vol 3: Loss, Sadness and Depression. London: Hogarth.

Brandchaft B (1994) To free the spirit from its cell. In Stolorow RD, Atwood GE, Brandchaft B (Eds) The Intersubjective Perspective. New York. Aronson.

Brandchaft B, Stolorow R (1984) The borderline concept: pathological character or iatrogenic myth? In Lichtenberg J, Bornstein M, Silver D, (Eds) Empathy II. Hillsdale, NJ: Analytic Press.

Brenman Pick I (1985) Working through in the countertransference. International Journal of Psychoanalysis 66: 157–66.

Brothers D (1995) Falling Backwards: An Exploration of Trust and Self Experience. Norton: New York.

Bruner J (1994) The view from the heart's eye: a commentary. In Niedentahl PM, Kiyayama S (Eds) The Heart's Eye: Emotional Influences in Perception and Attention. San Diego: Academic Press. pp 269–86.

Carpy DV (1989) Tolerating the countertransference: a mutative process. International Journal of Psychoanalysis 70: 287–94.

Carveth DL (1995) Self psychology and the intersubjective perspective. A dialectical critique. In Goldberg A (Ed) The Impact of New Ideas. Progress in Self Psychology II. Hillsdale, NJ: Analytic Press. pp 3–30.

Casement P (1985) On Learning From the Patient. London: Routledge.

Casement P (2000) Getting there: the unfolding potential of psychoanalysis, a personal view. The British Psycho-Analytical Society Bulletin 36(4): 1–9. (Restricted circulation)

Cavell M (1998a) Triangulation, one's own mind and objectivity. International Journal of Psychoanalysis 79: 449–68.

Cavell M (1998b) In response to Owen Renik's 'The analyst's subjectivity and the analyst's objectivity'. International Journal of Psychoanalysis 79: 1195–1202.

Cavell M (2000) Commentary on 'The analyst's witnessing and otherness' by WS Poland. Journal of the American Psychoanalytic Association 48(1): 48–57.

Chasseguet-Smirgel J (1985) Creativity and Perversion. London: Free Association Press.

Chiron JI, Nabbout R, Lounes R, Syrota A, Dulac O (1997) The right brain is dominant in human infants. Brain 120: 1057–65

Chodorow NJ (1986) Toward a relational individualism: the medium of self through psychoanalysis. Reprinted in (1999) Mitchell SA, Aron L, (Eds) Relational Psychoanalysis: The Emergence of a Tradition. Hillsdale, NJ: Analytic Press.

Clyman MA (1996) Autobiographical knowledge and autobiographical memories. In Rubin DC, (Ed) Remembering Our Past: Studies in Autobiographical Memory. New York: Cambridge University Press.

Cocks G (1994) The Curve of Life: The Correspondence of Heinz Kohut, 1923–1981. Chicago: University of Chicago Press.

Cooley CH (1902) Human Nature and the Social Order. New York: Schocken Books. (1964)

Cortina M, Maccoby M (1996) A Prophetic Analyst: Erich Fromm's Contributions to Psychoanalysis. Hillsdale, NJ: Aronson.

Damasio AR (1994) Descartes' Error. New York: Grosset/Putnam.

Damasio AR (1999) The Feeling of What Happens: Body, Emotion and the Making of Consciousness. London: Heinemann.

Darwin C (1872) The Expression of the Emotions in Man and Animals. Chicago: University of Chicago Press. (1965)

de Bono E (1967) The Use of Lateral Thinking. London: Jonathan Cape.

Denenberg VH, Garbanti J, Sherman G, Yutzey DA, Kaplan R (1978) Infantile stimulation induces brain lateralisation in rats. Science 201: 1150–52.

Deruelle C, De Schonen S (1988) Do the right and left hemispheres attend to the same visuospatial information within a face in infancy. Developmental Neuropsychology 14: 535–54.

Eigen M (1986) The Psychotic Core. New York: Jason Aronson.

Emde R (1983) The prerepresentational self and its affective core. The Psychoanalytic Study of the Child 38: 165–92.

Emde R (1988a) Development terminable and interminable, I. International Journal of Psychoanalysis 69: 23–42.

Emde R (1988b) Development terminable and interminable, II. International Journal of Psychoanalysis 69: 283–96.

Fairbairn WRD (1952) Psychoanalytic Studies of the Personality. London: Tavistock.

Feldman M (1992) The centrality of the oedipus complex. In Wallerstein RS, (Ed) The Common Ground of Psychoanalysis. Northvale, NJ: Aronson.

Feldman R, Greenbaum CW, Yirmiya N (1999) Mother–infant affect synchrony as an antecedent of the emergence of self-control. Developmental Psychology 35: 223–31.

Ferenczi S (1988) The Clinical Diary of Sandor Ferenczi. Cambridge, Mass: Harvard University Press.

Fonagy P (1991) Thinking about thinking. Some clinical and theoretical considerations in the treatment of a borderline patient. International Journal of Psychoanalysis 72: 1–18.

Fonagy P (1997) Attachment and theory of mind: overlapping constructs? Association for Child Psychology and Psychiatry Occasional Papers 14: 31–40.

Fonagy P (1999a) The process of change and the change of processes. What can change in a 'good analysis'? Keynote address to the Spring Meeting of Division 39 of the American Psychological Association, New York, 16 April.

Fonagy P (1999b) Memory and therapeutic action. Guest editorial. International Journal of Psychoanalysis 80: 215–23.

Fonagy P (1999c) An Open Door Review of Outcome Studies in Psychoanalysis. London: International Psychoanalytical Association.

Fonagy P (2000) Letter to the editor. International Journal of Psychoanalysis 81: 169.

Fonagy P, Steele M, Steele H, Moran GS, Higget AC (1991) The capacity for understanding mental states: the reflective self in parent and child and its significance for security of attachment. Infant Mental Health Journal 12: 201–18.

Fonagy P, Cooper A (1999) Joseph Sandler's intellectual contribution to theoretical and clinical psychoanalysis. In Fonagy P, Cooper A, Wallerstein RS, (Eds) Psychoanalysis on the Move: The Work of Joseph Sandler. London: Routledge.

Fonagy P, Target M (1996a) Playing with reality, I: Theory of mind and the normal development of psychic reality. International Journal of Psychoanalysis 77: 217–33

Fonagy P, Target M (1996b) Playing with reality, II: The development of psychic reality from a theoretical perspective. International Journal of Psychoanalysis 77: 459–79.

Fonagy P, Target M, Gergely G, Jurist EL (2000) Affect Regulation and Mentalization. London: Karnac.

Forgas JP (1982) Episode cognition: internal representations of interaction routines. In Berkowitz L (Ed) Advances in Experimental Psychology, Vol 15. New York: Academic Press.

Freud A (1937) The Ego and the Mechanisms of Defence. London: Hogarth.

Freud S (1900) The interpretation of dreams. Standard Edition of the Complete Psychological Works of Sigmund Freud, IV and V. London: Hogarth.

Freud S (1914) On narcissism. An introduction. Standard Edition of The Complete Psychological Works of Sigmund Freud, XIV. London: Hogarth.

Freud S (1916) Some character types met with in psycho-analytic work: the 'exceptions'. Standard Edition of the Complete Psychological Works of Sigmund Freud, XIV. London: Hogarth.

Freud S (1917) Mourning and melancholia. Standard Edition of the Complete Psychological Works of Sigmund Freud, XIV. London: Hogarth. pp 239–58.

Freud S (1920) Beyond the pleasure principle. Standard Edition of the Complete Psychological Works of Sigmund Freud, XVIII. London: Hogarth.

Freud S (1923) The ego and the id. Standard Edition of the Complete Psychological Works of Sigmund Freud, XIX. London: Hogarth.

Freud S (1924) The economic problem of masochism. Standard Edition of the Complete Psychological Works of Sigmund Freud, XIX. London: Hogarth.

Freud S (1926) Inhibitions, symptoms and anxiety. Standard Edition of the Complete Psychological Works of Sigmund Freud, XX. London: Hogarth.

Freud S (1940a) An outline of psycho-analysis. Standard Edition of the Complete Psychological Works of Sigmund Freud, XXIII. London: Hogarth.

Freud S (1940b) Splitting of the ego in the service of defence. Standard Edition of the Complete Psychological Works of Sigmund Freud, XXIII. London: Hogarth.

Freyd JJ (1996) Betrayal Trauma. The Logic of Forgetting Childhood Abuse. Cambridge, MA: Harvard University Press.

Fricchione G, Howantiz E (1985) Aprosodia and alexithymia – a case report. Psychotherapy and Psychosomatics 43: 156–60.

Fromm E (1965) The Heart of Man: Its Genius for Good and Evil. London: Routledge.

Frosch J (1983) The Psychotic Process. New York: International Universities Press.

Gabbard GO, Lester EP (1995) Boundaries and Boundary Violations in Psychoanalysis. Basic Books: New York.

Gabbard G (1997) A reconsideration of objectivity in the analyst. International Journal of Psychoanalysis 1: 15–26.

Gabbard G (2000) Disguise or consent: problems and recommendations concerning the publication and presentation of clinical material. International Journal of Psychoanalysis 81: 1071–86.

Gaensbauer TJ, Mrazek D (1981) Differences in the patterning of affective expression in infants. Journal of the American Academy of Child Psychiatry 20: 673–91.

Galin D (1974) Implications for psychiatry of left and right cerebral specialisation. Archives of General Psychiatry 31: 572–83.

Gedo J (1981) The psychoanalytic management of archaic transference. In (1984) Advances in Clinical Psychoanalysis. New York: Jason Aronson.

Gerhardt J, Beyerle S (1997) What if Socrates had been a woman? The therapist's use of acknowledgement tokens as a nonreflective means of intersubjective involvement. Contemporary Psychoanalysis 33: 367–410.

Ghent E (1992) Foreword. In Skolnick NJ, Warshaw SC, (Eds) Relational Perspectives in Psychoanalysis. Hillsdale, NJ: Analytic Press.

Glover E (1968) The Birth of the Ego. International Universities Press: New York.

Goffman E (1968) Stigma: Notes on the Management of Spoiled Identity. Pelican: Harmondsworth.

Goldberg A (1983) Self psychology and alternative perspectives on internalisation. In Lichtenberg JD, Kaplan S, (Eds) Reflections on Self Psychology. Hillsdale, NJ: Analytic Press.

Goldberg A (1994) Farewell to the objective analyst. International Journal of Psychoanalysis 75: 21–30.

Goldberg A (2000) Letter: Memory and therapeutic action. International Journal of Psychoanalysis 81(3): 593–94.

Green A (1983) The dead mother. In (1986) On Private Madness. London: Hogarth Press and Institute of Psychoanalysis.

Green A (1999) The Work of the Negative. London: Free Association Books.

Greenberg J, Mitchell S (1983) Object Relations in Psychoanalytical Theory. Cambridge, MA: Harvard University Press.

Greenwald AG (1980) The totalitarian ego: fabrication and revision of personal history. American Psychology 35: 603–8.

Groddeck G (1929) The Unknown Self. London: Daniel.

Grossman L (1996) 'Psychic reality' and reality testing. International Journal of Psychoanalysis 77: 509–15.

Grotstein JS (1977) The psychoanalytic concept of schizophrenia, II: reconciliation. International Journal of Psychoanalysis 58: 427–52.

Grotstein JS (1981) Who is the dreamer who dreams the dream and who is the dreamer who understands it? A psychoanalytic inquiry into the ultimate nature of being. In Grotstein JS (Ed) Do I Dare Disturb the Universe? A Memorial to Wilfred R. Bion. Beverly Hills, Calif: Caesura Press.

Grotstein JS (1983) Some perspectives on self psychology. In Goldberg A (Ed) The Future of Psychoanalysis. New York: International Universities Press.

Grotstein JS (1990) The 'black hole' as the basic psychotic experience: some newer psychoanalytic and neuroscience perspectives on psychosis. Journal of the American Academy of Psychoanalysis 18: 29–46.

Grotstein JS (1991) Nothingness, meaninglessness, chaos and the 'black hole', III. Self and interactional regulation and the background presence of primary identification. Contemporary Psychoanalysis 27: 1–33.

Grotstein JS (1994a) Comments on the cover of Ogden TH. Subjects of Analysis. New York: Jason Aronson.

Grotstein JS (1994b) Projective identification reappraised, part I: projective identification, introjective identification, the transference/countertransference neurosis/psychosis, and their consummate expression in the crucifixion, the Pieta and 'therapeutic exorcism'. Contemporary Psychoanalysis 30(4): 708–46.

Grotstein JS (1995) Projective identification reappraised, part II: the countertransference complex. Contemporary Psychoanalysis 31(3): 479–511.

Grotstein JS (1997a) Why Oedipus and not Christ? A psychoanalytic inquiry into innocence, human sacrifice, and the sacred – Part 1: innocence, sprituality, and human sacrifice. American Journal of Psychoanalysis 57(3): 193–220.

Grotstein JS (1997b) Foreword. Alexithymia: the exception that proves the rule – of the unusual significance of affects. In Taylor GJ, Bagby RM, Parker JDA, (Eds) Disorders of Affect Regulation. Cambridge: Cambridge University Press.

Grotstein JS (1997c) Bion: the pariah of 'O'. British Journal of Psychotherapy 14(1): 77–87.

Grunberger B (1971) Narcissism. New York: International Universities Press.

Guntrip H (1961) Personality Structure and Human Interaction. London: Hogarth.

Guntrip H (1968) Schizoid Phenomena, Object Relations and the Self. London: Hogarth.

Hamburg P (1991) Interpretation and empathy: reading Lacan with Kohut. International Journal of Psychoanalysis 72: 347–61.

Hartmann H (1939) Ego Psychology and the Problem of Adaptation. New York: International Universities Press. (Reprinted 1958)

Hartmann H (1950) Comments on the psychoanalytic theory of the ego. The Psychoanalytic Study of the Child 5: 74–96. New York: International Universities Press.

Hartmann H (1964) Essays on Ego Psychology. New York: International Universities Press.

Heidegger M (1927) Being and Time. New York: Harper and Row. (Reprinted 1962)

Heimann P (1950) On countertransference. International Journal of Psychoanalysis 31: 81–84.

Heimann P (1956) Dynamics of transference representations. International Journal of Psychoanalysis 37: 303–10

Hernandez M, Lemlij M (1999) Internal objects: theoretical perimeter and clinical contour. In Fonagy P, Cooper AM, Wallerstein R, (Eds) Psychoanalysis on the Move: The Work of Joseph Sandler. London: Routledge.

Hietanen JK, Surakka V, Linnankoski I (1998) Facial electromyographic responses to vocal affect expressions. Psychophysiology 35: 530–36.

Hinshelwood RD (1997) The elusive concept of 'internal objects' (1934–1943): its role in the formation of the Klein group. International Journal of Psychoanalysis 78: 877–97.

Hinshelwood RD (1999) Countertransference. International Journal of Psychoanalysis 80: 797–818.

Horton FC (1995) The comforting substrate and the right brain. Bulletin of the Menninger Clinic 59: 480–86.

Jackson JH (1931) Selected Writings of J.H. Jackson, Vol 1. London: Hodder and Stoughton.

Jacobson E (1964) The Self and the Object World. New York: International Universities Press.

Jacobson E (1967) Psychotic Conflict and Reality. New York: International Universities Press.

Jacobson E (1971) Depression: Comparative Studies of Normal, Neurotic and Psychotic Conditions. New York: International Universities Press.

Jaynes J (1976) The Origin of Consciousness in the Breakdown of the Bicameral Mind. Boston: Houghton Mifflin.

Joffe WG, Sandler J (1968) Comments on the psychoanalytic psychology of adaptation, with special reference to the role of affects and the representational world. International Journal of Psychoanalysis 49: 445–54.

Joseph B (1982) Addiction to near-death. International Journal of Psychoanalysis 63: 449–56.

Joseph B (1989) Psychic change and the psychoanalytic process. In Psychic Equilibrium and Psychic Change: Selected Papers of Betty Joseph. London: Routledge and the Institute of Psycho-Analysis.

Joseph R (1996) Neuropsychiatry, Neuropsychology, and Clinical Neuroscience. 2nd edn. Baltimore: Williams and Wilkins.

Kaplan-Solms K, Solms M (2000) Clinical Studies in Neuropsychoanalysis: Introduction to a Depth Neuropsychology. London: Karnac.

Kennedy R (1998) The Elusive Human Subject: A Psychoanalytic Theory of Subject Relations. London: Free Association Press.

Kernberg O (1975) Borderline Conditions and Pathological Narcissism. New York: Aronson.

Kernberg O (1976) Object Relations Theory and Clinical Psychoanalysis. New York: Aronson.

Kernberg O (1982) Review of Advances in Self Psychology. American Journal of Psychiatry 139: 374–75.

Kernberg O (1984) Severe Personality Disorders: Psychotherapeutic Strategies. New Haven, Conn: Yale University Press.

Kernberg O (1996) Thirty methods to destroy the creativity of psychoanalytic candidates. International Journal of Psychoanalysis 77: 1031–40

Kitterle FL (1995) Hemispheric Communication: Mechanism and Models. Hillsdale, NJ: Erlbaum.

Klein G (1976) Psychoanalytic Theory: An Exploration of Essentials. New York: International Universities Press.

Klein M (1946) Notes on some schizoid mechanisms. In (1975) Envy and Gratitude: The Writings of Melanie Klein, Vol III. London: Hogarth.

Klein M (1952) The emotional life of the infant. In (1975) Envy and Gratitude: The Writings of Melanie Klein, Vol III. London: Hogarth.

Kluft RP (1994) Multiple personality disorder: observations on the aetiology, natural history and recognition of a long neglected condition. In Klein RM, Doane BK, (Eds) Psychological Concepts and Dissociative Disorders. Hillsdale, NJ: Erlbaum.

Koestler A (1964) The Act of Creation. New York: Dell.

Kohon G (1999) The Dead Mother: The Work of Andre Green. London: Routledge.

Kohut H (1959) Introspection, empathy and psychoanalysis. An examination of the relation between mode of observation and theory. Journal of the American Psychoanalytic Association 7: 459–83. Reprinted in (1978) The Search for the Self: Selected Writings of Heinz Kohut, Vol 1. New York: International Universities Press.

Kohut H (1966) Forms and transformations of narcissism. Journal of the American Psychoanalytic Association 14: 243–72. Reprinted in (1978) The Search for the Self: Selected Writings of Heinz Kohut: 1950–1978, Vol 1. New York: International Universities Press.

Kohut H (1968a) Intropection and empathy. Further thoughts about their role in psychoanalysis. In (1990) The Search for the Self: Selected Writings of Heinz Kohut: 1978–1981, Vol 3. New York: International Universities Press.

Kohut H (1968b) The psychoanalytic treatment of narcissistic personality disorders: outline of a systematic approach. The Psychoanalytic Study of the Child 23: 86–113. Reprinted in (1978) The Search for the Self: Selected Writings of Heinz Kohut: 1950–1978, Vol 1. New York: International Universities Press.

Kohut H (1971) The Analysis of the Self: A Systematic Approach to the Psychoanalytic Treatment of Narcissistic Personality Disorders. New York: International Universities Press.

Kohut H (1972) Thoughts on narcissism and narcissistic rage. The Psychoanalytic Study of the Child 27: 360–400. Reprinted in (1978) The Search for the Self: Selected Writings of Heinz Kohut, Vol 2. New York: International Universities Press.

Kohut H (1977) The Restoration of the Self. New York: International Universities Press.

Kohut H (1978) Reflections on Advances in Self Psychology. In (1990) The Search for the Self: Selected Writings of Heinz Kohut 1978–1981, Vol 3. New York: International Universities Press.

Kohut H (1979) The two analyses of Mr Z. International Journal of Psychoanalysis 60: 3–27. Reprinted in (1991) The Search for the Self. Selected Writings of Heinz Kohut. Vol. 4. New York. International Universities Press.

Kohut (1981) The psychoanalyst and the historian. In (1985b) Self Psychology and the Humanities. New York: Norton.

Kohut H (1983) Selected problems of self psychological theory. In Lichtenberg J, Kaplan S, (Eds) Reflections on Self Psychology. Hillsdale, NJ: Analytic Press.

Kohut H (1984) How Does Analysis Cure? Chicago: University of Chicago Press.

Kohut H (1985a) On courage. In (1985b) Self Psychology and the Humanities. New York: Norton.

Kohut H (1985b) Self Psychology and the Humanities. New York: Norton.

Kohut H (1990a) From the analysis of Mr R. In (1990) The Search for the Self: Selected Writings of Heinz Kohut, 1978–1981, Vol 3. New York: International Universities Press.

Kohut H (1996) The Chicago Institute Lectures. (Tolpin P, Tolpin M, Eds) Hillsdale, NJ: The Analytic Press.

Kohut H, Seitz PFD (1963) Concepts and theories of psychoanalysis. In (1978) The Search for the Self, Vol 1: Selected Writings of Heinz Kohut: 1950–1978. New York: International Universities Press.

Kraemer GW, Ebert MH, Schmidt DE, McKinney WT (1991) Strangers in a strange land: a psychobiological study of infant monkeys before and after separation from real or inanimate mothers. Child Development 62: 548–66.

Kubie L, Israel H (1955) 'Say you're sorry!' Psychoanalytic Study of the Child 10: 289–99.

Lacan J (1948) Aggressivity in psychoanalysis. In (1977) Ecrits. London: Tavistock.

Lacan J (1949) The mirror stage as formative of the function of the I as revealed in psychoanalytic experience. In (1977) Ecrits. London: Tavistock.

Lacan J (1977) Ecrits: A Selection. London: Tavistock.

Langs R (1976) The Bipersonal Field. New York: Aronson.

Langs R (1997) Death Anxiety and Clinical Practice. London: Karnac.

Leader D (2000) Freud's Footnotes. London: Faber and Faber.

Leigh R (1998) Panel Report: Perversion. International Journal of Psychoanalysis 79: 1217–20.

Lewis E (1979) Two hidden predisposing factors in child abuse. Journal of Child Abuse and Neglect 3: 227–330.

Lewis E, Casement P (1986) The inhibition of mourning by pregancy: a case study. Psychoanalytic Psychotherapy 2(1): 45–52.

Locke JL (1997) A theory of language development. Brain and Language 58: 265–326.

Luria AR (1973) The Working Brain. New York: Basic Books.

Luria AR (1980) Higher Cortical Functions in Man. New York: Basic Books.

Main M (1991) Metacognitive knowledge, metacognitive monitoring, and singular (coherent) vs. multiple (incoherent) models of attachment: findings and directions for future research. In Parkes CM, Marris P, Stevenson-Hinde J, (Eds) Attachment Across the Life Cycle. New York: Routledge. pp 127–59.

Malcom RR (1986) Interpretation: the past in the present. International Review of Psycho-Analysis 13: 433–43.

Manning JT, Trivers RL, Thornhill R, Singh D, Denman J, Eklo MH, Anderton RH (1997) Ear asymmetry and left-side cradling. Evolution and Human Behaviour 18: 327–40.

Matte-Blanco I (1975) The Unconscious as Infinite Sets. London: Duckworth.

Matte-Blanco I (1988) Thinking, Feeling, Being: Clinical Reflections on the Fundamental Antinomy of Human Beings and the World. London: Routledge.

Meloy JR (1992) Violent Attachments. New York: Aronson.

Meltzer DW (1978) The Kleinian Development. Perthshire: Clunie Press.

Michels R (2000) The case history. Journal of the American Psychoanalytic Association 48(2): 355–75.

Mitchell S (1988) Relational Concepts in Psychoanalysis. Cambridge, MA: Harvard University Press.

Mitchell S (1997a) Influence and Autonomy in Psychoanalysis. Hillsdale, NJ: Analytic Press.

Mitchell S (1997b) Interaction in the Kleinian tradition. In: Influence and Autonomy in Psychoanalysis. Hillsdale, NJ: Analytic Press.

Mitchell SA, Aron L (1999) Relational Psychoanalysis: The Emergence of a Tradition. Hillsdale, NJ: Analytic Press.
Modell AH (1999) The dead mother syndrome and reconstruction of trauma. In Kohon G, (Ed) The Dead Mother: The Work of André Green. London: Routledge and the Institute of Psychoanalysis.
Mollon P (1986a) An appraisal of Kohut's contribution to an understanding of narcissism. British Journal of Psychotherapy 3: 151–61.
Mollon P (1986b) A note on Kohut and Klein: idealisation, splitting and projective identification. British Journal of Psychotherapy 3: 162–64.
Mollon P (1986c) Narcissistic vulnerability and the fragile self: a failure of mirroring. British Journal of Medical Psychology 59: 317–24.
Mollon P (1993) The Fragile Self: The Structure of Narcissistic Disturbance. London: Whurr.
Mollon P (1996) Multiple Selves, Multiple Voices: Working with Trauma, Violation and Dissociation. Chichester: Wiley.
Mollon P (1998) Remembering Trauma: A Psychotherapist's Guide to Memory and Illusion. Chichester: Wiley.
Mollon P (2000) Freud and False Memory Syndrome. Cambridge: Icon Books.
Money-Kyrle R (1956) Normal countertransference and some of its deviations. International Journal of Psychoanalysis 37: 360–66.
Money-Kyrle R (1971) The aim of psychoanalysis. In The Collected Papers of Roger Money-Kyrle. Strath Tay: Clunie Press.
Muller JP (1989) Lacan and Kohut. In Dietrich DW, Dietrich SP, (Eds) Self Psychology: Comparisons and Contrasts. Hillsdale, NJ: Analytic Press.
Nahum JP (1999) Review of 'Affect Regulation and the Origin of the Self' by Allan Schore. Neuro-Psychoanalysis 1(2): 258–63.
Nelson CA (1987) The recognition of facial expressions in the first two years of life: mechanisms of development. Child Development 58: 889–909.
Ogden TH (1989) The Primitive Edge of Experience. Northvale, NJ: Aronson.
Orange DM (1995) Emotional Understanding. New York: Guilford Press.
Orange DM, Atwood GE, Stolorow R (1997) Working Intersubjectively: Contextualism in Psychoanalytic Practice. Hillsdale, NJ: Analytic Press.
Ornstein P (1995) Critical reflections on a comparative analysis of 'Self Psychology and Intersubjectivity Theory'. In Goldberg A (Ed) The Impact of New Ideas. Progress in Self Psychology II. Hillsdale, NJ: Analytic Press.
Palef SR (1995) A self-psychological perspective on multiple personality disorder. In Goldberg A, (Ed) The Impact of New Ideas. Progress in Self Psychology II. Hillsdale, NJ: Analytic Press.
Panksepp J (2000) Concluding remarks: neuroscientific and psychoanalytic perspectives on emotion. Conference organised by the Anna Freud Clinic, London, 23 July.
Pao P-N (1979) Schizophrenic Disorders. New York: International Universities Press.
Parker J, Taylor G, (1997) The neurobiology of emotion, affect regulation and alexithymia. In Taylor GJ, Bagby RM, Parker JDA, (Eds) Disorders of Affect Regulation. Cambridge: Cambridge University Press.
Perlow M (1995) Understanding Mental Objects. London: Routledge.
Poland WS (1996) Melting the Darkness: The Dyad and Principles of Clinical Practice. Northvale, NJ: Aronson.

Poland WS (2000) The analyst's witnessing and otherness. Journal of the American Psychoanalytic Association 48: 17–34

Powell C (1995) Internal object relations as intersubjective phenomena. In Goldberg A (Ed) The Impact of New Ideas. Progress in Self Psychology, Vol 11. Hillsdale, NJ: Analytic Press.

Racker H (1957) The meanings and use of countertransference. In (1968) Transference and Countertransference. London: Hogarth.

Rayner E (1991) The Independent Mind in British Psychoanalysis. Northvale, NJ: Aronson.

Renik O (1993). Analytic interaction: conceptualizing technique in light of the analyst's irreducible subjectivity. Psychoanalytic Quarterly 62: 553–71. Reprinted in Mitchell SA, Aron L (1999) Relational Psychoanalysis. Hillsdale, NJ: Analytic Press.

Renik O (1996) The perils of neutrality. Psychoanalytic Quarterly 65: 495–517.

Renik O (1998) The analyst's subjectivity and the analyst's objectivity. International Journal of Psychoanalysis 79: 487–97.

Renik O (1999) Letter to the editor – Renik replies to Cavell. International Journal of Psychoanalysis 80: 382–83.

Ribble MA (1944) Infantile experience in relation to personality development. In Personality and the Behaviour Disorders, Vol II. London: Roland Press.

Rosenfeld H (1964) On the psychopathology of narcissism: a clinical approach. International Journal of Psychoanalysis 45: 332–37.

Rosenfeld H (1971) A clinical approach to the psychoanalytic theory of the life and death instincts: an investigation of the aggressive aspects of narcissism. International Journal of Psychoanalysis 52: 169–78.

Rosenfeld H (1987) Impasse and Interpretation: Therapeutic and Anti-therapeutic Factors in the Psychoanalytic Treatment of Psychotic, Borderline and Neurotic Patients. London: Tavistock and the Institute of Psychoanalysis.

Rothstein A (1980) The Narcissistic Pursuit of Perfection. New York: International Universities Press.

Rubovits-Seitz PFD (1999) Kohut's Freudian Vision. Hillsdale, NJ: Analytic Press.

Ryan RM, Kuhl J, Deci EL (1997) Nature and autonomy: an organisational view of social and neurobiological aspects of self-regulation in behaviour and development. Development and Psychopathology 9: 701–28.

Salter AC (1995) Transforming Trauma. Thousand Oaks, Calif: Sage.

Sandler J (1976) Countertransference and role responsiveness. International Review of Psycho-Analysis 3: 3–47.

Sandler J (1990) On internal object relations. Journal of the American Psychoanalytic Association 38: 859–80.

Sandler J, Dreher AH (1996) What Do Psychoanalysts Want? London: Routledge.

Sandler J, Rosenblatt B (1962) The concept of the representational world. Psychoanalytic Study of the Child 17: 128–45.

Sandler J, Sandler, A-M (1984) The past unconscious, the present unconscious and interpretation of the transference. Psychoanalytic Inquiry 4: 367–99.

Sandler J, Sandler A-M (1997) A psychoanalytic theory of repression and the unconscious. In Sandler J, Fonagy P, (Eds) Recovered Memories of Abuse: True or False? London: Karnac.

Scharff JS (2000) On writing from clinical experience. Journal of the American Psychoanalytic Association 48(2): 421–47.

Schore AN (1994) Affect Regulation and the Origin of the Self. Hillsdale, NJ: Erlbaum.
Schore AN (2000a) Attachment, the developing brain, and psychotherapy. Paper presented at Minds in the Making, The Bowlby Conference. London, 3–4 March.
Schore AN (2000b) Attachment and the regulation of the right brain. Attachment and Human Development. 2(1) 23–47.
Schore A (in press) Affect Regulation and the Repair of the Self. New York: Guilford Press.
Schumann JH (1997) The Neurobiology of Affect in Language. Malden, Mass: Blackwell.
Schwaber EA (1981) Empathy: a mode of analytic listening. Psychoanalytic Inquiry 1: 357–92.
Schwaber EA (1983a) Psychoanalytic listening and psychic reality. International Review of Psychoanalysis 10: 379–92.
Schwaber EA (1983b) Construction, reconstruction and the mode of clinical attunement. In Goldberg A (Ed) The Future of Psychoanalysis. New York: International Universities Press.
Schwaber EA (1983c) Psychoanalytic listening and psychic reality. International Review of Psychoanalysis 10: 379–92.
Schwaber EA (1986) Reconstruction and perceptual experience: further thoughts on analytic listening. Journal of the American Psychoanalytic Association 34: 911–32.
Schwaber EA (1990) Interpretation and the therapeutic action of psychoanalysis. International Journal of Psychoanalysis 71: 229–40.
Schwaber EA (1992a) Countertransference: the analyst's retreat from the patient's vantage point. International Journal of Psychoanalysis 73: 349–61.
Schwaber EA (1992b) Psychoanalytic theory and its relation of clinical work. Journal of the American Psychoanalytic Association 40: 1039–57.
Schwaber EA (1995a) The psychoanalyst's mind: from listening to interpretation – a clinical report. International Journal of Psychoanalysis 76: 271–81.
Schwaber EA (1995b) A particular perspective on impasses in the clinical situation: further reflections on psychoanalytic listening. International Journal of Psychoanalysis 76: 711–22.
Schwaber EA (1996a) The conceptualisation and communication of clinical facts in psychoanalysis: a discussion. International Journal of Psychoanalysis 77: 235–53.
Schwaber EA (1996b) Toward a definition of the term and concept of interaction: its reflections in psychoanalytic listening. Psychoanalytic Inquiry 16: 5–24.
Schwaber EA (1997a) Psychic reality and psychic testing. Letter to editor. International Journal of Psychoanalysis 78: 157–58.
Schwaber EA (1997b) A reconsideration of objectivity in the analyst. Letter to the editor. International Journal of Psychoanalysis 78: 1219–21.
Schwaber EA (1998) The non-verbal dimension in psychoanalysis: 'state' and its clinical vicissitudes. International Journal of Psychoanalysis 79: 667–79.
Schwalbe ML (1991) The autogenesis of the self. Journal of the Theory of Social Behaviour 21: 269–95.
Searles H (1959) The effort to drive the other person crazy: an element in the aetiology and psychotherapy of schizophrenia. In (1965) Collected Papers on Schizophrenia and Related Subjects. London: Hogarth.
Segal H (1973) Introduction to the Work of Melanie Klein. London: Hogarth.

Seganti A, Carnevale G, Mucelli R, Solano L, Target M (2000) From sixty-two interviews on 'the worst and the best episode of your life': relationships between internal working models and a grammatical scale of subject–object affective connections. International Journal of Psychoanalysis 81(3): 529–51.

Semrud-Clikeman M, Hynd GW (1990) Right hemisphere dysfunction in nonverbal learning disabilities: social, academic, and adaptive functioning in adults and children. Psychological Bulletin 107: 196–209.

Shane M, Shane E, Gales M (1997) Intimate Attachments: Toward a New Self Psychology. New York: Guilford Press.

Sinason V (in press) The Shoemaker and the Elves: Working with Multiplicity. London: Routledge.

Solms M (1999) The deep psychological functions of the right cerebral hemisphere. Bulletin of the British Psycho-Analytical Society 35(1): 9–29.

Solms M (2000) Freud, Luria and the clinical method. Psychoanalytic History 2: 76–109.

Spillius E (1988a) Introduction. In Spillius E (Ed) Melanie Klein Today, Vol 2. New Library of Psychoanalysis 8. London: Routledge.

Spillius E (1988b) Melanie Klein Today, Vols 1 and 2. New Library of Psychoanalysis 8. London: Routledge.

Spillius E, Feldman M (1989) Psychic Equilibrium and Psychic Change: Selected Papers of Betty Joseph. London: Routledge.

Springer SP, Deutsch G (1989) Left Brain, Right Brain. New York: Freeman.

Sroufe LA (1996) Emotional Development: The Organisation of Emotional Life in the Early Years. New York: Cambridge University Press.

Steiner J (1993) Psychic Retreats. New Library of Psychoanalysis 19. London: Routledge.

Stenberg G, Wiking S, Dahl M (1998) Judging words at face value: interference in a word processing task reveals automatic processing of affective facial expressions. Cognition and Emotion 12: 755–82.

Stern D (1985) The Interpersonal World of the Infant. New York: Basic Books.

Stern D (1995) The Motherhood Constellation. New York: Basic Books.

Stern D, Sander LW, Nahum JP, Harrison AM, Lyons-Ruth K, Morgan AC, Bruschweiller-Stern N, Tronick EZ (1998) Non-interpretive mechanisms in psychoanalytic therapy: the 'something more' than interpretation. International Journal of Psychoanalysis 79(5): 903–21.

Stewart H (1989) Technique at the basic fault regression. International Journal of Psychoanalysis 70: 221–30.

Stoller RJ (1976) Perversion: The Erotic Form of Hatred. Hassocks: Harvester Press.

Stoller RJ (1986) Sexual Excitement: Dynamics of Erotic Life. London: Karnac.

Stoller RJ (1991) Pain and Passion: A Psychoanalyst Explores the World of S and M. New York: Plenum.

Stoller RJ (1992) Observing the Erotic Imagination. New York: Yale University Press.

Stolorow R (1994) Subjectivity and Self Psychology. In Stolorow R, Atwood G, Brandchaft B, (Eds) The Intersubjective Perspective. Northvale, NJ: Jason Aronson.

Stolorow R, Atwood G (1979) Faces in a Cloud: Subjectivity in Personality Theory. New York: Jason Aronson.

Stolorow R, Atwood G (1992) Contexts of Being: The Intersubjective Foundations of Psychological Life. Hillsdale, NJ: Analytic Press.

Stolorow R, Atwood G (1997) Deconstructing the myth of the neutral analyst: an alternative from intersubjective systems theory. Psychoanalytic Quarterly 56: 431–49.

Stolorow R, Atwood G (1999) Afterword to 'Three realms of the unconscious'. In Mitchell SA, Aron L (Eds) Relational Psychoanalysis. Hillsdale, NJ: Analytic Press.

Stolorow R, Atwood G, Brandchaft B (1994) The Intersubjective Perspective. Northvale, NJ: Jason Aronson.

Stolorow R, Brandchaft B, Atwood G (1987) Psychoanalytic Treatment. An Intersubjective Approach. Hillsdale, NJ: Analytic Press.

Stone VE, Baron-Cohen S, Knight RT (1998) Frontal lobe contributions to theory of mind. Journal of Cognitive Neuroscience 10: 640–56.

Strachey J (1934) The nature of the therapeutic action of psychoanalysis. International Journal of Psycho-Analysis 15:117–26.

Sullivan HS (1956) Clinical Studies in Psychiatry. New York: Norton

Sulloway FJ (1979) Freud, Biologist of the Mind: Beyond the Psychoanalytic Legend. New York: Basic Books.

Taylor GJ (1987) Psychosomatic Medicine and Contemporary Psychoanalysis. Madison, CT: International Universities Press.

Taylor G (1997) Substance use disorders. In Taylor GJ, Bagby RM, Parker JDA, (Eds) Disorders of Affect Regulation. Cambridge: Cambridge University Press.

Taylor GJ, Bagby RM, Parker JDA (1997) Disorders of Affect Regulation. Cambridge: Cambridge University Press.

Teasdale JD, Howard RJ, Cox SG, Ha Y, Brammer MJ, Williams SCR, Checkley SA (1999) Functional MRI study of the cognitive generation of affect. American Journal of Psychiatry 156: 209–15.

Thompson C (1950) Psychoanalysis: Evolution and Development. New York: Hermitage House.

Tolpin PH (1969) Some psychic determinants of orgastic dysfunction. Presented to the Chicago Psychoanalytic Society, October 1969 (unpublished).

Trevarthen C (1993) Brain science and the human spirit. In Ashbrook JB (Ed) Brain, Culture and the Human Spirit. Lanham, Md: Univ. Press America. pp 129–81.

Tronick EZ (1998) Interactions that effect change in psychotherapy: a model based on infant research. Infant Mental Health Journal (special issue) 19(3).

Trop JL (1995a) Self psychology and intersubjectivity theory. In Goldberg A (Ed) The Impact of New Ideas. Progress in Self Psychology 11. Hillsdale, NJ: Analytic Press.

Trop JL (1995b) Reply to Ornstein. In Goldberg A (Ed) The Impact of New Ideas. Progress in Self Psychology 11. Hillsdale, NJ: Analytic Press.

Tustin F (1981) Autistic States in Children. London: Routledge.

Tustin F (1986) Autistic Barriers in Neurotic Patients. London: Karnac.

Ulman R, Brothers D (1988) The Shattered Self: A Psychoanalytic Study of Trauma. Hillsdale, NJ: Analytic Press.

van der Kolk B, Pelcovitz D, Roth S, Mandel FS, Mcfarlane A, Herman J (1996) Dissociation, somatization, and affect regulation: the complexity of adaptation to trauma. American Journal of Psychiatry 153(7): 83–93.

Vermetten E, Douglas-Bremner D, Spiegel D (1998) Dissociation and hypnotizability: a conceptual and methodological perspective on two distinct concepts. In

Douglas-Bremner J, Marmar C, (Eds) Trauma, Memory and Dissociation. New York: American Psychiatric Press.

Voeller KS (1986) Right-hemisphere deficit syndrome in children. American Journal of Psychiatry 143: 1004–9.

Walker M, Antony-Black J (1999) Hidden Selves: An Exploration of Multiple Personality. Buckingham: Open University Press.

Wallerstein RS (1992) The Common Ground of Psychoanalysis. Northvale, NJ: Aronson.

Weintraub S, Mesulam MM (1983) Developmental learning disabilities of the right hemisphere. Archives of Neurology 40: 463–68

Wilshire B (1982) Role Playing and Identity: The Limits of Theatre as Metaphor. Bloomington: Indiana University Press.

Wilson A, Passik SD, Faude JP (1990) Self-regulation and its failures. In Masling J, (Ed) Empirical Studies of Psychoanalytic Theory, Vol 3. Hillsdale, NJ: The Analytic Press. pp 149–213.

Winnicott DW (1947) Further thoughts on babies as persons. In (1964) The Child, the Family, and the Outside World. Harmondsworth: Penguin.

Winnicott DW (1958) The capacity to be alone. In (1965) The Maturational Processes and the Facilitating Environment. London: Hogarth.

Winnicott DW (1960) Ego distortion in terms of true and false self. In (1965) The Maturational Processes and the Facilitating Environment. London: Hogarth.

Winnicott DW (1962) Ego integration in child development. In (1965) The Maturational Processes and the Facilitating Environment. London: Hogarth.

Winnicott DW (1963) The development of the capacity for concern. In (1965) The Maturational Processes and the Facilitating Environment. London: Hogarth.

Winnicott DW (1967) Mirror role of mother and family in child development. In Playing and Reality. Harmondsworth: Penguin.

Winnicott DW (1988) Human Nature. London: Free Association Books.

Wolf ES (1994) Selfobject experiences: development, psychopathology, treatment. In Kramer S, Akhtar S, (Eds) Mahler and Kohut. New York: Aronson.

Wright K (1991) Vision and Separation: Between Mother and Baby. Northvale, NJ: Aronson.

Zeanah CH, Barton ML (1989) Introduction: internal representations and parent-infant relationships. Infant Mental Health Journal 10: 135–41.

Index

Note: 'n.' after a page reference refers to a footnote.

abandonment
　anxiety, 159
　depression, 179–180
acknowledgment tokens, 111
action-thoughts, 76–78
addiction, 202
　selfobject dysfunction, 203–205
Adler, G., 114
adversarial selfobject, 23
affect attunement, 90
affective arousal, mother–infant attunement, 194
affectivity, 98
affect regulation, x, 202
　childhood trauma, 213
aggression
　depression, 86
　schizophrenia, 175–176
Aichhorn, August, 24, 247
Alexander, Franz, 24, 247
alexithymia, 202, 204
alienating mirror, 225–226
alpha function
　presymbolic dread, 7–8
　representation and illusion, 12–13
　selfobject, 202–203, 224
ambivalence
　fears of encountering, 170
　towards reality, 171–172
American Psychoanalytic Association (APA), 247

anality
　self psychology, 69–70
　traditional psychology, 65–66
anti-selfobjects, 59
　childhood trauma, 213
　freeing the patient, 225
　internalized relationships, 119
　pathogenic selfobjects, 58–59
　selfobject catastrophes, 192
art, 185
attachment, x, 84, 191, 206
Atwood, G. E.
　impasse, 160
　intersubjectivity, 87, 88, 110
　　criticisms of self psychology, 88–91
　　intrapsychic psychoanalysis, 104–105
　　Kohut's concept of self, 91, 95–96
　　transference and the unconscious, 100–101, 102, 125
autoeroticism, 5, 32
　schizophrenia, 165
autohypnosis, 212
autonomy
　alienating mirror, 226
　cognitive imperialism, 229
　and depression, 181–183
　mother's respect for infant's, 200
　nuclear self, 36–37

Baars, B. J., 224
Baker, R., 107
Balint, M., 2, 130, 211
Bateman, A. W., 38

Printed and bound by CPI Group (UK) Ltd, Croydon, CR0 4YY

09/06/2025

14685974-0002
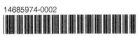